Health Policy and Ethics

Introduction to the Pharmacy Business Administration Series

Books in the Pharmacy Business Administration Series have been prepared for use in university level graduate and professional level courses, as well as for continuing education and self-study uses. The series includes books covering the major subject areas taught in Social and Administrative Pharmacy, Pharmacy Administration, and Pharmacy MBA programs.

World-class authors with well-regarded expertise in the various respective areas have been selected and the book outlines as well as the books themselves have been reviewed by a number of other experts in the field. The result of this effort is a new integrated and coordinated series of books that is up to date in methodology, research findings, terminology, and contemporary trends and practices.

This is one book in that series of about 12 subjects in total. It is intended that each of the books will be revised at least every 5 years. Although the books were intended for the North American market, they are just as relevant in other areas.

Titles in the series currently include:

Health Economics
Health Policy and Ethics
Principles of Good Clinical Practice
Strategic Pharmaceutical Marketing: A Practical Guide
Financial Analysis in Pharmacy Practice
Research Methods for Pharmaceutical Practice and Policy

The series editor-in-chief is Professor Albert Wertheimer, PhD, MBA, of Temple University School of Pharmacy, Philadelphia.

Suggestions and comments from readers are most welcome and should be sent to the Commissioning Editor, Pharmaceutical Press, 1 Lambeth High Street, London SE1 7JN, UK.

Health Policy and Ethics

Jack E Fincham PhD, RPh

Professor of Pharmacy Practice and Administration
School of Pharmacy, University of Missouri-Kansas City, Kansas City,
Missouri, USA

Adjunct Professor of Health Administration
Henry W Bloch School of Management
University of Missouri-Kansas City, Kansas City, Missouri

Adjunct Professor of Health Policy and Management
The University of Georgia, College of Public Health, Athens, Georgia, USA

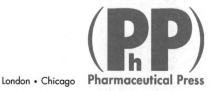

London • Chicago   **Pharmaceutical Press**

Published by Pharmaceutical Press

1 Lambeth High Street, London SE1 7JN, UK
1559 St Paul Avenue, Gurnee, IL 60031, USA

© Royal Pharmaceutical Society of Great Britain 2011

(**PP**) is a trade mark of Pharmaceutical Press

Pharmaceutical Press is the publishing division of the
Royal Pharmaceutical Society

First published 2011

Typeset by Thomson Digital, Noida, India
Printed in Great Britain by TJ International, Padstow, Cornwall

ISBN 978 0 85369 838 8

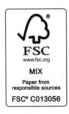

Dedication

To Meg, always marvelous and magical

Contents

Foreword

Definition of "health" from the World Health Organization:

> Health is a state of complete physical, mental and social well-being and not merely the absence of disease or infirmity (World Health Organization 2010).

It should be noted that this widely quoted and used definition has not been updated or altered in any sense since 1946. Much health policy (local, national, regional, global) has been crafted since this decree; it has indeed stood the test of time in fine fashion. The oppressive burdens of vastly differing incomes, unequal access to care, disparity of sophistication, and variance in quality have led to disturbingly large differences between those with care options and those with none.

Reference

World Health Organization (2010). Frequently asked questions. What is the WHO definition of health? Available online at: http://www.who.int/suggestions/faq/en/ (accessed 17 December 2010).

Preface

Health policy can be defined as regulations, legislations, rules, and other structures that guide how health issues and/or health care are structured, delivered, and provided. Using American departments or regulatory agencies, these influencers can be local (municipal health departments), state (health departments, community and public health departments, environmental protection agencies), federal (Environmental Protection Agency, Food and Drug Administration, Health Care Financing Administration, Occupational Health and Safety Administration, Centers for Disease Control and Prevention, Drug Enforcement Administration), or international (World Health Organization (WHO)). The perplexing part is that in some cases these regional/national/international agencies overlap in oversight. The WHO, a well-known international organization, while global in scope of activities, does not have power (other than referent power) to provide edicts on health policy in specific regions or countries.

In the UK, nationally the National Health Service (NHS) exerts influence upon health care matters, and local and regional primary care trusts monitor services and options for patients and providers. The UK National Institute for Health and Clinical Excellence (NICE) monitors spending and costs within the NHS. NICE controls about 4% of the NHS outlays, but monitors prescription drug approval for use within the NHS, as well as new technologies (e.g., cardiac stents). Within this 4% of NHS outlays, NICE controls which drugs can be added to formularies. Within the primary care trusts, specific drugs or technologies can be provided if funding balances allow for payment despite NICE disapproval at the national level.

In Canada, Health Canada controls drugs and drug approvals at the national level. Individual provinces provide coverage within provinces, but health care insurance is universally available and transferable from one Canadian province to the other.

Elsewhere (Vietnam), Ministries of Health control health care services at the national level, with provinces and communes providing care at local and regional levels. Health workers and health professionals provide varying levels of care at each level of service provision.

How health care systems are structured and how funds are allocated require a synergism between local, state, regional, national, and sometimes international planning and policy implementations. How these policies are developed is of interest to many, whether patient, provider, or payer. Health policy deliberations and implementations are subject to partisan, political, religious, and societal influence. Perhaps this is how it should be: health and its ramifications affect all, so all should be involved in all aspects that are pertinent. Voices are heard and some are ignored in these discussions. Some have enormous power and influence, but many are powerless and have no voice or advocacy. External influences that cannot be predicted – war, acts of God (floods, fires, natural disasters), acts of terrorism and bioterrorism – can also have unanticipated damaging effects on the best-laid plans affecting health policy and its crafting. In addition, pandemics that quickly spread through person-to-person transmittal as a result of the immediacy of travel, widespread food distribution, or animal disease vector transmission can overtake previous health policy planning.

While cultural aspects of health impact all, the inclusion of cultural dimensions has not always been a part of health care policy deliberations or implementation. Culture, experiences, beliefs, and expectations all color health care outcomes with varying hues. Future planning must recognize the importance of culture on many segments of health care. We will explore this component of health policy in this book.

The ethics of health care delivery, planning, and utilization has always been debated extensively. Why should the ethics of health care be infused into a book dealing with health policy and analysis? It is not unusual for health policy experts and bioethicists to be diametrically opposed to one another (Emanuel 2002). These disciplines often look at the same issue from different perspectives, for example, managed care, comparative effectiveness research, and/or health care financing.

Ethics is an influencer of much of what we do or should do regarding health and health care delivery and systems. Health care and health policy need strong doses of ethics to center our compass when it comes to how we structure health care – locally, regionally, nationally, and globally. References to ethics and ethical components are referred to frequently in this text. Ethical issues are embedded in numerous chapters.

We live in an ever-increasing climate of extreme disparity. The separation of "haves" and "have nots" in economic, health care use, and health care outcomes is becoming split by chasms. Funding for improving health care in developing countries has increased from $6.4 billion (1997) to $8.16 billion (2002) (Anonymous 2006). How this money has been assigned leads to ethical challenges. The funding stream in many cases has a predetermined focus, e.g., HIV-AIDS, tuberculosis, malaria. While these specifically focused programs have been seen to make wonderful impacts, other primary care basic health care has continued to struggle for sustainment. A recent proposed effort, the 15 by 2015 initiative (De Maeseneer *et al.* 2008a) has included a suggestion that 15% of donated funds, regardless of intended use, be applied to initiate or support primary care programs. This disparity between vertical services (funding for all health care services within a provided amount) and horizontal services (providing coverage for many types of services across the board) has left many without basic primary care services. In a separate paper, De Maeseneer and colleagues (2008b) suggest a "new global strategy is needed" to bolster community-focused care in the developing world.

The issues of health, health access, insurance coverage for health care services, and planning for health care services are universal concerns shared by all. Regions of the world, and sometimes even within countries, contain disparate systems for health care delivery, financing, and health care utilization opportunities. Each of these components of a health care system, regardless of location, needs to be served by appropriate health care planning and policies. Unfortunately, this demand is not met in many locations, developing world and developed world alike. The lack of proper planning and health policy analyses costs time and many other resources, and unfortunately affects patient outcomes deleteriously.

Gostin and Powers (2006) posit "that a commitment to social justice lies at the heart of public health" (p. 1060). They suggest that justice in public health deserves more attention than the political process has allowed. Kenny and Giacomini (2005) point to the need for a new ethics field for health policy analysis. Further, they suggest that a need exists for robust, high-quality ethical analysis for the purpose of public policy-making.

Focus of this book

The goal of this book is to put heath policy and ethics into a universal context that has global applicability. Much of this book has a focus on the USA, but there are numerous references and case studies that are solely focused on the international aspects of health policy. I feel it is so vital for all to understand the macro effects of health policy as they relate to structure, financing, and delivery of health care. In addition, the micro elements of outcomes and health improvement are directly affected by health policy.

Regardless of where we end up living, working, or using health care, it is hoped that this book will shed light on, and promote an understanding of, health policy, its influencers, and how policy directly affects health and health care.

References

Anonymous (2006). *Engaging for Health. Eleventh General Programme of Work 2006–2015*. Geneva: World Health Organization.

De Maeseneer J, van Weel C, Egilman D, *et al.* (2008a). Strengthening primary care: addressing the disparity between vertical and horizontal investment. *Br J Gen Pract* 58: 3–4.

De Maeseneer J, van Weel C, Egilman D, *et al.* (2008b). Funding for primary health care in developing countries: money from disease specific projects could be used to strengthen primary care. *Br Med J* 336: 518–519.

Emanuel E (2002). Foreword. In: Danis M, Clancy C, Churchill L (eds) *Ethical Dimensions of Health Policy.* New York: Oxford University Press.

Gostin LO, Powers M (2006). What does social justice require for the public's health? Public health ethics and policy imperatives. *Health Affairs* 25: 1053–1060.

Kenny N, Giacomini M (2005). Wanted: a new ethics field for health policy analysis. *Health Care Anal* 13: 247–260.

About the author

Dr. **Jack E Fincham** is a graduate of the University of Nebraska College of Pharmacy, and was a Kellogg Pharmaceutical Clinical Scientist Fellow at the University of Minnesota where he obtained his PhD in Social and Administrative Pharmacy. He received a Post-Graduate Degree in Health Economics at the University of Aberdeen (UK). Dr. Fincham has researched varying topics pertaining to health economics, international health, patient compliance, public health, medication management, pharmaceutical marketing, avoiding medication risks, the Medicare Part D Drug Benefit, and drug use in the elderly.

Dr. Fincham has teaching and research expertise in research designs and methodology, statistical analyses, discrete choice experiments, economic evaluations, grant writing, and outcomes evaluations. Dr. Fincham has led teaching and research programs for undergraduate and graduate students in Vietnam.

Dr. Fincham has written over 200 refereed and professional papers and has made over 200 professional and research presentations to varying health professional groups from Asia, Australia, Canada, the Republic of China, continental Europe, Turkey, Vietnam, the UK, and the USA. Dr. Fincham has written 12 books. He is an Associate Editor for the *American Journal of Pharmaceutical Education*. From 1994 to 2004, Dr. Fincham served as dean of the University of Kansas School of Pharmacy.

Dr. Fincham has been frequently interviewed for newspaper, radio, and television programs on topics related to prescription and over-the-counter medication use, pharmacy and medical services, public health issues, health care reform, and quality of care concerns.

He currently serves as Professor of Pharmacy Practice and Administration, the University of Missouri-Kansas City, School of Pharmacy; as Professor Public Affairs and Administration, UMKC Bloch School of management; and as Adjunct Professor of Health Policy and Management at the University of Georgia, College of Public Health.

Contributor

Arif Ahmed, BDS, PhD, MSPH
Assistant Professor of Health Administration, Department of Public Affairs, Henry W Bloch School of Management, University of Missouri-Kansas City, Kansas City, Missouri 64110-2499, USA

Adjunct Assistant Professor, School of Dentistry, University of Missouri-Kansas City, Kansas City, Missouri, USA

Glossary

AAFDA	Arthur Ashe Foundation to Defeat AIDS: foundation developed by tennis great Arthur Ashe in the 1990s
AARP	American Association of Retired Persons: advocacy organization for seniors in the USA
ABC	Abstinence, Be faithful, and, as appropriate, correct and consistent use of Condoms
ACIP	Advisory Committee on Immunization Practices
ADR	adverse drug reaction
AHRQ	Agency for Healthcare Research and Quality: US agency overseeing comparative effectiveness, quality improvement, and health services-related federal government-sponsored research
AIDS	acquired immune deficiency syndrome
AMP	average manufacturer price: proposed payment-based data point for the reimbursement of outpatient prescription programs such as Medicare at present, and potentially Medicaid in the future. Payment is based on actual manufacturer-provided data as opposed to factitiously derived average wholesale price (AWP) mechanism for reimbursement.
APhA	American Pharmacists Association: umbrella pharmacy association in the USA representing various types of pharmacy interests
AR-DRG	Australian refined diagnosis-related groups: Australian prospective payment system (PPS) set in play to group like diseases in a similar pay scheme to pay prospectively for institutional health services
ARRA	American Recovery and Reinvestment Act: US federally funded stimulus program to jumpstart the US economy
ARV	antiretroviral

AWP	average wholesale price: since 1965 the payment list base price for reimbursement for outpatient prescription drug benefit programs. This value is a moving target, and has been manipulated illegally to increase pharmacy reimbursement and pharmaceutical company profits. AWP has been referred to as "ain't what's paid"
BNDD	Bureau of Narcotics and Dangerous Drugs: US predecessor of the Drug Enforcement Administration
CA-MRSA	community-acquired methicillin-resistant *Staphylococcus aureus*
CDC	Centers for Disease Control and Prevention: US agency that monitors and responds to disease outbreaks in the USA and globally
CDSS	clinical decision support system
CER	comparative effectiveness research: also known as patient-centered outcomes research
CHAI	Clinton Health Access Initiative: William J. Clinton foundation addressing global health initiatives
CMS	Centers for Medicare and Medicaid Services: division of the US Department of Health and Human Services that oversees the Medicaid and Medicare social insurance programs of the US government
CPI-M	consumer price index for medical care
CPI-U	consumer price index for urban consumers
CSDH	Commission on Social Determinants of Health: World Health Organization committee examining means to: improve daily living conditions; tackle the inequitable distribution of power, money, and resources; measure and understand the problem and assess the impact of actions that may be implemented
DEA	Drug Enforcement Administration
DESI	Drug Efficacy Study Implementation
DMF	deltoid muscle fibrosis
DO	doctor of osteopathy: osteopathic physician
DoD	Department of Defense: US department overseeing logistics, health care services, and all other factors relating to US military functions at home and abroad
DRG	diagnosis-related group: begun in the USA in the early 1980s, this classification of diseases into similar groupings allowed for prospective reimbursement for institutionally delivered health care services as opposed to after-the-fact, retrospective reimbursement for health services provided

DTCA	direct-to-consumer advertising: controversial advertising of prescription medications directly to consumers, allowed only in the USA and New Zealand
DUR	Drug Utilization Review
EIS	Epidemiologic Intelligence Service: Centers for Disease Control and Prevention service from which physician-epidemiologists track and monitor disease outbreaks worldwide, often from unknown or unrecognized causative agents
e-prescribing:	electronic prescribing: digital transfer of prescription from physician to pharmacist or pharmacy for processing
FDA	Food and Drug Administration: US federal agency that oversees the manufacturing, channels of distribution and market entry, marketing, and promotion of brand-name and generic medications in the USA
FDC	Food, Drug, and Cosmetic
FMI	Food Marketing Institute: trade advocacy group representing the interests of supermarket outlets in the USA
FSS	Federal Supply Schedule: pharmaceutical drug pricing level for federally qualified entities to purchase pharmaceuticals at vastly reduced price levels over other pricing levels in the USA
FUL	federal upper limit: upper payment price for Medicaid drugs (generic)
G8	Group of Eight countries (Canada, France, Germany, Italy, Japan, Russia, UK, and the USA)
GAVI	Global Alliance for Vaccines and Immunizations
H1N1	swine influenza
H1N5	avian influenza
HAART	highly active antiretroviral therapy: prescription medication treatment for HIV/AIDS
HHS	Department of Health and Human Services: cabinet-level department in the US government executive branch that oversees health care programs of the US federal government
HIT	health information technology
HIV	human immunodeficiency virus: causative virus leading to acquired immunodeficiency syndrome (AIDS)
HMO	health maintenance organization: a managed care entity
HR-QOL	health-related QOL: a self-assessed measure of overall health and well-being

HRSA	Health Resources and Services Administration: federal agency examining health profession shortage areas in the USA
ICD-10	*International Classification of Disease*, version 10
IED	improvised explosive device
MAIC	maximum allowable ingredient cost
MA-PDPs	Medicare Advantage prescription drug plans: Medicare Advantage plans, Medicare Part C, provide prescription drug coverage as part of a package for eligible Medicare enrollees. The profitability and expense of these plans for consumers have served as a lightning rod for debate regarding the affordability of these plans
MD	medical doctor: allopathic physician
MDGs	Millennium Development Goals
MMA	Medicare Prescription Drug, Improvement, and Modernization Act of 2003: federal legislation that initiated the Medicare Drug Discount Program in 2004, and the Medicare Prescription Drug Program on January 1, 2006
MRSA	methicillin-resistant *Staphylococcus aureus*: strain of bacterium that is resistant to traditional antibiotic therapies
MSF	Médecins Sans Frontières (Doctors Without Borders): non-profit humanitarian relief efforts coordinated by international physicians globally
MTMS	medication therapy management services: pharmacist or other directed review of patient
NACDS	National Association of Chain Drugstores: trade advocacy group representing the interests of the chain pharmacy industry in the USA
NCMS	New Cooperative Medical Scheme: revised health care delivery scheme instituted in the People's Republic of China
NCPA	National Community Pharmacists Association: advocacy group for pharmacy owners in the USA
NGO	non-governmental organization: non-government-sponsored group working within national and international frameworks
NHS	British National Health Service: begun in 1948, often referred to as the Beveridge model of a health care system
NICE	National Institute for Health and Clinical Excellence: comparative effectiveness center in the UK

NIDA	National Institute on Drug Abuse: monitors drug abuse with prescription medications along with illicit drugs of abuse
NIH	National Institutes of Health: US federal institute that provides funding for basic and applied science health-related research
OBRA '90	Omnibus Budget Reconciliation Act of 1990: sweeping budget reconciliation act passed in 1990 that instituted mandatory drug regimen reviews for outpatient Medicaid patients, patient counseling requirements, and Medi-Gap insurance regulations, among other items
PBMs	pharmacy benefit managers: companies in the USA that manage the "carve out" prescription drug benefits for large insurers. PBMs negotiate with pharmacies to provide prescriptions for insured patients, specifying the cost parameters for prescription drugs and the dispensing fee paid to pharmacies
PDPs	Medicare Part D prescription drug plans: private plans providing insurance coverage for a portion of Medicare-eligible enrollee outpatient prescription medications. Approximately 50 PDPs are available for Medicare enrollees regardless of where they live in the USA
PEPFAR	President's Emergency Plan for AIDS Relief: program started within President George W. Bush's administration to address the global needs for assistance in treating HIV/AIDs
PhRMA	Pharmaceutical Research and Manufacturers Association: the lobbying and promotion component of the research-intensive brand-name drug industry in the USA
PMSI	Programme de Médicalisation du Système d'Information: the French version of diagnosis-related group; prospective reimbursement for health care services delivered within institutions
PPACA	Patient Protection and Affordable Care Act: sweeping health care reform legislation passed in 2010 in the USA
PRC	People's Republic of China
QALYs	quality-adjusted life-years: estimating the life-enhancing aspects of a medical or health care technology by placing a value on years that would benefit an individual for the intervention in question
QOL	quality of life: self-assessed measure of overall well-being

SAMHSA	Substance Abuse and Mental Health Services Administration: US federal agency examining drug abuse and mental health services
SCHIP, S-CHIP, or CHIP	State Children's Health Insurance Program: begun in 1997, states not initially choosing to participate could defer for 3 years without penalty. This program provided Medicaid coverage for children of low-income families who were otherwise not eligible for Medicaid coverage
Taiwan	Republic of China
TCM	traditional Chinese medicine: also called eastern medicine
TJC	Joint Commission for the Accreditation of Hospital Organizations (The Joint Commission): reviews and accredits health care organizations in the USA. TJC accreditation is required in order to receive federal funds for services provided for Medicare clients
UK	United Kingdom (England, Northern Ireland, Scotland, and Wales)
UNESCO	United Nations Educational, Scientific and Cultural Organization
VA	Veterans Affairs: US federal department that oversees benefits provided for US war veterans. The mission statement of the VA department is: To fulfill President Lincoln's promise "To care for him who shall have borne the battle, and for his widow, and his orphan" by serving and honoring the men and women who are America's veterans
VIPPS	Verified Internet Pharmacy Practice Sites: verification process for internet pharmacies to reduce the scourge of illicit online unscrupulous pharmacies
VRSA	vancomycin-resistant *Staphylococcus aureus*: strain of bacterium that is resistant to traditional antibiotic therapies
WHO	World Health Organization: the directing and coordinating authority for health within the United Nations system
WTP	willingness to pay: a health economic measure examining the decisions individuals make when considering several competing options

1

Introduction: the growing disparity of excess and deprivation in health care

Introduction

Through the examination of how health care access, status, and quality change from one part of the world to another, or within countries, one can gauge the influence, efforts, and success (or lack thereof) of health policy. Depending on the site of interest, these efforts may be local, regional, national, or international. These advocacy efforts may be spurred on by any number of players, but the issue of the disparity between those who have access to the finest of health care resources and those who do not seems to become more prominent as time progresses.

Health policy and questions to ask

When considering decisions that are made concerning health policy, it is important to analyze several questions concerning the issues and subsequent decisions. The questions are:

1 What are the issues involved?
2 Who is affected? (Patients are the most important participating party in health policy impacts.)
3 Who are the influencers that have a vested interest in decisions that are made?
4 What is the decision?
5 What are the outcomes?
6 If things need to be changed after a health policy decision is made, how would changes be made and at what level?

These six questions are crucial when considering health policy decisions, no matter where health policy is focused: local, regional, national, and/or international.

Political change and resultant health policy effects on health care systems

Issues related to disparities in health care and access to care affect health policy discussions in virtually every country in the world. With or without extensive coverage for care, disparities exist and inadequacies are ubiquitous. Those who are disadvantaged have an effect on costs both individually and collectively. How those without care are covered impacts every facet of health care delivery and delivery systems.

US experiences

Calls for health care reform of the US health care system were heard and a landmark bill was passed in 2010. The Patient Protection and Affordable Care Act (PPACA) was signed into law in the spring of 2010. After this bill was signed, and as midterm elections were completed in the USA in 2010, calls for further changes in the PPACA have increased and will increase in both frequency and intensity. Some will call for repeal of the recently passed bill and other calls will go out seeking expansion of benefits by special-interest groups seeking specific goals. This is the reality of health policy and its influence on health care systems and societies: health policy is not static and will not be in the future.

Pharmaceuticals

Pharmaceuticals are a frequent focus of health policy debates and deliberations. There may be calls for more expeditious approval of brand-name drugs, or allowing easier entry for generic drugs for market entry, or perhaps for disease-specific coverage for of out-of-reach treatments. For example, swift approval for cancer treatments and human immunodeficiency virus (HIV) therapies for autoimmune deficiency disease have been advocated for decades now. Biosimilar generics in competition with brand-name biotechnologically derived drugs are now being considered via submitted applications for approval by the US Food and Drug Administration.

State Children's Health Insurance Program (SCHIP)

Expanded eligibility for specific programs has been advocated as well. In late 2007, President George W. Bush stalled efforts to enhance eligibility for SCHIP. These benefits were subsequently increased and expanded in the Patient Protection and Affordable Care Act. Advocacy groups helped steer this focus back to the need for children to have access to health and health care insurance.

In a paper examining the effects of expanding public health insurance eligibility for older children, Currie et al. (2008) found that, while eligibility for public health insurance unambiguously improves current utilization of preventive care, it has little effect on current health status. They also found evidence that Medicaid eligibility in early childhood has positive effects on future health. They conclude by suggesting that adequate early medical care puts children on a better health trajectory, resulting in better health as they grow.

Grassroots movements

Hoffman (2003) suggests calls for health care reform have come from grassroots sources, and have contained an initiation of a wider critique of the American health care system, leading some movements to adopt calls for universal coverage. This did not happen in 2010, and whether or not a single-payer approach will ever be approved in the USA is debatable. But efforts to foster a favored view from health policy advocates of many differing points of view will continue to be discussed, debated, and possibly enacted.

UK experiences

How dramatically the landscape of health care changes with elections at a national level is apparent when looking at recent experiences in the UK. The UK, with a one-payer, national health care service, provides cradle-to-grave health care coverage for British citizens. Recent controversies have arisen in Britain regarding the access to medicines that varies within the primary care trust system. At present in the UK, the Pharmaceutical Price Regulation Scheme regulates profits, not prices, on sales to the state health service (Hirschler 2010). In the UK, the National Institute for Health and Clinical Excellence (NICE) assesses cost-effective comparisons of compet-ing drugs. It has been proposed that components of this may change. In its *Programme for Government* document (http://www.direct.gov.uk/en/Nl1/Newsroom/DG_187877) the newly elected coalition government said it would "reform NICE and move to a system of value-based pricing" (Hirschler 2010).

Hirschler (2010) notes:

> Loss of free pricing could also have a knock-on impact, since companies can currently use Britain to set a high price point for reference pricing in the rest of the European Union and other countries, such as Japan.

The Association of the British Pharmaceutical Industry said it was keeping an open mind ahead of talks with government. "Value-based pricing is one way of doing it," said spokesman Richard Ley. "We are not opposed to the principle. It is a question of how it is achieved to get it right."

This focus away from concentration on profits to so-called value-based pricing for drug prices would fundamentally change how drugs are priced in the UK and beyond. This may serve as an entrée for price controls in the UK for pharmaceuticals. Along with the USA, the UK is currently one of only several countries where markets exist with free drug pricing (Hirschler 2010).

Negative economic impact of lack of insurance

The impact of the insured on health care costs and the ethics of care provided to some but not others, solely dependent upon their insurance status, is garnering ever-more increasing attention. The numbers at risk obviously contain those without health insurance, but there remain a large number of underinsured individuals in the USA. Some may have health insurance as an employee benefit, yet need to attain out-of-reach co-payments of $1000 or more before insurance coverage is available. Having to spend this amount as a co-payment or as a deductible before receiving health insurance benefits leaves many with the equivalent of no insurance whatsoever. Even with the enactment of health reform legislation in the USA, uninsured individuals and families will be commonplace in the USA. In a study examining uncompensated care for individuals without health insurance, Hadley and colleagues (2008) note:

> People uninsured for any part of 2008 spend about $30 billion out of pocket and receive approximately $56 billion in uncompensated care while uninsured. Government programs finance about 75% of uncompensated care. If all uninsured people were fully covered, their medical spending would increase by $122.6 billion. The increase represents 5% of current national health spending and 0.8% of gross domestic product. However, it is neither the cost of a specific plan nor necessarily the same as the government's costs, which could be higher, depending on plans' financing structures and the extent of crowd-out (p. 399).

Hadley *et al.* (2008), examining out-of-pocket and total costs, point to the uninsured, who are that way for the year, and who end up paying 35% out of pocket for their care, with the balance being subsidized from one source or another. The updated study also examines total and out-of-pocket spending for the uninsured. People who are uninsured for a full year receive less than half as much care as the insured and pay 35% ($583) out of pocket towards average health costs of $1686 per uninsured person.

The passage of the Patient Protection and Affordable Care Act in 2010 in the USA is a dramatic opportunity to provide health insurance for many in the USA. Some of those eligible for insurance coverage will not choose to acquire insurance, and the expansion of opportunities will not be in play until several years have passed. Thus, the problem of uninsurance in the USA will remain an obstacle for many.

Ubiquitous nature of health disparities

Disparities are not just a facet of the US health care system. The view that disparities are uniquely American, to be solved by universal health care coverage, is simply not the case. Hussey and colleagues (2008) point to the occurrence of disparities in a variety of indicators in four different health systems in Canada, the UK, New Zealand, and the USA. Payment for components of health services, such as drugs, varies within come countries as well. Krobot *et al.* (2004) found in a study of differences between private and state (statutory)-provided insurance coverage that disparities exist. They note:

> Even though virtually everyone in Germany has health insurance and drug coverage, use of new and recommended migraine medicines was less common among those with SHI [statutory health insurance] compared with their privately insured counterparts (p. 491).

Within the USA, disparities occur based upon differences between knowledge bases of groups of community-based directors with more advanced knowledge of behavior and outcomes as opposed to those with less knowledge about the influence of behavior and health outcomes for disadvantaged populations (Dearing *et al.* 2004). Gaps between what is known about behavior change and what is actually practiced in social programs grow larger, especially for community-based programs intended to help minority populations, the poor, and those living in inner-city and rural areas (Dearing *et al.* 2004).

The poor are at a distinct disadvantage worldwide

In a global assessment of the impact of disparities on health outcomes, the World Health Organization (WHO) Commission on Social Determinants of Health (CSDH) (2008) released a report (*Closing the Gap in a Generation: Health Equity through Action on the Social Determinants of Health*) that examines disparities around the world. Among numerous findings, the report includes these examples of health differences around the world: 4/5 of persons with diabetes live in the developing world; and currently in Afghanistan the lifetime risk of maternal death is 1 in 8, whereas in Sweden, it is 1 in 17 400. In the USA alone, close to 900 000 deaths would have been prevented in the 1990s if mortality rates were equal between whites and African-Americans. In its summary, the commission (World Health Organization 2008) outlines a three-pronged approach to addressing health inequities, which includes three overarching recommendations to remove health disparities globally in a generation:

- Improve the conditions of daily life – the circumstances in which people are born, grow, live, work, and age.
- Tackle the inequitable distribution of power, money, and resources – the structural drivers of those conditions of daily life – globally, nationally, and locally.
- Measure the problem, evaluate action, expand the knowledge base, develop a workforce that is trained in the social determinants of health, and raise public awareness about the social determinants of health (p. 10).

The final assessment of this report (World Health Organization 2008) is that "social injustice is killing people on a grand scale" (p. 10).

Dor and colleagues (2008) have found Medicaid and uninsured patients treated in health centers are significantly poorer, in significantly worse health, and if uninsured, more likely to be members of racial and ethnic minorities. These groups were compared with those treated by other sources of primary care.

Colorectal cancer incidence rates in American Indians and Alaska Natives vary dramatically between regions (Perdue *et al.* 2008). Perdue *et al.* suggest that efforts are needed to make screening a priority, to overcome access barriers to endoscopic screening, and to engage communities in culturally appropriate ways to participate in prevention and early detection programs for colorectal cancer.

Kasturi and Ruth (2000) point to impressive improvements that have occurred in global health status in the past century. They suggest these improvements have not been universal within and between countries. Gains have been offset by response to economic, political, and social changes and disruptions. They call for enhanced surveillance systems to underpin efforts to address old and newer health impacts.

In a concept paper examining definitions of health disparities, inequalities, and health equity, Braveman (2006) concluded that health disparities/inequalities include differences between the most advantaged group in a given category, e.g., the wealthiest, the most powerful racial/ethnic group, and all others, not only between the best- and worst-off groups. Pursuing health equity means pursuing the elimination of such health disparities/inequalities.

Corso *et al.* (2002), in a study examining consumer preferences for payment for prevention versus payment for treatments found that willingness to pay (WTP) for treatment was significantly greater than WTP for prevention. WTP significantly increased with age and household income in the full sample but was not significantly affected by gender or educational attainment. They conclude that a better understanding is needed of the discrepancy between citizens' stated preferences for prevention (e.g., through polling) and the findings that they were willing to pay substantially more for treatment than for prevention.

Many disease states are influenced by racial and ethnic inequities (Oliver and Muntaner 2005). Blacks suffer from an increased burden of illness, with higher incidence and mortality rates and more severe morbidity in cerebrovascular disease, heart disease, cancer, diabetes, and many other ailments. *Healthy People 2010*, the federal government's health plan, called for eliminating health disparities by race, ethnicity, gender, education, income, disability, geographic location, or sexual orientation (US Department of Health and Human Services 2000); this has been reiterated in the *Healthy People 2020* document (US Department of Health and Human Services 2010).

Lack of access or lack of empowerment?

Marmot (2006) has suggested that it is not only the lack of access to material resources that leads to poor health, but also the overt lack of empowerment. This lack of a feeling of ownership over health care access and outcomes can lead to a diminished health status in and of itself (Gwatkin 2007).

Changes in types of services available

Certainly, health policy will play a major role in the coming months and years. Borger *et al.* (2006) suggest stable trends in spending through 2015 may be obscured by dramatic changes in health care in the next decade. The impending entry of many baby-boomers into the Medicare program, and continued increased in the growth of Medicaid, may change the type of care consumed. The advent of the Medicare Part D drug benefit in 2006 ushered in continually increasing participation by seniors and spending on prescription medications. Other shifts may also occur in spending categories of institutional care and physician services.

Borger *et al.* (2006) conclude:

> Given this confluence of changes for both public and private payers and our projection that health care spending growth will outpace the growth of the economy, we anticipate that society will again need to confront the underlying questions about the supply of and demand for health care services, as we anticipate that one in every five dollars will be devoted to this sector by 2015 (p. w73).

Referring to the issue of burden of disease globally and requirements for reimbursement for varying disease categories, Widdus (2001) suggested that the burden of disease, influenced by infectious diseases, disproportionately affects populations in developing countries. Widdus noted that lack of access to pharmaceuticals and/or vaccinations diverts expenditures that may be necessary for other diseases that could be positively influenced by provision of basic primary care services. He concluded by calling for partnerships between public and private entities, specifically the pharmaceutical industry, to work to solve the disparities caused by excess funding for one problem (infectious diseases) over other basic needs.

How underreporting affects disparities and consideration

Call *et al.* (2007), from findings of a study examining differences in uninsured estimates, suggest that state surveys of health insurance coverage are less than the estimates provided through the US Census Bureau's Current Population Survey Annual Social and Economic Supplement (http://www. census.gov/apsd/techdoc/cps/cpsmar05.pdf). The study brings into question reported rates of uninsurance and changes over time. Sen and Bonita (2000) point to impressive gains in global health status, yet inadequate regional and national health surveillance systems undermine efforts to address the complex mixture of old and new health concerns. Sen and Bonita (2000) conclude:

> Impressive improvements have occurred in global health status in the past century. Unfortunately, these improvements have not been shared equally and health inequalities within and among countries are entrenched. The fragility of health gains has been seen in response to economic, political, and social changes, and civil disruption (p. 577).

Influence of health literacy upon health outcomes and lessons for health policy considerations

Schillinger *et al.* (2006) studied a sample of persons with diabetes to determine whether literacy mediates the relationship between education and glycemic control: they indeed found this to be the case. This finding indicated that health policy discussions should address not only health disparities, but also the effects that health illiteracy has upon health outcomes.

World Health Organization and disparity concerns

In May 2008, the 61st session of the World Health Assembly was held in Geneva. The assembly was attended by close to 3000 participants from almost 200 countries (World Health Organization 2008). Among others, health policy-related endorsements from this meeting included (World Health Organization 2008):

- calls for a 6-year action plan to tackle non-communicable diseases, now the leading threats to human health
- the adoption of a resolution urging Member States to take decisive action to address health impacts from climate change
- the commitment of Member States to accelerating action towards eliminating the practice of female genital mutilation through laws and educational and community efforts
- directing WHO to help countries in reaching higher coverage of immunization and encouraging the development of new vaccines
- requesting WHO to assess the health aspects in migrant environments and to explore options to improve the health of migrants.

Apart from these important suggestions, there need to be rigorous, ongoing examinations of how disparities and deprivation impact the achievement of these lofty goals. Interventions must be thoroughly evaluated for effectiveness and intended impact.

The impact of the ethical dimension of uninsurance and health

Although this is the final segment of this chapter, it is not the least important. There is a focal ethical dimension to the impact of health disparities and lack of insurance or availability of health care resources for the USA. The USA is not isolated in these disparities, but for the sake of example, US data will be presented here. The discussion is limited to the following topics:

- infant, neonatal, and postneonatal mortality rates
- chronic conditions among adults and influence of poverty
- health insurance coverage for non-seniors
- uninsured population under 65 years
- cost-prohibitive nature of health services
- access to care and *Healthy People 2010* goals.

Infant, neonatal, and postneonatal mortality rates

The most vulnerable population in any country is the infant and neonatal subgroup. The inability to have a voice or input into health care choices is the hallmark of this group of society. Figure 1.1 shows the great gains in mortality rates for infants, neonatal, and postneonatal groups in the USA. It is readily apparent that there have been tremendous gains in saving lives in these subgroups. Each of these categories now has less than 10% mortality rate. But, by combining these values across the groupings, there remains a greater than 10% mortality rate for perinatal mortality. In a country with the vast

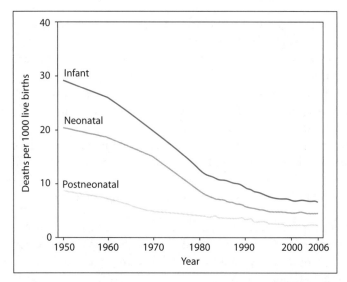

Figure 1.1 Infant, neonatal, and postneonatal mortality rates. Source: CDC/NCHS, Health, United States, 2009, Figure 17. Data from the National Statistics System. National Center for Health Statistics; Health, United States, 2009 With Chartbook on Trends in the Health of Americans, Hyattsville, MD: 2010.

resources and availability of specialized services, is it ethical to have these figures, although diminishing, remain at the level they have been between 1995 and the present?

Chronic conditions among adults and influence of poverty

Figure 1.2 presents a cross-tabulation of numbers of chronic diseases by age and by percentage of poverty level. The pervasively negative impact of poverty (here stratified by four quartiles) upon the number of chronic diseases (three or more) and age groupings is depicted, although not especially in the 75+ age grouping. This is the fastest-growing segment of the population in the USA, and upwards of 30–40% of these individuals have three or more chronic conditions. We may be living longer as a society on average, but the influence of disease morbidity upon individuals as they age is significant. Of further interest is the availability of health insurance coverage, or lack thereof, for individuals and subsequent influence upon disease occurrence and chronicity.

Health insurance coverage for non-seniors

Figure 1.3 shows the various categories of health insurance for individuals other than seniors. The percentage of the uninsured in the USA has remained fairly stable, hovering around 15–17% of the population over a 20-year

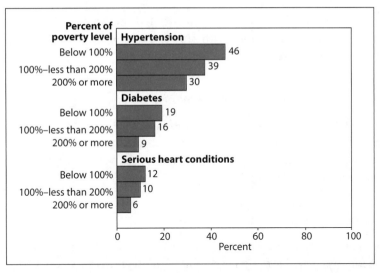

Figure 1.2 Chronic conditions among adults and influence of poverty. Respondent-reported conditions among adults aged 45–64, 2007. Source: CDC/NCHS, Health, United States, 2009, Figure 10. Data from the National Health Interview Survey. National Center for Health Statistics; Health, United States, 2009 With Chartbook on Trends in the Health of Americans, Hyattsville, MD: 2010.

period. Over this same period the percentage of the population less than age 65 has dropped. Since most private insurance is employer-provided (and for the most part with employee cost-sharing), this decrease portends a growing phenomenon of full-time employment but without health benefits. The

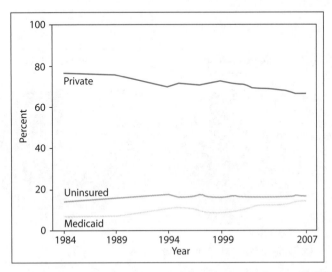

Figure 1.3 Health insurance coverage among people under age 65. Source: CDC/NCHS, Health, United States, 2009, Figure 19. Data from the National Health Interview Survey. National Center for Health Statistics; Health, United States, 2009 With Chartbook on Trends in the Health of Americans, Hyattsville, MD: 2010.

percentage of the population covered through the Medicaid program has doubled in a 20-year period, with slower rates of increase for the years 2005–2009, which are not shown in this figure.

Uninsured population under 65 years

Uninsured individuals and health care insurance are disproportionately affected by variables of age, race, marital status, and poverty level. The influence of each of these is apparent, but the influence of race, poverty level, and marital status is telling.

Cost-prohibitive nature of health services

Figure 1.4 shows how costs make the access of basic health services out of reach for so many. Particularly telling is the segment of seniors (theoretically covered under Medicare) who are unable to access services due to costs. Despite the vast sums spent on health care in the USA – more in total and per capita than anywhere else in the world – associated benefits do not match the money spent. Table 1.1 presents a WHO ranking carried out in 2000 examining how countries measure against each other. Sadly, the USA ranks 37 out of the 191 countries examined. This reinforces the point that money spent is not necessarily a good estimator of overall health. It is also a telling assessment of the impact of the uninsured or underinsured subpopulations in the USA.

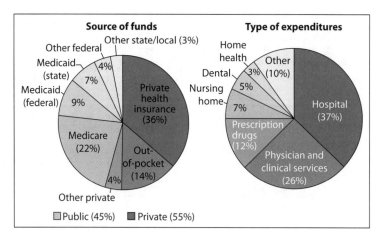

Figure 1.4 Cost centers for costs associated with health services. Personal health care expenditures, 2007. Expenditures: $1.9 trillion. Source: CDC/NCHS, Health, United States, 2009, Figure 21. Data from the Centers for Medicare & Medicaid Services. National Center for Health Statistics; Health, United States, 2009 With Chartbook on Trends in the Health of Americans, Hyattsville, MD: 2010

Table 1.1 World Health Organization health care rankings

Ranking	Country
1	France
2	Italy
3	San Marino
4	Andorra
5	Malta
6	Singapore
7	Spain
8	Oman
9	Austria
10	Japan
11	Norway
12	Portugal
13	Monaco
14	Greece
15	Iceland
16	Luxembourg
17	Netherlands
18	UK
19	Ireland
20	Switzerland
21	Belgium
22	Colombia
23	Sweden
24	Cyprus
25	Germany
26	Saudi Arabia
27	United Arab Emirates
28	Israel

(continued overleaf)

Table 1.1 *(continued)*	
Ranking	**Country**
29	Morocco
30	Canada
31	Finland
32	Australia
33	Chile
34	Denmark
35	Dominica
36	Costa Rica
37	USA
38	Slovenia

Source: World Health Organization (2000). *The World Health Report*. Geneva: WHO.
A total of 191 countries were evaluated, not just the 38 listed here.

Access to care and *Healthy People 2010* goals

Figure 1.5 provides a picture of three basic components of the *Healthy People 2010* goals which indicate the status of American health care indices of well-being. Each of the histograms presented provides data indicating that much remains to be achieved regarding the adequacy and ethics of the care provided in the USA:

- persons under age 65 with health care coverage
- persons of all ages with a specific source of ongoing primary care
- females who received prenatal care in the first trimester of pregnancy.

Sources of data regarding health policy considerations

In order to make informed decisions about health policy pertaining to populations, subpopulations, at-risk groups, and/or disproportionately disadvantaged groups, access to current and relevant data that can be trusted as being accurate is crucial. In this regard, data are certainly powerful. Table 1.2 provides a listing of data sources that provide reliable health statistics, and other information, that can be of use for health policy considerations.

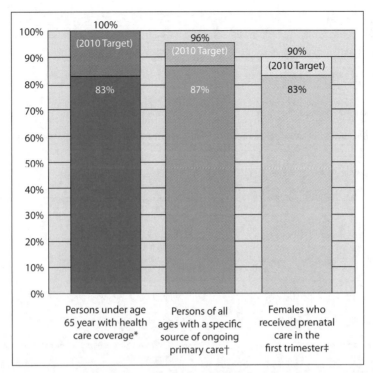

Figure 1.5 Access to care and Healthy People 2010 goals. Sources: Centers for Disease Control and Prevention, National Center for Health Statistics. National Health Interview Survey. *1997 and †1998. Centers for Disease Control and Prevention, National Center for Health Statistics. National Vital Statistics System. ‡1998.

Ethical considerations

We as a society are short-changing vulnerable populations on the provision of basic services. Ethically we are not meeting our responsibilities to provide for those without appropriate access. During an election period, much is laid out, debated, and promised if certain election outcomes are realized. What is necessary is for those elected, those within federal and state bureaucracies, and all others influencing health policy to put remedies in place to impact health outcomes that remain unachieved at present. If there are inadequate segments of recently passed legislation (e.g., the Patient Protection and Affordable Care Act), health policy discussions and advocacy must continue to carry the mantle until more equitable components are included via further regulations or additive legislation.

Table 1.2 Data sources for health policy analyses

Data source	Website
Behavioral risk factor surveillance system	http://apps.nccd.cdc.gov/s_broker/htmsql.exe/weat/index.hsql
Communicable diseases data	http://apps.who.int/globalatlas
Comprehensive list of health data, tools, and statistics	http://www.nlm.nih.gov/hsrinfo/datasites.html
Demographic and health survey data	http://www.measuredhs.com
General demographics and US facts	http://factfinder.census.gov/home/saff/main.html?_lang=en
Health data tools and statistics library	http://phpartners.org/health_stats.html
Mortality, morbidity, risk factors, and health systems data	http://www.who.int/research/en
Research tools on KaiserEDU.org	http://www.kaiseredu.org/research_index.asp
State health facts	http://www.statehealthfacts.org
The World Factbook	https://www.cia.gov/library/publications/the-world-factbook
US global health policy	http://www.globalhealthfacts.org
US expenditures and utilization	http://www.meps.ahrq.gov/mepsweb/data_stats/meps_query.jsp

Discussion questions

1 Assuming that there are racial differences in how health care is provided in the USA, what health policy influences can remedy this situation?
2 What can be done to influence rates of uninsurance and the impact this has upon health status?
3 Why do disparities in health care exist throughout the world? Why do well-intentioned health professionals treat different groups in a disparate fashion?
4 What influence does poverty have upon health care?
5 What effect do you feel the 2010 UK elections will have on drug pricing not only in the UK, but also elsewhere?
6 Why is there a positive correlation between health status and socioeconomic class/status?

7 List several social determinants of health and explain their influence upon health. What health policy impacts can influence these social determinants?

8 What disease states are influenced to a different degree due to racial differences?

9 What health policy decisions will need to be made to deal with increasing US Medicaid and Medicare enrollments in the next several decades?

10 Is it ethical for Medicare Part D enrollees to pay premiums and increasing co-payment amounts for prescription medications while drug company profits continue to increase?

11 Why do infectious diseases seem to affect disproportionately developing countries in the Third World?

12 What influence does a varying level of health literacy have upon patient subgroups?

13 Why do neonatal mortality rates differ so much internationally?

14 What influence can health policy have upon *Healthy People 2020* goals and objectives?

References

Borger C, Smith S, Truffer C, *et al.* (2006). Health spending projections through 2015: changes on the horizon. *Health Aff* 25: w61–w73.

Braveman P (2006). Health disparities and health equity: concepts and measurement. *Ann Rev Pub Health* 27: 167–194.

Call KT, Davern M, Blewett LA (2007). Estimates of health insurance coverage: comparing state surveys with the current population survey. *Health Aff* 26: 269–278.

Commission on Social Determinants of Health (CSDH) (2008). *Closing the Gap in a Generation: Health Equity through Action on the Social Determinants of Health. Final Report of the Commission on Social Determinants of Health.* Geneva: World Health Organization.

Corso PS, Hammitt JK, Graham JD, *et al.* (2002). Assessing preferences for prevention versus treatment using willingness to pay. *Med Decision Making* 22(suppl): S92–S101.

Currie J, Decker S, Lin W (2008). Has public health insurance for older children reduced disparities in access to care and health outcomes? *J Health Econ* 27: 1567–1581.

Dearing JW, Full N, Dearing W (2004). Improving the state of health programming by using diffusion theory. *J Health Commun* 9(suppl1): 21–36.

Dor A, Pylypchuck Y, Shin P, *et al.* (2008). *Uninsured and Medicaid Patients' Access to Preventive Care: Comparison of Health Centers and Other Primary Care Providers.* Research Brief 44. Washington, DC: Geiber/Gibson Program RCHN Community Health Foundation Research Collaborative, 2008.

Gwatkin DR (2007). 10 best resources on . . . health equity. *Health Aff* 26: 269–278.

Hadley J, Holahan J, Coughlin T, *et al.* (2008). Covering the uninsured in 2008: current costs, sources of payment, and incremental costs. *Health Aff* 27: w399–w415.

Hirschler B (2010). UK coalition govt. could end free drug pricing. Available online at: http://www.reuters.com/article/idUSLDE64O05G20100525?type=marketsNews (accessed 25 May 2010).

Hoffman B (2003). Health care reform and social movements in the United States. *Am J Public Health* 93: 75–85.

Hussey P, Anderson G, Berthelot JM, *et al.* (2008). Trends in socioeconomic disparities in health care quality in four countries. *Int J Qual Health Care* 20: 53–61.

Kasturi S, Ruth B (2000). Global health status: two steps forward, one step back. *Lancet* 356: 577–582.

Krobot KJ, Miller WC, Kaufman JS, *et al.* (2004). The disparity in access to new medication by type of health insurance: lessons from Germany. *Med Care* 42: 487–491.

Marmot M (2006). Health in an unequal world. *Lancet* 368: 2081–2094.

Oliver MN, Muntaner C (2005). Researching health inequities among African Americans: the imperative to understand social class. *Int J Health Serv* 35: 485–498.

Perdue DG, Perkins C, Jackson-Thompson J, *et al.* (2008). Regional differences in colorectal cancer incidence, stage, and subsite among American Indians and Alaska Natives, 1999–2004. *Cancer* 113: 1179–1190.

Schillinger D, Barton LR, Karter AJ, *et al.* (2006). Does literacy mediate the relationship between education and health outcomes? A study of a low-income population with diabetes. *Public Health Rep* 121: 245–254.

Sen K, Bonita R (2000). Global health status: two steps forward, one step back. *Lancet* 356: 2195.

US Department of Health and Human Services (2000). *Healthy People 2010: Understanding and Improving Health*, 2nd edn. Washington, DC: US Government Printing Office, 2000.

US Department of Health and Human Services, Office of Disease Prevention and Health Promotion (2010). *Healthy People 2020*. Available online at: http://www.healthypeople. gov/Default.htm (accessed 29 April 2010).

Widdus R (2001). Public–private partnerships for health: their main targets, their diversity, and their future directions. *Bull WHO* 79: 713–720.

World Health Organization (2008). Sixty-first World Health Assembly. Available online at: http://www.who.int/mediacentre/events/2008/wha61/en/index.html (accessed 9 September 2008).

Further reading

Abercrombie DD (2008). Health disparities. In: Ballweg R, Sullivan EM, Brown D, *et al. Physician Assistant*, 4th edn. Philadelphia: WB Saunders, pp. 739–748.

Apter AJ, Casillas AM (2009). Eliminating health disparities: What have we done and what do we do next? *J Allergy Clin Immunol* 123: 1237–1239.

Brownell P (2010). Social issues and social policy response to abuse and neglect of older adults. In: Gloria G, Charmaine S (eds) *Aging, Ageism and Abuse*. London: Elsevier, pp. 1–15.

Carter SL (2010). Improving the importance of treatment effects. *The Social Validity Manual*. San Diego: Academic Press, pp. 175–208.

Cox KJ (2009). Midwifery and health disparities: theories and intersections. *J Midwifery Women's Health* 54: 57–64.

Feisullin K, Westhoff C (2010). Contraception. In: Legato MJ (ed.) *Principles of Gender-Specific Medicine*, 2nd edn. San Diego: Academic Press, pp. 357–365.

Hightower J (2010). Abuse in later life: When and how does gender matter? In: Gloria G, Charmaine S (eds) *Aging, Ageism and Abuse*. London: Elsevier, pp. 17–29.

Messinger-Rapport B (2009). Disparities in long-term healthcare. *Nurs Clin North Am* 44: 179–185.

Narva AS, Sequist TD (2010). Reducing health disparities in American Indians with chronic kidney disease. *Semin Nephrol* 30: 19–25.

Smith DL (2008). Disparities in health care access for women with disabilities in the United States from the 2006 National Health Interview Survey. *Disability Health J* 1: 79–88.

Steinberg ML (2008). Inequity in cancer care: explanations and solutions for disparity. *Semin Radiat Oncol* 18: 161–167.

Yamada A-M, Brekke JS (2008). Addressing mental health disparities through clinical competence not just cultural competence: The need for assessment of sociocultural issues in the delivery of evidence-based psychosocial rehabilitation services. *Clin Psychol Rev* 28: 1386–1399.

Case Study

OBRA '90 (USA)

Introduction

The Omnibus Budget Reconciliation Act of 1990 (OBRA '90), passed and signed into law, is a startling example of health policy being driven by federal legislation. Among other measures dealing with health and many non-health-related matters, it is safe to say OBRA '90 has had a major influence on health care and health care delivery. Its passage was significant, from the range of activities affected within health professions, the pharmaceutical industry, and the insurance industry. This act has changed the landscape of health care and health care delivery in the USA. Within this bill, the following components were included:

- regulation of Medi-Gap insurance policies for Medicare-eligible seniors
- requirements for patient counseling in the pharmacy setting
- providers are required to provide information to patients and caregivers on advance directives and living wills
- Medicaid coverage is expanded to all children living in households living below the poverty level
- stipulated how drugs are reimbursed and for the first time required rebates from pharmaceutical manufacturers for participation within the Medicaid program in the USA (since Medicaid programs are jointly financed by the state and federal government, this has impacted every pharmacy and every Medicaid patient within each of the 50 states).

Medi-Gap insurance policies

According to the US Centers for Medicare and Medicaid Services (CMS), Medi-Gap (Medicare Supplement Insurance) policies are in place to fill the gaps left by Medicare insurance coverage for seniors. These policies, which are sold by private insurance companies and which require monthly premium payments, are regulated via requirements initially specified within OBRA '90 and by federal and state laws. OBRA '90 put the parameters in place that stipulate benefits within Medi-Gap policies. Medi-Gap policies are for individuals only; spouses must purchase their own policies.

Medicaid Drug Rebate Program

Created by the OBRA '90, the Medicaid Drug Rebate (2010) Program requires a drug manufacturer to enter into and have in effect a national rebate agreement with the Secretary of the Department of Health and Human Services (HHS) for states to receive federal funding for outpatient drugs dispensed to Medicaid patients. The Medicaid Drug Rebate Program, as a part of OBRA '90, was placed in this bill as a compromise between interests representing the US pharmaceutical industry and representatives from the US CMS. The Drug Rebate Program is administered by the CMS Center for Medicaid and State Operations. The Drug Rebate Program was amended by the Veterans Health Care Act (VHCA) of 1992. Under VHCA, drug manufacturers are required to enter into a pricing agreement with HHS for the Section 340B Drug Pricing Program, which is administered by the Health Resources and Services Administration.

Approximately 550 pharmaceutical companies currently participate in this program. Forty-nine states (Arizona is excluded) and the District of Columbia cover drugs under the Medicaid Drug Rebate Program.

As of January 1, 1996, the rebate for covered outpatient drugs is as follows: for innovator drugs, the larger of 15.1% of the average manufacturer price (AMP) per unit or the difference between the AMP and the best price per unit, adjusted by the consumer price index for urban consumers based on launch date and current quarter AMP. And for non-innovator drugs, the rebate required is 11% of the AMP per unit.

This agreement, to require a rebate to be paid based on the amount of drugs used within individual state Medicaid programs, was a compromise that was instituted in exchange for individual state Medicaid programs not to place restrictive formularies as a requirement for the drug component of Medicaid. State Medicaid programs operate with guidance from federal edicts (via CMS). Medicaid programs are financed from joint state and federal funding sources. Thus the overarching guidance from CMS with broad guidelines influences state level programs. The allowance of open formularies (almost any drug can be prescribed, dispensed, and reimbursed within Medicaid programs across the country) in exchange for requiring rebates is a lasting component of OBRA '90.

This compromise may be considered to be a "pact with the devil" which avoids at all costs any negotiation between the federal government and the pharmaceutical industry for coverage of drugs within Medicaid and Medicare programs. Despite the fact that the federal government has negotiated with pharmaceutical companies for decades for drugs procured for use in the Veterans Administration, Public Health Clinics (so called 340B programs), and other federal programs through the federal supply schedule pricing, Medicare and Medicaid programs do not benefit from potential negotiated savings for drugs within these massive federal and state programs.

Medicaid drug utilization review programs

This segment of OBRA '90 required patient counseling for outpatients receiving Medicaid prescriptions to be provided for every prescription. From OBRA '90, specific guidelines regarding how to counsel patients were detailed. Topics that pharmacists need to address with patients included, but were not limited to, the following:

- name and description of the medication
- route of administration
- dose
- dosage form
- duration of drug therapy
- special directions and precautions for preparation of drugs
- administration and use by the patient
- common severe side-effects/adverse effects
- interactions and therapeutic contraindications that may be encountered (including their avoidance and the action required if they occur)
- techniques for self-monitoring drug therapy
- proper storage
- refill information
- appropriate action in case of a missed dose.

This act sparked increased national interest in the need for patient counseling, and was the result of the awareness that patients were not receiving adequate counseling on their prescriptions, and subsequently led to the passing of legislation mandating the need to counsel all patients from various states across the USA. In effect, how could counseling be specified for one "class of patients" – Medicaid patients – but not for others? So, a piece of federal legislation changed health policy for Medicaid patients, and subsequently State Board of Pharmacy rules and regulations were changed in all states mandating that these OBRA '90 initially directed drug utilization review activities now be regulated by board edict in all states.

Discussion questions

1 Why do you feel OBRA '90 has had as many, varied health policy impacts as it has? Name two of these and explain why you consider them to be significant.
2 What influence have Medicaid rebates had upon health care utilization in the USA?
3 Do you feel the creators of the OBRA '90 envisioned the impact drug use/utilization review requirements of OBRA '90 would have on every patient receiving outpatient prescriptions in the USA?
4 Why have Medi-Gap insurance policies for seniors had such an impact upon Medicare enrollees in the USA?
5 What are the health policy implications of open formularies within Medicaid programs throughout the USA?
6 Why would pharmaceutical companies challenge closed formularies as a health policy option?
7 Why have state pharmacy boards of pharmacy incorporated OBRA '90 components into state pharmacy rules and regulations?
8 From a health policy and outcomes perspective, does it matter that OBRA '90 drove patient counseling regulations as opposed to a professional effort to enhance patient counseling for patients receiving outpatient prescription medications? Does it really matter what the means are, or is the end result the important point to consider?
9 Discuss the ethics of receiving patient counseling for prescription medications for patients on one type of insurance as opposed to requirements for all patients.
10 Do you feel OBRA '90 legislative and regulatory requirements could have been instituted via other means? If yes, how could this have been accomplished?

References

Medicaid Drug Rebate (2010). Available online at: http://www.cms.hhs.gov/MedicaidDrugRebateProgram/ (accessed 21 January 2010).
The Standard of Practice – OBRA '90. Citation: Public Law 101-508, S4401, 1927(g) (November 5, 1990) and OBRA '90 Regulations. Federal Register November 2, 1992; 57FR(212):49397-49401.

Further reading

Blake KB, Madhavan SS, Scott VG, *et al.* (2009). Medication therapy management services in West Virginia: Pharmacists' perceptions of educational and training needs. *Res Soc Admin Pharm* 5: 182–188.

Clark BE (2009). Corporate control and professional prerogative: An unresolved tension for pharmacists. *Res Soc Admin Pharm* 5: 299–301.

Guo JJ, Gibson JT, Hancock GR, *et al.* (1995). Retrospective drug utilization review and the behavior of Medicaid prescribers: an empirical marginal analysis. *Clin Ther* 17: 1174–1187.

Guo JJ, Gibson JT, Barker KN (1996). P10. Economic evaluation of drug utilization review on Medicaid pharmacy dispensing behavior: an empiric marginal analysis. *Clin Ther* 18(suppl1): 50.

Guo JJ, Hancock GR, Gibson JT, *et al.* (1996). P11. Effects of drug utilization review on Medicaid prescriber behavior: a latent means modeling analysis. *Clin Ther* 18(suppl1): 50–51.

Gupta S, Rappaport HM, Bennett LT, *et al.* (1996). Inappropriate drug prescribing and related outcomes for elderly Medicaid beneficiaries residing in nursing homes. *Clin Ther* 18: 183–196.

Kamble P, Chen H, Sherer J, *et al.* (2008). Antipsychotic drug use among elderly nursing home residents in the United States. *Am J Geriatr Pharmacother* 6: 187–197.

Lakey SL, Gray SL, Sales AE, *et al.* (2006). Psychotropic use in community residential care facilities: A prospective cohort study. *Am J Geriatr Pharmacother* 4: 227–235.

McKercher PL (1997). Pharmaceuticals in Medicare reform. *Clin Ther* 19: 1426–1432.

Puspitasari HP, Aslani P, Krass I, *et al.* (2009). A review of counseling practices on prescription medicines in community pharmacies. *Res Soc Admin Pharm* 5: 197–210.

Roberts AS, Benrimoj SI, Chen TF, *et al.* (2005). Understanding practice change in community pharmacy: A qualitative study in Australia. *Res Soc Admin Pharm* 1: 546–564.

Sewak SS, Wilkin NE, Bentley JP, *et al.* (2005). Direct-to-consumer advertising via the internet: The role of website design. *Res Soc Admin Pharm* 1: 289–309.

Shah B, Chewning B (2006). Conceptualizing and measuring pharmacist–patient communication: a review of published studies. *Res Soc Admin Pharm* 2: 153–185.

Touré JT, Brandt NJ, Limcangco MR, *et al.* (2006). Impact of second-generation antipsychotics on the use of antiparkinson agents in nursing homes and assisted-living facilities. *Am J Geriatr Pharmacother* 4: 25–35.

Trygstad TK, Christensen DB, Wegner SE, *et al.* (2009). Analysis of the North Carolina Long-Term Care Polypharmacy Initiative: A multiple-cohort approach using propensity-score matching for both evaluation and targeting. *Clin Ther* 31: 2018–2037.

2

Health care systems and health policy

Introduction

Although there are four main systems for providing health care insurance and coverage, there are many nuanced differences in these basic plans based on country-specific factors. Throughout the world there are hundreds of independent countries with differing health care system models in place that globally affect how health care is structured, delivered, and paid for. Differing societal expectations, mores, culture, history, and needs all play into how health care systems are structured. These structures drive health policy, and certainly vice versa as well.

Influencing health care systems via health policy

Figure 2.1 is a schematic representation of varying points of influence for health policy: these segments influence health policy and in turn are influenced by health policy. The processes in play are never static; there is constant movement to and fro and between these influencers.

The recent passage of health care reform legislation (Patient Protection and Affordable Care Act (PPACA)) will provide health insurance coverage options for additional Americans who currently do not have health insurance, but it is incomplete in providing coverage for all who currently lack insurance. In a Congressional Budget Office (CBO) assessment in April, 2010, there will be about 3 million individuals required to pay fines in 2016. These assessed fines will be for individuals with incomes below $59 000 and $120 000 for families of four, according to the CBO projections. The other 900 000 people who must pay the fine will have higher incomes. The collection of $4 billion from such fines will be used to partially subsidize other insurance offerings within the health care reform legislative package (PPACA). Fines will be in the range of $1000. It is noted in this CBO report that the US government will collect about $4 billion a year in fines from 2017 through 2019.

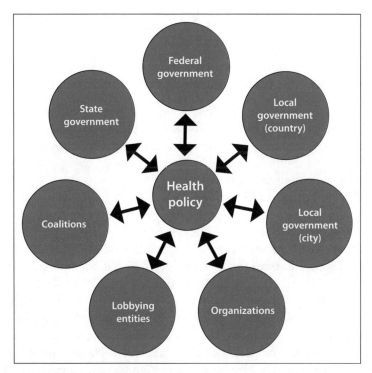

Figure 2.1 Influencers of health policy.

The PPACA will increase spending by $938 billion over 10 years (The Staff of the Washington Post 2010a). These increases will come from providing:

- tax credits
- subsidies to help small businesses and consumers to buy insurance
- government increases in Medicaid coverage expansion.

Spending cuts that are projected at this point will total $1 trillion (The Staff of the Washington Post 2010a). These cuts are from the following sources:

- reduction in spending within Medicare
- new taxes and penalties for non-purchase of insurance.

It is difficult at this time to assess this massive bill and its purported successes accurately (The Staff of the Washington Post 2010b). Difficulties with the PPACA stem from the fact that the largest provision for individual coverage mandate, insurance exchange, and the subsidies do not take hold until 2014 (The Staff of the Washington Post 2010b). Challenges to the success of this bill include the effects of inflation over a 10-year period, and predicting what will happen to physicians' charges, hospital charges, and pharmaceutical costs. The experience to date in the USA with universal coverage lies in the state of Massachusetts. And the Massachusetts experience is that these costs have increased and not been affected by the universal coverage requirements that were put into place.

Models of health care delivery and financing systems

In *The Healing of America: A Global Quest for Better, Cheaper, and Fairer Health Care,* author TR Reid (2009) describes the methods that other industrialized democracies have used to provide health care for citizens for far less than what is spent on health care in the USA. These countries provide universal coverage for all their citizens.

Reid (2009) describes his purpose in writing this book as to "search the developed world for effective health care systems and take lessons from the ones that work best." Not surprisingly, Reid finds positives and negatives in many of the systems he evaluates in an unbiased fashion. His conclusion that all spend less administratively than the USA, gain better outputs than the US system, and cover all citizens within countries is irrefutable (Reid 2009).

Reid couches the issue in terms of a fundamental moral decision to provide health care coverage to all citizens or not. Other democracies have embraced providing universal coverage for citizens, and in doing so, they outperform the US health care system on indices of cost, quality, and choice – three key focal points for discussion in the book. Reid (2009) notes that over 20 000 Americans die each year because they cannot afford to see a doctor, and quotes that 700 000 individuals must declare bankruptcy due to mounting bills arising from a lack of health insurance coverage.

Four basic models of health care delivery and insurance

Four basic models of health care delivery and insurance have evolved over time. As was noted above, these models have been adapted and combined for country-specific necessities. The four models are as follows:

1 Beveridge model
2 Bismarck model
3 national health insurance model
4 out-of-pocket model.

The Beveridge model

The Beveridge model, named for William Beveridge (1879–1963), describes the British National Health Service (NHS) (http://www.bbc.co.uk/history/historic_figures/beveridge_william.shtml). William Beveridge was an economist and social reformer in the UK. In 1941, the British government commissioned a report to detail how the UK should be rebuilt after World War II (Anonymous 2010). The report, issued in 1942, detailed five "giant evils" in need of being addressed: want, disease, ignorance, squalor, and idleness. This report served as the basis for the UK to address health care problems, the health care delivery system, and payment for health care in the UK (Anonymous 2010).

The British NHS was begun in 1948, and its initiation was based upon the work of William Beveridge and the model he proposed. As an appointed peer in the British Parliament, Beveridge was a leader of the Liberals in the British House of Lords (Anonymous 2010). Although the model was named in honor of William Beveridge, Aneurin Bevan, government Minister of Health at the time, was the chief architect of the British NHS (Klein 2006).

The British NHS is truly a cradle-to-grave insurance and health delivery system covering all British citizens (Klein 2006). In his historical treatise on the politics of the decision to form the NHS Klein (2006) noted:

> Britain's National Health Service (NHS) came into existence on 5 July 1948. It was the first health system in any western society to offer free medical care to the entire population. It was, furthermore, the first comprehensive system to be based not on the insurance principle, with entitlement following contributions, but on the national provision of services available to everyone. It thus offered free and universal entitlement to state-provided medical care (p. 1).

Delamothe (2008) notes that, in addition to the above, quality and equity should be added to this descriptor of the British NHS, since these tenets have been key segments of the NHS from its inception. Other countries have applied the Beveridge model to health care systems and include Italy, Spain, and Cuba. The Medicaid program in the USA is a Beveridge model for those with coverage, with the exception that hospitals, providers, and associated allied health providers who provide Medicaid services are not owned by the US government.

US Department of Veterans Affairs (VA) health care – similar to the Beveridge model

The VA health care system in the USA is probably the most exact duplicator of the British NHS, as is the US Indian health service (care provided to Native Americans) and the US Department of Defense (active-duty military personnel and their families through the Tricare managed care program within the Department of Defense).

VA health care issues

The number of US veterans is depicted in Figure 2.2. Also shown is the number of veterans with service-connected disabilities. The number of service-connected disabilities has increased recently as more advanced methods of treating battlefield traumas have emerged, saving many soldiers. Also, as shown in Figure 2.2, the numbers of US veterans has decreased from 1980 (elevations

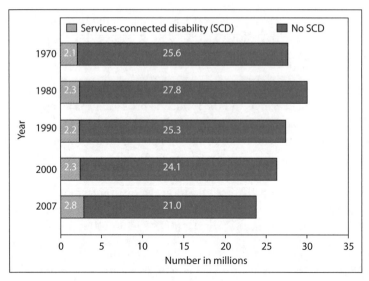

Figure 2.2   Living US military veterans in the USA. Source: CDC/NCHS, Health, United States, 2009, Figure 3. Data from the US Department of Veterans Affairs and the US Census Bureau. National Center for Health Statistics; Health, United States, 2009 With Chartbook on Trends in the Health of Americans, Hyattsville, MD: 2010.

due to the number of US veterans from the Vietnam War) through the first decade of the 2000s. However, with wars under way in both Iraq and Afghanistan at present, the numbers of individuals expected to seek care from VA facilities will no doubt increase in the near and long-term future. The individuals currently receiving care through the US Department of Defense will increase the numbers treated within the VA system. Care provided within the VA system is considered to be good in comparison with that received elsewhere in the US system.

Service-related concerns within the VA system
The access to care and treatment of long-term consequences of war injuries or exposures has long been a sore point for US veterans. The health effects of exposure to Agent Orange by Vietnam veterans (Schuck 1987), Gulf War syndrome for the first Iraq War veterans (Taylor and Stephenson 2007), improvised explosive device-related traumas and need for subsequent rehabilitation (Gondusky and Reiter 2005), and posttraumatic stress disorder for many veterans from many wars have long been controversial and contentiously debated syndromes (Seal *et al.* 2007). Posttraumatic stress disorder among US veterans is not something that just occurred with veterans from World Wars I and II or the Vietnam War. Similarly occurring symptoms experienced by Civil War veterans were

called "soldiers' heart," referring to a rapid heart rate that occurred with veterans. Within other wars, veterans of those wars spoke of shell shock or battle fatigue.

The Bismarck model

The Bismarck model of health care structure, financing, and delivery is named in honor of Prussian Chancellor Otto von Bismarck, who unified Germany in the 19th century. As a component of unification, Bismarck oversaw the creation of the first western welfare state. This system incorporates "sickness funds" which are jointly financed by employers and employees via payroll deductions. In this instance, the Bismarck model represents what is available to employees via employer-sponsored health insurance coverage. The major difference in the German system is that the "sickness funds" companies (e.g., health insurance companies) are not profit-generating entities. These "sickness fund" companies do not make a profit.

This Bismarck model of health care can be found in Germany, France, Belgium, the Netherlands, Japan, Switzerland, and in some cases in Latin America (Reid 2009). It is also, as noted, available in the USA as employer–employee-partnered insurance for many employed Americans less than 65 years of age.

The national health insurance model

The Canadian system of health care approximates a national health insurance model. The Canadian system originated in Saskatchewan in the late 1940s. Saskatchewan Premier Tommy Douglas was the architect of the plan, providing public coverage for residents through the Saskatchewan Hospitalization Act. On January 1, 1947, hospital care became free for residents of Saskatchewan (Reid 2009). Through debate, short-term strikes by the medical community, rancor and discussion, the will of the Canadian people remained steadfast for a health care system nationwide. The Canadian Health Act, providing for a universal plan throughout Canada, was passed by the Canadian Parliament in 1984 (Reid 2009). Each of the 10 Canadian provinces and three territories administers its own plan (Reid 2009). This model of structure, delivery, and financing contains elements of both the Beveridge and Bismarck models. This system uses private-sector care providers coupled with universal coverage with one payer – the Canadian government. The Canadian system is a true national health insurance model, and is guided by five principles:

1 publicly administered throughout all provinces
2 comprehensive coverage for all services
3 universal, home jurisdiction covers the individual until residency status is settled during any waiting periods

4 portable (coverage is available for Canadians regardless of the province they are in or travel to or move to, e.g., moving from Ontario to British Columbia). However the Ontario Health Insurance Plan (OHIP) will not pay for services deemed not medically necessary.

5 accessibility: all insured Canadians have reasonable access to health care facilities. Also, health providers (physicians, pharmacies, hospitals, and other providers) must be reasonably compensated for provision of health care services.

The Taiwanese (Republic of China), when constructing a revised health care system in the 1990s, chose a model most like the national health insurance model, with elements of the Beveridge model. The South Koreans did likewise. Those patients in the USA with Medicare coverage find their health care insurance plan is most like a national health insurance model, e.g., Canada's. The formula for payment to physicians and the process for paying physicians on behalf of Medicare clients are in need of alteration. Three times in 2010 before the end of the fiscal year, stop-gap intercessions were made to stem the implementation of a 21–23% decrease in payments to physicians. In 1997, as part of the budget reconciliation, the US Congress passed a balanced budget law that put the current formula in place, determining how doctors will be paid.

The out-of-pocket model

Until health care reform package (PPACA) was passed, the US system was partially an out-of-pocket model for the 45–47 million uninsured in the USA. Precisely how many will become insured, and thus lose the out-of-pocket status, remains to be seen over the 10-year phase-in of the health care reform package (PPACA), and perhaps alteration based on changes in the US House of Representatives, the US Senate, and presidential elections to be conducted between now and 2014. The lack of a system, or an amalgamated series of differing plans which was and is such a patchwork of a system, has beget a legacy of currently 700 000 medical bankruptcies in the USA each year.

The additional segments which will now eliminate exclusion of pre-existing conditions for insurance eligibility, removal of insurance caps on payments over a lifetime, expansion of coverage for many currently uninsured, provision of Medicaid to more individuals due to reduction in the income eligibility ceiling, and coverage for children under their parents' insurance plans through age 26, will be a hoped-for tremendous help for many currently desperate individuals in the USA.

Rural India, Burkina Faso, and Cambodia all have out-of-pocket models of health care system structure, delivery, and payment for health care in play. This system of out-of-pocket care may also be referred to as a market-driven process of health care delivery.

Socialized medicine

The term "socialized medicine" dates back to the 1940s, 12 US presidential eras back in the past, when there was a backlash against then President Harry Truman's efforts to sponsor a reorganization of the US health care system to provide universal health care insurance for all Americans. Then, the American Medical Association used "socialized medicine" as a "red herring" to avert the American public's eye away from the beneficial segments of a national health insurance for all program. In Reid's treatise, the myth of many foreign (to the USA) systems as all being "socialized medicines" is debunked (Reid 2009). In Chapter 13 of his book, Reid explodes various myths surrounding foreign health care systems, namely:

* "It's all socialized medicine out there."
* "They ration care with waiting lists and limited choice."
* "They are wasteful systems run by bloated bureaucracies."
* "Health insurance companies have to be cruel."
* "Those systems are too foreign to work in the USA."

Not every one of these comparator systems is perfect and to his credit Reid (2009) points out flaws consistently and fairly. For example, he finds long queues in Canada, poorly paid physicians in Japan, undertreated patients in the UK, and challenging facilities in France. Reid interviews physicians, hospital administrators, governmental regulators, international health care experts, and finally patients receiving care.

Influence of lobbyists and special-interest groups on health policy

It is certainly not a surprise to anyone that the influence of lobbyists on many pieces of legislation is significant, pervasive, and effective in achieving specific goals of special-interest groups. One can guess as to the influence the contributions have on many aspects of what extends into laws affecting many aspects of our lives. These resultant effects (of perhaps funding shifts to other items) on health care, health care systems, health insurance programs, health professions, health professionals, and health professional educational programs are blatant and oppressive because of neglect of other worthy funding points.

Follow the money

The passage of the Medicare Prescription Drug, Improvement, and Modernization Act of 2003 (MMA) (Pub. L. 108-173) is a case in point of how funding follows lobbyists' collective activities. The Medicare Part D drug program as a part of this legislation overtly favored pharmaceutical manufacturers, insurers, and pharmacy benefit management companies in an egregious fashion. Pharmaceutical companies were and are allowed to do business as usual with multiple pricing levels, and retain the ability to raise prices at will. The MMA legislation specifically prohibits the Centers for Medicare and Medicaid Services (CMS) from negotiating with pharmaceutical companies for advantageous prices that these same companies provide freely elsewhere. The Federal Supply Schedule pricing has allowed the VA to purchase drugs at reduced prices and the federal 340B Drug Pricing Program provides access to reduced-price prescription drugs to over 12 000 health care facilities certified in the USA. Pharmaceutical companies remain profitable even with these reduced pricing programs, partly due to their ability to shift price hikes elsewhere in a multilayered process of drug pricing.

To provide for optimum participation by Medicare Part D prescription drug plans (PDPs) and Medicare Advantage (MA-PDPs, as a component of managed care Medicare Part C) drug plans, a component of the MMA legislation provided PDPs and MA-PDPs with significant subsidies containing upfront funding, allowing these companies to participate with an assurance of profitability (Levinson 2007). In effect, participating plans were given a profitability fallback regardless of what happened with enrollment into their plans by eligible seniors, and were thus risk-averse from a lack of enrollment and/or profitability with their proffered plans.

As the legislation was written and enabled, for the first year of the program, due to overpayment to PDP and MA sponsors, Part D plan sponsors owed Medicaid a net total of $4.4 billion for the year 2006. This amount of overpayment has been reduced to $600 million for 2007, a significant reduction, but this amount remains sizeable. These overestimated payments provided to plans were to be returned to Medicare. However, to complicate this matter further, CMS had no mechanisms in place to collect funds from such overpayments. This was finally set up and accomplished well into 2007 for the 2006 payments; as such, sponsors held significant amounts of money for an extended period of time. Lobbyists exerted pressure to pass the MMA in the form in which it was enacted.

The health care lobbyist influence on health care matters is significant (Heid and Sook 2009). According to Northwestern University's Medill News Service, the number of former House and Senate key staffers turned lobbyists is significant (Heid and Sood 2009). There are 14 former chiefs of staff and four former deputy chiefs of staff among the more than 200 former congressional aides now working as lobbyists and registered in 2008–2009 (Heid and Sood 2009).

These are US Senators and they work at a federal level and greatly impact health policy. Funding scenarios by these vested interests may be less intense in terms of dollar volumes in various state legislatures, but these groups in the health sector, providing funding at the federal level, also fund state legislators in each state. Here the competing interests for funding affecting state Medicaid programs most definitely intersect with state funding for other worthy entities.

Changing health care systems is contentious

The structures of a country's health care systems are a complex amalgamation of influences, patterns, and societal expectations. Changing a system dramatically becomes more difficult as health policy influences from insurers, providers, patient advocacy groups, state and federal government entities, and society bear down on health care systems. Efforts to pass enabling legislation in the UK in 1948, in Canada in 1984, in Taiwan and Switzerland in the 1990s, and in the USA in 2010 were all contentious processes.

Key points of stress for the future US health care system and health care policy applications

With the passage of PPACA in March 2010, one inclination is to rest easy; problems currently in the USA health care system will now be fixed. This is far from the true state of affairs both at present and in the future. Small steps of success often herald the major cliffs yet to be surmounted. For example, the passage of health care reform legislation earlier in 2010 was heralded by suggestions of an immediate impact on public health as a result, while others suggest this bill is flawed and incomplete. Perhaps these views may both be correct. Regardless, the major influences on the health care system and patients remain to be seen and may be decades away. Oftentimes pundits will suggest that it was important to get something passed, even if not the most appropriate bill possible. In the future, problems currently in place can be readily fixed when improvements are made on the passed bill. This did not occur with the passage of PPACA and the Medicare Part D program, flawed in design and implementation from the outset.

Initial problems with the Medicare Part D drug benefit included:

- "doughnut hole" period of lack of coverage after initial co-insurance requirements met, targeted to be reduced over a 10-year period with the enactment of PPACA and specific components dealing with the "doughnut hole"
- pricing increases
- many competing plans with many choices

- access to CMS website by seniors: the website has recently been updated, but readability concerns may still exist
- readability of materials supplied to seniors.

This program, which began on January 1, 2006, was not significantly altered by the passage of the PPACA. Tinkering with the benefit might be the best consideration of the passage of PPACA and subsequent effects on the Part D drug benefit. A sum of $250 was provided to Medicare Part D recipients in 2010 to cover some of the "doughnut hole" gap in coverage for eligible seniors. With average prescriptions costing in the range of $70–75, roughly a 160% increase over costs in 1982, this $250 amount will not help many in a significant way. The "doughnut hole" gap is set to shrink over a 10-year phase-in of decreases in costs shared by generic and brand-name drug manu-facturers. However, as optimistic as this sounds, the reality is that prices can still be increased at will by both generic and brand-name manufacturers during this period, as they have done over the years in which Medicare Part D has been in existence (since January 1, 2006). A recent analysis by the Kaiser Family Foundation (Hoadley *et al.* 2010) found that, between 2009 and 2010, monthly prices in the coverage gap increased by 5% or more for half of the top 10 brand-name drugs, while the consumer price index for urban consumers (CPI-U) increased by 2.7% and the CPI for medical care (CPI-M) increased by 3.5% between January 2009 and January 2010.

Competing plans are still numerous – less so with Medicare Advantage plans, which were targeted by the PPACA. The www.medicare.gov website was recently upgraded, but the site is still difficult for many seniors to wade through. Part of this difficulty rests with the degree of readability of Medicare materials: this makes understanding difficult for many, not just seniors.

When examining what lies ahead in the USA, one factor is the rapid numerical rise of the population. From the projections seen in the population growth figure estimated through the year 2050 (Figure 2.3), the number of US citizens is projected to increase dramatically over the next decades. A signif-icant increase in those over the age of 65 is apparent. This projected increase of around 50% in the US population between the years 2010 and 2050 will be impacted by health care costs and availability of coverage, but such a large population increase will surely dramatically influence the US health care system. The true effects of the passage of PPACA upon the population remains to be seen: what can be estimated with certainty is that the system of care, insurance for care, payment levels for care, demand for health services, and the availability of health care will all be significantly challenged in the years ahead.

Individuals are covered under Medicare immediately upon reaching the age of 65 years. But approximately 15% of Medicare recipients are less than age 65 years; they may be disabled or eligible for end-stage renal disease

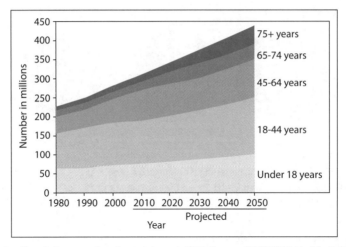

Figure 2.3 Population growth estimates through 2050. Source: CDC/NCHS, Health, United States, 2009, Figure 1A. Data from the US Census Bureau. Source: National Center for Health Statistics; Health, United States, 2009 With Chartbook on Trends in the Health of Americans, Hyattsville, MD: 2010.

services under Medicare. Even with coverage under Medicare, there are gaps in insurance for necessary health expenditures for recipients. This coverage gap will remain significant for several reasons: more seniors will be eligible for Medicare, and this number will not decrease; expenditures will no doubt increase – there has not been an overall decrease in health expenditures for as long as can be remembered; and the types of services, scope, and intensity will increase with advancements, profitability of such, and demand for more advanced treatments.

Medicare does not pay for many services that are required by recipients. For example, long-term care that is custodial in nature is not covered, whether this is home care or care in a long-term care facility. Dental services are not covered under Medicare, including dentures or routine dental care. Vision services, such as routine examinations, eyeglasses and refractions, are not covered by Medicare plans. Also, hearing aids or hearing examinations are not covered under Medicare. There are no limits (ceilings) for out-of-pocket costs on a yearly basis for Medicare enrollees – many private health insurance plans have such limits for out-of-pocket payments. Many seniors purchase Medi-Gap coverage plans to cover non-covered expenses, but these premiums can be expensive and further out-of-pocket payments are additionally required for the most part.

As can readily be discerned from Figure 2.4, the proportion of the population between the ages of 65 and 74 years is estimated to increase by 50% (from 6% to 9%) by 2050, and the population aged 75 and older will virtually double from 6% of the population in 2007 to 11% in 2050. A key point is that the proportion of those between ages 45 and 64 years, as well as between 18

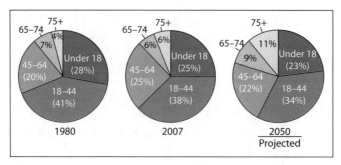

Figure 2.4 Selected population percentages categorized by age. Source: CDC/NCHS, Health, United States, 2009, Figure 1A. Data from the US Census Bureau. National Center for Health Statistics; Health, United States, 2009 With Chartbook on Trends in the Health of Americans, Hyattsville, MD: 2010.

and 44 years, are both decreasing during this projection. The number of eligible individuals requiring Medicare services is increasing dramatically and the proportion of those who will carry the heaviest burden of financing the Medicare program is shrinking as a percentage of the population. These are estimates, it should be noted, but sobering estimates nonetheless. The US CBO provides frequent projections for spending in coming periods. The latest projections point to a projected federal spending in 2020 with a comparison of Medicaid and Medicare percentage of total spending (Congressional Budget Office 2010). Medicare is projected to account for 17% of total federal spending, and Medicaid 8% of total federal spending.

Figure 2.5 provides a view of seniors' longevity in the USA, and the life expectancy for additional years once reaching the age of 65 years. These

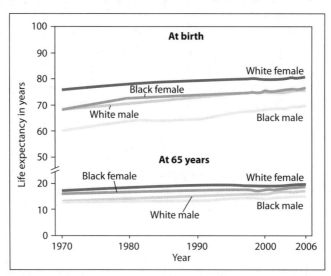

Figure 2.5 Life expectancy. Source: CDC/NCHS, Health, United States, 2009, Figure 16. Data from the National Vital Statistics System. National Center for Health Statistics; Health, United States, 2009 With Chartbook on Trends in the Health of Americans, Hyattsville, MD: 2010.

figures are broken down further, showing differences between blacks, whites, and gender-specific trends within the two races. People are living longer regardless of race; a more pronounced increase for whites than blacks and gender separation is apparent across the two racial groupings. These trend lines again show the pervasively negative influence of race on aging. But the data indicate above other differences that Americans are living longer, and to ages never reached (on average) before. This will have significant societal ramifications in the long term, not only for health care and health care utilization but for other tangents as well.

Figure 2.6 shows that the proportion of the US population accounted for by African-Americans and Hispanic-Americans is increasing. These increases are noteworthy in that data indicate both groups receive disparate care when compared with whites in the USA. How future health care is delivered more equitably will rest on the shoulders of health professionals, health systems, insurers, and the expectations of all these and the recipients of that care.

The percentage breakdown of those living in poverty in the USA is presented in Figure 2.7 and by race and/or ethnicity in Figure 2.8. A significant number of Americans live in poverty in the USA, and minority populations suffer to a significant degree in comparison with whites. Those with fewer resources, economic and otherwise, do not fare as well as those who are better off in the US health care system. The segments of the elderly living in poverty and children living in poverty are both of considerable concern at present and certainly in the future as well. The dramatic decrease in seniors living in

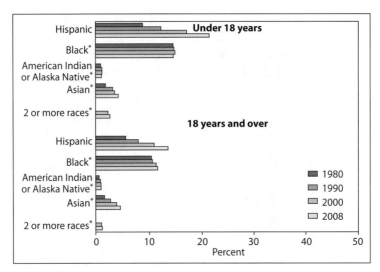

Figure 2.6   Breakdown of population by race/ethnicity. Source: CDC/NCHS, Health, United States, 2009, Figure 2. Data from the Census Bureau. National Center for Health Statistics; Health, United States, 2009 With Chartbook on Trends in the Health of Americans, Hyattsville, MD: 2010. *Not Hispanic.

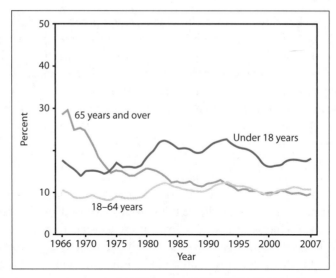

Figure 2.7 Poverty percentages in the USA. Source: CDC/NCHS, Health, United States, 2009, Figure 4. Data from the Census Bureau. National Center for Health Statistics; Health, United States, 2009 With Chartbook on Trends in the Health of Americans, Hyattsville, MD: 2010.

poverty that is seen in Figure 2.7 in 1966 is directly due to the passage of Medicare legislation in 1965 along with Medicaid. These social health insurance programs dramatically affected the levels of poverty (decreasing) and health status (increasing) at that point in the USA.

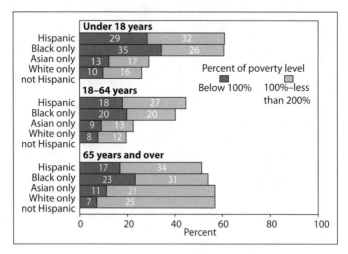

Figure 2.8 Low-income population in 2007 in the USA. Source: CDC/NCHS, Health, United States, 2009, Figure 5. Data from the Census Bureau.National Center for Health Statistics; Health, United States, 2009 With Chartbook on Trends in the Health of Americans, Hyattsville, MD: 2010.

Jones (2010) suggests that health disparities exist along lines of race/ethnicity and socioeconomic class in US society. These disparities are a moral, ethical, and class example of the shortcomings of the US health care system. As with any systemic problem within health care systems and insurance coverage for such, moral courage will be called upon to address these differences in unequal treatment for segments of the US population.

Senior-specific health care issues and future concerns

Figure 2.9 presents interesting data regarding vaccinations and rates for influenza and pneumococcal pneumonia vaccinations by varying age groups. The relatively low rates of vaccinations for both are startling. The rate for pneumococcal pneumonia vaccination is around 60% across all age groupings. It is lowest for those between the ages of 65 and 74 years. This is discouraging since this is a covered benefit within Medicare with no out-of-pocket expenditure required of patients. Providers of care for seniors (physicians, nurses, pharmacists) should be much more proactive in ensuring seniors receive this vaccination. Pneumonia, often a sequela after hip fracture, is a predominant cause of death for seniors. This vaccine can save untold morbidity and postpone mortality to a significant degree. Similarly, the lack of influenza vaccinations by younger as well as older seniors is troubling. Both of the rates of vaccinations (influenza and pneumococcal pneumonia) are low and indicative of serious quality issues for care provided to seniors in the USA.

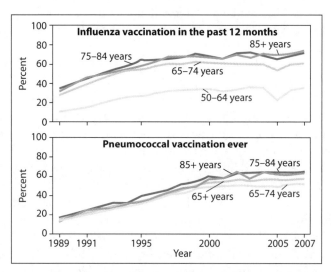

Figure 2.9   Vaccinations and seniors in the USA: influenza and pneumoccal vaccination. Source: CDC/NCHS, Health, United States, 2009, Figure 9. Data from the National Health Interview Survey. National Center for Health Statistics; Health, United States, 2009 With Chartbook on Trends in the Health of Americans, Hyattsville, MD: 2010.

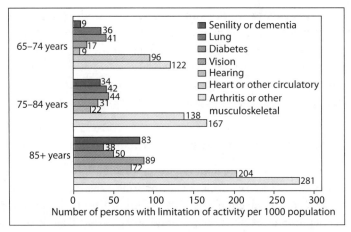

Figure 2.10   Activity limitations due to chronic conditions in seniors. Source: CDC/NCHS, Health, United States, 2009, Figure 9. Data from the National Health Interview Survey. National Center for Health Statistics; Health, United States, 2009 With Chartbook on Trends in the Health of Americans, Hyattsville, MD: 2010.

Figure 2.10 shows the impact that chronic health conditions have upon activities of individuals. Not surprisingly, these data point to decreasing levels of activities as individuals age. By far and away the largest limiter of activity occurs with arthritis and musculoskeletal ailments, more than doubling in its intensity from the age of 65–74 years to 85 years and older. Medicare-related expenses for each of these ailments are significant at present and will increase dramatically as the numbers of individuals in Medicare-eligible coverage continue to increase. Also several ailments, e.g., vision and hearing, are not covered items under Medicare.

Figure 2.11 provides a view of how precipitously personal health expenditures have risen over a 20-year period. Rising health care costs drive each of these trend lines forward. Private health insurance payments on behalf of individuals outpace spending from these other sources. Insurance premiums for private health insurance on the part of both employers providing insurance and employees with coverage have increased by over 130% in the past 10 years in the USA. One additional reason for the rise in personal health costs is that, as Medicare and Medicaid (government-sponsored coverage) have attempted to stem health care cost increases, costs have shifted from providers (hospitals, physicians) to the private sector (private health insurance payments) (Chernichovsky and Leibowitz 2010). Medicare and Medicaid have also increased both in terms of numbers of covered individuals as well as the expenditures paid on their behalf. Examples of this cost shifting include private out-of-pocket payments for deductibles, co-payments, co-insurance, and/or payment for items not covered under health insurance plans such as over-the-counter drug products, eyeglasses, and dentures.

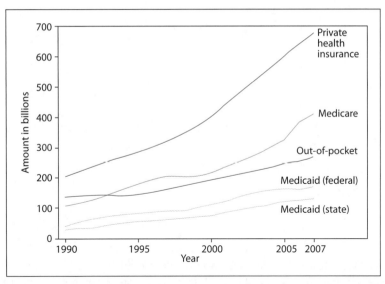

Figure 2.11 Increases in personal health expenditures in the USA. Source: CDC/NCHS, Health, United States, 2009, Figure 22. Data from the Centers for Medicare and Medicaid Services. National Center for Health Statistics; Health, United States, 2009 With Chartbook on Trends in the Health of Americans, Hyattsville, MD: 2010.

Medicare payments for each of the six principal procedures tracked in Figure 2.12 are increasing, as are expenditures for all methods of payment for these health services. Let's focus on Medicare alone and payment for percutaneous transluminal coronary angioplasty (PTCA). These costs are profiled in Figure 2.13, showing PTCA/stent procedures with segmentation by age

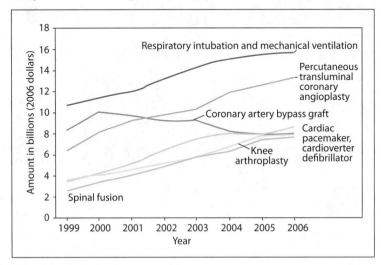

Figure 2.12 Costs for hospital stays for the six most expensive principal procedures. Source: CDC/NCHS, Health, United States, 2009, Figure 36. Data from the Agency for Healthcare Research and Quality. National Center for Health Statistics; Health, United States, 2009 With Chartbook on Trends in the Health of Americans, Hyattsville, MD: 2010.

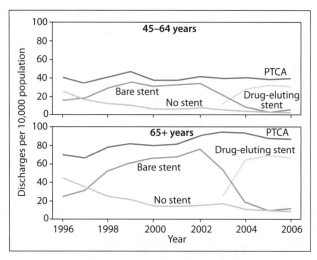

Figure 2.13 Hospital discharges for percutaneous transluminal coronal angioplasty (PTCA) procedures. Source: CDC/NCHS, Health, United States, 2009, Figure 28. Data from the National Hospital Discharge Survey. National Center for Health Statistics; Health, United States, 2009 With Chartbook on Trends in the Health of Americans, Hyattsville, MD: 2010.

differentiation – 45–64 years and 65 years plus. The numbers of PTCA and drug-eluting stent procedures have significantly increased in the Medicare-eligible age group, 65 years plus. Payments for these expensive procedures are partially responsible for the increase in Medicare expenditures.

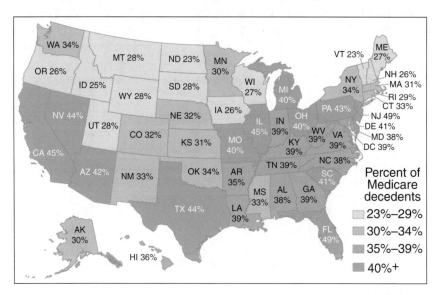

Figure 2.14 Medicare decedents over age 65 with intensive care unit (ICU)/coronary care unit (CCU) stays. Source: CDC/NCHS, Health, United States, 2009, Figure 31. Data from the Dartmouth Atlas of Health Care. National Center for Health Statistics; Health, United States, 2009 With Chartbook on Trends in the Health of Americans, Hyattsville, MD: 2010.

For Medicare recipients another unfortunate aspect of living and dying is hospitalization in an intensive care unit or cardiac care unit during the last 6 months of life (Figure 2.14). Regional differences are evident. These geographic differences may be partially explained by examining the map and considering where the major metropolitan areas are in the USA, coupled with population density data for where seniors live and where they need to seek tertiary care at the end of life. It has been estimated that upwards of 80% of what Medicare patients use in the form of health care services occurs in the last 6 months of life.

Summary

This chapter explored the relationships between various forms of health care systems and countries of origin. Many of the systems in play have evolved over time (German system since the late 19th century; British system since 1948), whereas some were recently put in place (Canada in the 1980s; Taiwan and Switzerland in the 1990s). The reform of the US system in the 2010s will await the test of time to determine its ultimate effects. What can be examined in the US context is the trends in spending for the multilayered system of care provided in the USA. Through replicating the various subsystems of care in a revised health care system, estimates of costs can be placed in debate.

The influencers of many segments impacting health policy are evident when examining each of the different forms of health care systems presented in this chapter.

Discussion questions

1   Under the PPACA, passed in 2010, fines will be levied against those who fail to purchase health insurance as stipulated in the bill. Is this fair, ethical, or feasible? Why or why not?

2   In his book, *The Healing of America: A Global Quest for Better, Cheaper, and Fairer Health Care*, author TR Reid couches the issue of health care as a moral imperative for countries. Do you agree? Why or why not?

3   Oftentimes people point to the UK system (an example of a Beveridge system) as an estimable system to replicate. Do you feel that this system could be implemented in the USA? Do you feel it could be instituted for the first time in the UK today, over 60 years after its formation?

4   The US VA health care system is similar to the UK NHS system. Has this system of care for veterans of US military service worked positively for US veterans?

5   Ethically, what does the US government owe Vietnam War veterans exposed to Agent Orange during the war?

6   Could Medicare patients be effectively treated in US VA health care facilities? Would this be a cost-effective method of treating Medicare patients?

7   Does the passage of PPACA in the USA mean that the US health care system is now a socialized medicine system?

8   Should the influence of lobbyists on health care issues in the USA be limited in some fashion? If so, how would you implement this?

9   What would you do to improve the Medicare Part D drug plan immediately?

10 Why do you think the "doughnut hole" segment was initially placed within the Medicare Part D Drug Benefit program? Who would have advocated for this inclusion?

11 If you examine the population increase trends described in this chapter, what impact do you feel these projected increases will have on social insurance programs in the USA?

12 Why do you feel the vaccination rates for pneumococcal pneumonia for seniors is as low as it is in the USA? What are the ethical implications of this low rate?

13 With Medicare and Medicaid projected to account for 25% of total federal government spending in the USA, how do you see cost-cutting strategies meshing with increasing potential for enhanced use of pharmaceuticals?

References

Anonymous (2010). http://www.bbc.co.uk/history/historic_figures/beveridge_william.shtml (accessed 24 April 2010).

Chernichovsky D, Leibowitz AA (2010). Integrating public health and personal care in a reformed US health care system. *Am J Public Health* 100: 205–211.

Congressional Budget Office (CBO) (2010). Budget and economic information. Available online at: www.cbo.gov/budget/budget.cfm (accessed 22 May 2010).

Delamothe T (2008). NHS at 60, founding principles. *Br Med J* 336: 1216–1218.

Gondusky MC, Reiter MP (2005). Protecting military convoys in Iraq: an examination of battle injuries sustained by a mechanized battalion during Operation Iraqi Freedom II. *Milit Med* 170: 546.

Heid M, Sood K (2009). The behind-the-scenes battle over health care reform in the US. MedillWashington, Medill News Service, Northwestern University. Available online at: http://medilldev.net/2009/12/army-of-influence-the-behind-the-scenes-battle-over-health-care-reform/ (accessed 28 December 2009).

Hoadley J, Summeri L, Elizabeth H, *et al.* (2010). Medicare Part D, data spotlight, Medicare prescription drug plans in 2010 and key changes over five years: Summary of findings. Available online at: http://www.kff.org/medicare/upload/8096.pdf (accessed 17 December 2010).

Jones CM (2010). The moral problem of health disparities. *Am J Public Health* 100(suppl. 1): S47–S51.

Klein R (2006). *The New Politics of the NHS: From Creation to Reinvention.* Abingdon: Radcliffe.

Levinson DR (2007). *Medicare Part D Sponsors: Estimated Reconciliation Amounts for 2006.* OEI-02-07-00460. Washington, DC: US Department of Health and Human Services, Office of the Inspector General.

Reid TR (2009) *The Healing of America: A Global Quest for Better, Cheaper, and Fairer Health Care.* New York: Penguin Press.

Schuck PH (1987) *Agent Orange on Trial: Mass Toxic Disasters in the Courts.* Cambridge, MA: Belknap-Harvard University Press.

Seal KH, Bertenthal D, Miner CR, *et al.* (2007). Bringing the war back home: Mental health disorders among 103 788 US veterans returning from Iraq and Afghanistan seen at Department of Veterans Affairs facilities. *Arch Intern Med* 167: 476–482.

Taylor MV, Stephenson PL (2007). Gulf war syndrome. *J Consumer Health Internet* 11: 49–60.

The Staff of the Washington Post (2010a). Paying for it: taxes, penalties and spending cuts. In: *Landmark, The Inside Story of America's New Health-Care Law and What it Means for us All.* New York: Public Affairs Reports, pp. 169–182.

The Staff of the Washington Post (2010b). Conclusion, judging success. In: *Landmark, The Inside Story of America's New Health-Care Law and What it Means for us All.* New York: Public Affairs Reports, pp. 191–194.

Further reading

Albreht T, Klazinga N (2009). Privatisation of health care in Slovenia in the period 1992–2008. *Health Policy* 90: 262–269.

Apter AJ, Casillas AM (2009). Eliminating health disparities: What have we done and what do we do next? *J Allergy Clin Immunol* 123: 1237–1239.

Bankauskaite V, O'Connor JS (2008). Health policy in the Baltic countries since the beginning of the 1990s. *Health Policy* 88: 155–165.

Bryant JH, Richmond JB (2008). Alma-Ata and primary health care: an evolving story. In: Kris H (ed.) *International Encyclopedia of Public Health.* Oxford: Academic Press, pp. 152–174.

Caussy D, Sein T (2008). East Asia and Pacific states, health systems of. In: Kris H (ed.) *International Encyclopedia of Public Health.* Oxford: Academic Press, pp. 267–276.

Cavagnero E (2008). Health sector reforms in Argentina and the performance of the health financing system. *Health Policy* 88: 88–99.

Cox KJ (2009). Midwifery and health disparities: theories and intersections. *J Midwifery Women's Health* 54: 57–64.

Jatrana S, Crampton P (2009). Primary health care in New Zealand: Who has access? *Health Policy* 93: 1–10.

Kennedy J, Morgan S (2009). Cost-related prescription nonadherence in the United States and Canada: A system-level comparison using the 2007 international health policy survey in seven countries. *Clin Ther* 31: 213–219.

Kruk ME, Freedman LP (2008). Assessing health system performance in developing countries: A review of the literature. *Health Policy* 85: 263–276.

Messinger-Rapport B (2009). Disparities in long-term healthcare. *Nurs Clin North Am* 44: 179–185.

Murthy VNR, Okunade AA (2009). The core determinants of health expenditure in the African context: Some econometric evidence for policy. *Health Policy* 91: 57–62.

Narva AS, Sequist TD (2010). Reducing health disparities in American Indians with chronic kidney disease. *Semin Nephrol* 30: 19–25.

Prata N (2008). Sub-Saharan Africa, health systems of. In: Kris H (ed.) *International Encyclopedia of Public Health.* Oxford: Academic Press, pp. 250–257.

Ramesh M, Wu X (2009). Health policy reform in China: Lessons from Asia. *Soc Sci Med* 68: 2256–2262.

Short NM (2009). Influencing health policy: strategies for nursing education to partner with nursing practice. *J Profession Nurs* 24: 264–269.

Smith DL (2008). Disparities in health care access for women with disabilities in the United States from the 2006 National Health Interview Survey. *Disabil Health J* 1: 79–88.

Steinberg ML (2008). Inequity in cancer care: explanations and solutions for disparity. *Semin Radiat Oncol* 18: 161–167.

Toth F (2010). Healthcare policies over the last 20 years: Reforms and counter-reforms. *Health Policy* 95: 82–89.

Wang H (2008). Comparative health systems. In: Kris H (ed.) *International Encyclopedia of Public Health*. Oxford: Academic Press, pp. 799–806.

Xu J, Yang Y (2009). Traditional Chinese medicine in the Chinese health care system. *Health Policy* 90: 133–139.

Yamada A-M, Brekke JS (2008). Addressing mental health disparities through clinical competence not just cultural competence: The need for assessment of sociocultural issues in the delivery of evidence-based psychosocial rehabilitation services. *Clin Psychol Rev* 28: 1386–1399.

Case Study

Medicare Part D (USA)

This case study is an example of a health policy program component that might be termed a type of incrementalism (Callahan and Wasunna 2006). This refers to a health program that is designed to meet a specific need that exists in the health care system of a country. However, the program is not designed to address the problem to the extent that it perhaps could. This is certainly the case with Medicare Part D, a prescription drug outpatient benefit for Medicare enrollees in the USA. The program only partially covers the expense of outpatient drug therapy in the USA for eligible enrolled seniors.

Introduction commentary regarding health care reform

The addition of the Medicare Part D Drug Benefit in January 2006 is an interesting and revealing health policy impact worth close examination. The discussion of health care reform in the USA has been carried out in a uniquely American context. It has been a parochial discussion, and examining systems in place internationally seems not to have been an option. Curiously, successful options for care in the UK, Canada, Australia, or elsewhere are not seriously considered. A change in options was feasible if and only if current systems or insurers were retained in a "new" system. Table 2.1 provides a listing of the various Medicare programs and what items the Medicare part will cover.

When other countries revised their health care systems, systems existing elsewhere are considered in crafting a new delivery and insurance structure. For example, Taiwan looked at the best options available in numerous systems when reforming the Taiwanese system of insurance and delivery of care (Reid 2009). This process was not undertaken in the USA, which could be considered detrimental to those who need the most assistance, i.e., patients and families.

Table 2.1 Medicare insurance programs

Medicare component (Part)	What does it cover?	What types of service are included?	Do you need to sign up for the plan?
Part A	Hospital insurance	Inpatient hospital services, skilled nursing facilities, home care	Eligible at age 65 years. Payroll taxes finance the plan so you pay no premiums
Part B	Supplemental medical insurance	Physician and other health care provider office visits, outpatient services, drugs administered in an outpatient clinic	Pay by premiums which vary per month, and the rates are raised each year. You sign up for Part B Medicare
Medicare Advantage	Medicare Advantage (managed care) formerly Medicare Choice, or Medicare Part C	Medicare Parts A, B, and D provided through a private health plan such as a managed care organization (health maintenance organization: HMO)	You sign up for this plan which is paid for by a combination of payroll taxes and premiums
Part D	Prescription drug insurance	Outpatient prescription drugs such as those purchased in a community pharmacy or from an outpatient hospital pharmacy	Premiums vary depending on which plan you choose. You sign up for coverage

Source: adapted from Medicare Part D information sections, available online at www.medicare.gov.

Medicare Part D and health care reform

Some of the materials presented in this case study have been adapted from Fincham (2009, 2010). Elements of health care reform receiving attention in past debates regarding potential changes in the US health care system have included elements of the following:

- universal coverage (horizontal equity in health economics terms)
- placing a cap on the amount insurance companies can spend administratively
- somehow limiting insurance company profits
- no elimination of coverage for patients with pre-existing health conditions
- standardizing care coverage at different levels (vertical equity in health economics terms)
- ensuring that all plans cover a range of benefits
- allowing for comparisons between plans by consumers in an easier fashion than currently available

- eliminating premium markups based on differing levels of health status
- minimizing premium variations based on age.

The passage of health care reform in the USA (PPACA) will no doubt change how health care is delivered and financed in the USA. Changes suggested to be possible include eliminating the taxfree status of health insurance coverage, reduced profits for providers and institutions, expansion of coverage for the current underinsured and uninsured, and penalties for corporate businesses that do not participate in the revised plans.

Congressional debate and subsequent plans for health care reform in both the House of Representatives and the Senate were not necessarily bipartisan in nature; this alone has been suggested to be extremely problematic (Iglehart 2009). With the Obama administration intent on passing legislation reforming the US health care system, how specific patients, providers, and insurers will eventually fare is anyone's guess. Estimates placing the cost of a revised health care system amounting to $1.2 trillion or more over a 10-year period seem to lead to the conclusion that hospitals, providers, and the health professions will see unprecedented turmoil in the future.

As the health care reform debate continues after passage of health reform in the USA (PPACA), it may be instructive to consider the most recent major health care insurance proposal enacted in the past 5 years. This is the Medicare Part D Drug Benefit. Constructed during the administration of President George W. Bush and in place since January 1, 2006, the Medicare Part D program has a muddled track record of outcomes. In many ways, it provides an excellent case study of how not to implement a change in health care insurance. The Medicare Part D program is a market-based model of a government-subsidized health insurance program component.

This program was enacted with much hype and high expectations. The program helped many Medicare recipients, provided a much-needed impetus for pharmacy education and pharmacists to focus on outpatient pharmacy services necessary for patients, and was an incredibly profitable program for health insurance companies providing Medicare Part D and/or Medicare Advantage plans.

Pharmacy participation

The percentage of pharmacy participation in Medicare Part D has been high; however, not all pharmacies are participants in each of the

Medicare Part D prescription drug plans. The relatively low reimbursement rate, coupled with delays in payments for services provided, has challenged participating pharmacies (Spooner 2008).

Patient benefit

For the period of 2006–2009, the median premiums paid by beneficiaries increased by 35% (Hargrave *et al.* 2009). Between 2008 and 2009 alone premiums increased by 17% (Hargrave *et al.* 2009). Cost-sharing requirements for recipients also increased by 35% over the 3-year period (Hargrave *et al.* 2009).

Fiscal impact

The release of the latest Medicare Annual Report indicates the Medicare hospital insurance (HI) trust fund is projected to be exhausted by the year 2017 (CMS 2009). The annual updating report of 2008 indicated solvency of the HI trust fund through 2019, so in a 1-year period, a 2-year decrease has now been projected. Medicare Part D, along with Medicare Part B, is funded through a supplementary medical insurance (SMI) fund, which is separate from HI; the SMI is projected to be solvent over the same time period. However, the state of the economy, increased demand for services, and looming health care reform could quickly change the metrics of SMI. Considering the viability of Medicare Part D in the context of the current health care milieu is one thing; with the prospects of health care reform moving forward at an accelerated pace, current funding and future funding options may be dramatically challenged.

The passage of the MMA is a case in point of how funding follows lobbyists' collective activities. As previously noted, the Medicare Part D Drug Program as a part of this legislation significantly favored pharmaceutical manufacturers, insurers, and pharmacy benefit management companies in an egregious fashion. Pharmaceutical companies were and are allowed to do business as usual with multiple pricing levels, and retain the ability to raise prices at will. The MMA legislation specifically prohibits the CMS from negotiating with pharmaceutical companies for the advantageous prices that these same companies provide freely elsewhere. The Federal Supply Schedule pricing has allowed the VA to purchase drugs at reduced prices and the federal 340B Drug Pricing Program provides access to reduced price prescription drugs to over 12 000 health care facilities certified in the USA. Pharmaceutical companies remain profitable even with these reduced pricing programs, partly due to their ability to shift price hikes elsewhere in a multilayered process of drug pricing.

As noted in the main part of this chapter, in order to provide for optimum participation by Medicare Part D PDPs and MA-PDPs, a component of the MMA legislation provided PDPs and MA-PDPs with significant subsidies containing upfront funding, allowing for these companies to participate with an assurance of profitability (Levinson 2007). In effect, participating plans were given a profitability fallback regardless of what happened with enrollment into their plans by eligible seniors, and were thus risk-averse from a lack of enrollment and/or profitability with their proffered plans.

As the legislation was written and enabled, for the first year of the program, due to overpayment to PDP and MA sponsors, Part D plan sponsors owed Medicaid a net total of $4.4 billion for the year 2006. This amount of overpayment has been reduced to $600 million for 2007, a significant reduction, but this amount remains sizeable. These overestimated payments provided to plans were to be returned to Medicare. However, to complicate this matter further, CMS had no mechanisms in place to collect funds from such overpayments. This was finally set up and accomplished well into 2007 for the 2006 payments; as such, sponsors held significant amounts of money for an extended period of time. Lobbyists exerted pressure to pass the MMA in the form in which it was enacted.

With the passage and signing into law of the health care reform bill (PPACA), several key changes to the Medicare Part D drug benefit are in place to reduce Part D enrollees' out-of-pocket payments when they reach the drug coverage gap, known as the "doughnut hole."

Since 2006, beneficiaries enrolled in Part D plans have been required to pay 100% of their prescription drug costs for the vast majority of patients after their total drug spending exceeded an initial coverage limit. Then patients qualified for what is termed catastrophic coverage. The coverage gap was $3610 in 2010 and is projected to exceed $6000 by 2020. As noted, the vast majority of Part D plans have a coverage gap. It has been estimated that, in 2007, an estimated 3.4 million Part D enrollees (14% of all enrollees) reached the coverage gap (www.kff.org).

The recently passed health reform legislation reduces the amount that Medicare Part D enrollees are required to pay for their prescriptions when they reach the coverage gap. The gap is being phased out with differing levels of subsidies for brand-name and generic drugs in the gap, starting in 2011.

For the next few years, the follow enhancements have been codified:

- In 2010, Part D enrollees with spending in the coverage gap received a $250 rebate.
- Beginning in 2011, Part D enrollees who reach the coverage gap receive a 50% discount on the total cost of their brand-name drugs in the gap, as agreed by brand-name pharmaceutical manufacturers.
- Then in succeeding years Medicare gradually phases in additional subsidies in the coverage gap for brand-name drugs (starting in 2013) and generic drugs (starting in 2011), reducing the beneficiary co-insurance rate in the "doughnut hole" gap from 100% to 25% by 2020.
- Then by 2020, for brand-name drugs, Part D enrollees receive the 50% discount from pharmaceutical manufacturers, in addition to a 25% federal subsidy (starting in 2013). Part D subscribers would be responsible for only 25% of the total cost of their drugs out of pocket.
- Then by 2020, 75% of the cost of generic drugs in the gap would be subsidized by Medicare (starting in 2011), while beneficiaries would pay the remaining 25% out of pocket.
- Also, from 2014 to 2019, the bill reduces out-of-pocket amounts that qualify a subscriber for catastrophic coverage, further reducing out-of-pocket costs for those with relatively high prescription drug expenses. Starting in 2020, the level would revert to what it would have been without the reductions in the intervening years.

Summary

As can be deduced from the above discussion regarding the Medicare Part D program, a number of "players" interacted significantly in the passing of the legislation that enabled an outpatient drug therapy payment for Medicare recipients to be started in 2004 with a Medicare Drug Discount Card program, and in January 2006 with the Medicare Part D Drug Benefit program. These "players" included: lobbying entities representing the health insurance and pharmaceutical industries; seniors' advocacy groups such as the American Association of Retired Persons; professional pharmacy groups such as the American Pharmacists Association; the National Community Pharmacists Association; and trade groups such as the National Association of Chain Drugstores, and the Food Marketing Institute, representing food market-based pharmacies.

Discussion questions

1   Some people suggest the Medicare Part D Drug Benefit was heavily influenced by lobbyists advocating positions favorable to the pharmaceutical industry. From a health policy perspective, how do you appraise this situation?

2   The Medicare Advantage Plans (Medicare Part C) have been successful in promoting an umbrella approach to incorporating a drug benefit plan within other coverage. What are the benefits and downsides to this approach to providing Medicare coverage?

3   Do you feel that the "doughnut hole" approach used within Medicare Part D has been successful in this approach to influence utilization by Medicare Part D enrollees?

4   The US CMS has provided a website (www.medicare.gov) to guide consumers regarding Medicare Part D plans, options, and formulary options within drug plans. From a health policy perspective, what are the benefits and disadvantages of such an approach?

5   Medicare Part D PDPs negotiate on prices directly and individually with pharmaceutical companies for preferential pricing for drugs available within plan formularies. What are the benefits of this approach?

6   Should CMS negotiate directly with pharmaceutical companies for drugs used within Medicare Part D drug plans?

7   What influence do you feel Medicare Part D drug plans have had on enrollee patient compliance with medications?

8   From a health policy perspective, what changes would you make in Medicare Part D drug plans and the benefit provided to Medicare enrollees?

9   The "doughnut hole" segment of Medicare Part D drug plans is planned to be phased out over a decade. How will this benefit patients?

10 What can pharmaceutical manufacturers implement to influence their profitability within product lines available within Medicare Part D drug plan formularies?

References

Callahan D, Wasunna AA (2006). *Medicine and the Market: Equity v. Choice*. Baltimore, MD: The Johns Hopkins University Press.

CMS (2009). US Centers for Medicare and Medicaid Services, Department of Health and Human Services, 2009. Annual Report of the Boards of Trustees of the Federal Hospital Insurance and Federal Supplementary Medical Insurance Trust Funds. Available online at: http://www.cms.hhs.gov/reportstrustfunds/downloads/tr2009.pdf (accessed 18 June 2009).

Fincham JE (2009). Medicare Part D in the face of health care reform. *Am J Pharm Ed* 73: Article 112.

Fincham JE (2010). Financial realities affect political support for health care reform. *Am J Pharm Ed* 74: Article 1.

Hargrave E, Haodley J, Cubanski J, *et al.* (2009). New analysis reveals rising costs for Medicare Part D enrollees over time. Available online at: http://www.kff.org/medicare/upload/7917.pdf (accessed 11 June 2009).

Iglehart JK (2009). Congressional action on health care reform – an update. *N Engl J Med* 360: 2593–2595.

Levinson DR (2007). *Medicare Part D Sponsors: Estimated Reconciliation Amounts for 2006*. OEI-02-07-00460. Washington, DC: US Department of Health and Human Services, Office of the Inspector General.

Reid TR (2009). Sick around the world. Available online at: http://www.pbs.org/wgbh/pages/frontline/sickaroundtheworld/etc/notebook.html (accessed 18 June 2009).

Spooner JJ (2008). A bleak future for independent community pharmacy under Medicare Part D. *J Manag Care Pharm* 14: 878–881.

Further reading

Centers for Medicare and Medicaid Services (2010). Available online at: www.medicare.gov (accessed 2 May 2009).

Finkelstein A, McKnight R (2008). What did Medicare do? The initial impact of Medicare on mortality and out of pocket medical spending *J Publ Econom* 92: 1644–1668.

Goedken AM, Urmie JM, Farris KB, *et al.* (2010). Impact of cost sharing on prescription drugs used by Medicare beneficiaries. *Res Soc Admin Pharm* 6: 100–109.

Lundy J, Craig BM (2006). The use of disease-modifying agents among multiple sclerosis patients enrolled in Medicare from 1995 to 2002 and the impact of Medicare Part D: Analysis of claims data from the Medicare current beneficiary survey. *Clin Ther* 28: 140–145.

Meissner B, Harrison D, Carter J, *et al.* (2006). Predicting the impact of Medicare Part D implementation on the pharmacy workforce. *Res Soc Admin Pharm* 2: 315–328.

Radford A, Mason M, Richardson I, *et al.* (2009). Continuing effects of Medicare Part D on rural independent pharmacies who are the sole retail provider in their community. *Res Soc Admin Pharm* 5: 17–30.

Simonson W (2005). The Medicare Modernization Act of 2003, Part D. *J Am Med Directors Assoc* 6: 231–232.

St Peter WL (2008). Potential impact of Medicare Part D in the end-stage renal disease population. *Adv Chron Kidney Dis* 15: 140–146.

Stefanacci RG (2006). Implications of Medicare Part D in CKD anemia treatment. *J Am Med Directors Assoc* 7 (suppl. 1): S13–S16.

3

Quality issues

The issue of quality is not new to health, health care, or health care policy. With fewer resources to be allocated for more specific needs and applications, the issue of quality has taken on greater importance. If we consider that inefficient delivery of care leads to lower quality of care, and if errors in health care have an inverse correlation with quality, then quality becomes an increasingly important concept.

Quality of life (QOL) has been a health economic construct used to assess how patients view their health and health care, and measuring QOL has been used as a construct for evaluating health care resources and their application.

Introduction

QOL is a popular concept referring to how individuals view their overall health status or health status within a specific health condition. An individual disease-specific QOL measure is a health-related QOL (HR-QOL). The HR-QOL would be used with patients with cancer, hypertension, or diabetes. Analyses of QOLs and HR-QOLs can be accomplished using either non-parametric or parametric statistical tests to analyze potential differences. Various types of QOL assessment have been defined and validated by academicians, researchers, governmental, and pharmaceutical company personnel. While this concept may be quantifiable, the definition of QOL is really an individual-specific construct. Nevertheless, two types of QOL assessment have emerged over the decades since first use: general and disease-specific.

Early in the 1970s, researchers attempted to develop instruments that would enable the quantification of how individuals view their health status. Measurement of well-being via a scale assessing QOL began in earnest in the 1970s (Patrick *et al.* 1973). QOL and HR-QOL contain domains incorporating physical, psychological, and social domains. These specific domains are individually evaluated according to individuals' own experiences, beliefs, expectations, and perceptions of health (Brook *et al.* 1979, 1983). A general overall QOL measure was initially developed; the initial validated measure was the short-form 36 or SF-36, developed by Ware and colleagues (Brook *et al.* 1979; Testa and Simonson 1996). These varying domains were considered to be affected by experiences, beliefs, expectations for health, and perceptions (Brook *et al.* 1979, 1983; Testa and Simonson 1996).

Since the 1970s, a plethora of QOL measures have been developed. Conventional wisdom suggests that two QOL measures should be applied. The first is a general QOL measure which can be used as a baseline determination for evaluating QOL. The second is an HR-QOL measure. As an example, the general QOL would be administered annually, and the HR-QOL more frequently, perhaps quarterly or semiannually.

A newer standalone QOL measure is the EQ-5D. The five domains of the EQ-5D are: mobility, self-care, usual activities, pain/discomfort, and anxiety/depression. This scale is a product of the EuroQol organization (www.euroqol.org). In 1987, the EuroQol Group was formed, and developed a standardized instrument that was initially simultaneously available in Dutch, English, Finnish, Norwegian, and Swedish. It is now universally available in many languages. The EQ-5D has been used as both a general and a disease-specific measure of QOL. This instrument has been validated by many researchers in many settings. Interestingly, the EQ-5D has been suggested to have specificity for both general and disease-specific measurement of QOL (Nowels *et al.* 2005). The EQ-5D has served as a common metric to determine reference points in repeated evaluations of QOL.

Assessment of outcomes of drug therapy

Outcomes associated with drug therapy have been evaluated through clinical, economic, and humanistic outcomes of care. Evaluating clinical outcomes has remained the foremost method of assessing the worth of medications. Various compendia are available to consider numerous comparative outcomes of QOL in an unbiased fashion. The Cochrane Collaboration is an independent, not-for-profit international organization that maintains a database of evaluations of clinical outcomes incorporating QOL assessments (http://www.cochrane.org/index.htm). Also, the University of York (UK) Centre for Reviews and Dissemination (http://www.crd.york.ac.uk/crdweb/) contains an amalgam of three databases examining outcomes: (1) Database of Abstracts of Reviews of Effects; (2) the UK National Health Service (NHS) Economic Evaluation Database; and (3) Health Technology Assessment database. Each of these databases contains international comparators.

Points to note regarding the appropriate use of quality-of-life measures

When reviewing QOL studies, several key elements need to be considered. Initially, has the measure been validated? Has the measure been analyzed statistically (reliability, factor analysis, and/or other psychometric evaluations)? In the validation process, have appropriate sample sizes and relevant groups been evaluated? QOL measures lack credibility if they have not been fully analyzed for validity or sources of invalidity (Hjermstad *et al.* 1995).

It is also instructive to evaluate the study in which QOL measures have been used to determine if there appears to be a bias on the part of the researchers. Key questions to consider are: Who funded the study? Do the study findings appear to favor a particular drug or event outcome? Do the authors of papers emanating from QOL studies overreach in their conclusions?

QOL or HR-QOL instruments need to be culturally relevant. If a measure has been developed for use with patients with a specific disease, and yet is applied to individuals from another country with differing cultural norms, or perhaps to individuals for whom a disease may be rare, the results simply are not considered credible (Sperber 2004). Even within a country with subpopulations, results can be confounded by lack of cultural sensitivity (Sperber 2004). For example, if a sample is predominantly Hispanic with Spanish as a native tongue, instruments need to be written in Spanish.

Disease-specific measures need to be initially developed, assessed for reliability and validity with samples of patients with a specific disease or health condition of interest, and then applied for use with similar homogenous patients (Blazeby *et al.* 2003). To fail to accomplish these basic objectives would render a measure with the lack of these basic qualifiers meaningless.

Summary regarding quality of life

In summary, in three decades, measurement of QOL has become commonplace and utilized extensively by researchers in academia and the pharmaceutical industry to examine the humanistic outcomes of medication therapy. Currently the UK applies QOL in quality-adjusted life-years (QALYs) to assess the worthiness of adding specific drugs to the NHS formulary. Similar applications of QALYs will no doubt be applied elsewhere, including the USA, as scarce resources are perhaps further reduced and yet additionally requested for expenditures for drug therapies.

Comparative effectiveness research

Comparative effectiveness research is not new, but with the passage of the Patient Protection and Affordable Care Act (PPACA), the concept and potential uses of comparative effectiveness research have taken on added significance.

What is comparative effectiveness research?

According to the US Agency for Healthcare Research and Quality (AHRQ), comparative effectiveness research is designed to inform health care decisions by providing evidence on the effectiveness, benefits, and harms of different treatment options. The evidence is generated from research studies that compare drugs, medical devices, tests, surgeries, or ways to deliver health care. There are two ways that this evidence is found:

1 Researchers look at all the available evidence about the benefits and harms of each choice for different groups of people from existing clinical trials, clinical studies, and other research. These are called research reviews, because they are systematic reviews of existing evidence.
2 Researchers conduct studies that generate new evidence of effectiveness or comparative effectiveness of a test, treatment, procedure, or health care service.

Comparative effectiveness research requires the development, expansion, and use of a variety of data sources and methods to conduct timely and relevant research and disseminate the results in a form that is quickly usable by clinicians, patients, policymakers, and health plans and other payers. Several steps are involved in conducting this research and in ensuring continued development of the research infrastructure to sustain and advance these efforts:

• Identify new and emerging clinical interventions.
• Review and synthesize current medical research.
• Identify gaps between existing medical research and the needs of clinical practice.
• Promote and generate new scientific evidence and analytic tools.
• Train and develop clinical researchers.
• Translate and disseminate research findings to diverse stakeholders.

Use in evaluating differing drug therapies

Comparative effectiveness research revolutionizes how drug therapies are evaluated from an outcomes standpoint. The gold standard for evaluating the quality and effectiveness of particular therapies has been randomized controlled clinical trials evaluating drugs versus placebo for the most part. The head-to-head evaluation of therapies against other therapies is different and, many would argue, much more valuable in assessing drug therapies.

Use in the UK

Comparative effectiveness research has been prominently used in the UK through the National Institute for Health and Clinical Excellence framework.

It has not been prominently applied broadly across governmental agencies in the USA as a framework for evaluating therapies and interventions until now. The recently passed American Recovery and Reinvestment Act has an allocation of $1.2 billion for comparative effectiveness research. This type of research provides information on the relative strengths and weaknesses of various medical interventions. Such research will give clinicians and patients valid information to make decisions that will improve the performance of the US health care system. The Recovery Act authorized $300 million for the AHRQ, $400 million for the National Institutes of Health, and $400 million for the Secretary of Health and Human Services to support comparative effectiveness research.

Use in USA and guidance

Set to guide comparative effectiveness research in the US federal government, the Secretary of the Department of Health and Human Services (HHS), Kathleen Sebelius, has been charged to appoint a council to guide federal comparative effectiveness research. The council will not recommend clinical guidelines for payment, coverage, or treatment. The council will consider the needs of populations served by federal programs and opportunities to build and expand on current investments and priorities. It will also provide input on priorities for the $400 million fund from the Recovery Act that the Secretary will allocate to advance this type of research. Council members include:

- Chief Policy Officer, Office of Strategy and Innovation, Centers for Disease Control and Prevention
- Senior Advisor, Center for Medicare Management, Centers for Medicare and Medicaid Services (CMS)
- Director, Office of Applied Studies, Substance Abuse and Mental Health Services Administration
- Director, AHRQ, HHS
- Associate Administrator, HIV/AIDS Bureau Health Resources and Services Administration
- Chief Medical Officer, Office of the National Coordinator of Health Information Technology Adoption
- Assistant Secretary for Planning and Evaluation
- Director, National Heart, Lung, and Blood Institute, National Institutes of Health
- Deputy Assistant Secretary, Office of Minority Health at the HHS
- Acting Chief Medical Officer, Food and Drug Administration (FDA) Director, Center for Biologics Evaluation and Research, FDA centers
- Acting Deputy Director for Office on Disability/Office of the Secretary, HHS
- Counselor for Health Reform at HHS Office of the Secretary, HHS

- Chief Research and Development Officer, Veterans Administration
- Director of Strategic Communications for the Military Health System, Department of Defense
- Special Advisor for Health Policy, Office of Management and Budget.

This new council will help coordinate research and guide investments in comparative effectiveness research funded by the Recovery Act. Council members represent a diverse set of individuals and agencies; most of its members are clinicians.

Summary

Health policy influences have placed comparative effectiveness research as a key component of the recently passed PPACA in the USA: its long-term influence on governmental programs (Medicare and Medicaid) remains to be seen. The influence of comparative effectiveness research in the UK via the National Institute for Health and Clinical Excellence has been most influential regarding not only pharmaceutical use, but also cost–benefit analyses regarding optimum use of scarce health resources.

Discussion questions

1 Why does quality continue to be such a major issue in the delivery of health care services in the USA?
2 What have been the symptoms of reduced levels of quality in health care delivery of services both in the USA and abroad?
3 Describe the uses of the quality of life (QOL) construct in health care policy decisions.
4 What is the difference between a general QOL and a health-related QOL (HR-QOL) measure? Why are measures of QOL important?
5 How can entities such as the Cochrane Collaboration aid health policy decisions?
6 Discuss the need for QOL measures to be culturally relevant.
7 How do you see comparative effectiveness research informing health policy decisions?
8 How will comparative effectiveness research interact with randomized clinical trials in evaluating drug therapies? How are the two similar? How are they different?
9 Discuss where else in the world comparative effectiveness research has been used and what its impact has been.
10 Discuss the makeup of the council to guide the US federal government efforts pertaining to comparative effectiveness research.

References

Blazeby JM, Conroy T, Hammerlid E, *et al.* (2003). Clinical and psychometric validation of an EORTC questionnaire module, the EORTC QLQ-OES18, to assess quality of life in patients with oesophageal cancer. *Eur J Cancer* 39: 1384–1394.

Brook RH, Ware JE Jr, Davies-Avery A, *et al.* (1979). *Conceptualization and Measurement of Health for Adults in the Health Insurance Study*, vol. VIII, overview. Publication no. R-1987/3-HEW. Santa Monica, CA: Rand Corporation, 1979.

Brook RH, Ware JE, Jr Rogers WH, *et al.* (1983). Does free care improve adults' health? Results from a randomized controlled trial *N Engl J Med* 309: 1426–1434.

Hjermstad MJ, Fossa SD, Bjordal K, *et al.* (1995). Test/retest study of the European organization for research and treatment of cancer core quality-of-life questionnaire. *J Clin Oncol* 13: 1249–1254.

Nowels D, McGloin J, Westfall M, *et al.* (2005). Validation of the EQ-5D quality of life instrument in patients after myocardial infarction. *Qual Life Res* 14: 95–105.

Patrick DL, Bush JW, Chen MM (1973). Toward an operational definition of health. *J Health Soc Behav* 14: 6–23.

Sperber AD (2004). Translation and validation of study instruments for cross-cultural research. *Gastroenterology* 128: S124–S128.

Testa MA, Simonson DC (1996). Assessment of quality-of-life outcomes. *N Engl J Med* 224: 835–840.

Further reading

Barber SL, Gertler PJ (2008). Strategies that promote high quality care in Indonesia. *Health Policy* 88: 339–347.

Barber SL, Gertler PJ (2009). Health workers, quality of care, and child health: Simulating the relationships between increases in health staffing and child length. *Health Policy* 91: 148–155.

Boland MC, Daly L, Staines A, *et al.* (2009). Self-rated health and quality of life in adults attending regional disability services in Ireland. *Disabil Health J* 2: 95–103.

Brunton M, Jordan C, Fouche C, *et al.* (2008). Managing public health care policy: Who's being forgotten? *Health Policy* 88: 348–358.

Charyton C, Elliott JO, Lu B, *et al.* (2009). The impact of social support on health related quality of life in persons with epilepsy. *Epilepsy Behav* 16: 640–645.

Elliott JO, Lu B, Shneker B, *et al.* (2009). Comorbidity, health screening, and quality of life among persons with a history of epilepsy. *Epilepsy Behav* 14: 125–129.

Finn M, Sarangi S (2008). Quality of life as a mode of governance: NGO talk of HIV 'positive' health in India. *Soc Sci Med* 66: 1568–1578.

Gené-Badia J, Ascaso C, Escaramis-Babiano G, *et al.* (2008). Population and primary health-care team characteristics explain the quality of the service. *Health Policy* 86: 335–344.

Giacomini M, Kenny N, DeJean D, *et al.* (2009). Ethics frameworks in Canadian health policies: Foundation, scaffolding, or window dressing? *Health Policy* 89: 58–71.

Gravelle H, Siciliani L (2008). Optimal quality, waits and charges in health insurance. *J Health Econ* 17: 663–674.

Gulley SP, Altman BM (2008). Disability in two health care systems: Access, quality, satisfaction, and physician contacts among working-age Canadians and Americans with disabilities. *Disabil Health J* 1: 196–208.

Hu SW, Holt EW, Husni ME, *et al.* (2010). Willingness-to-pay stated preferences for 8 health-related quality-of-life domains in psoriatic arthritis: A pilot study. *Semin Arthritis Rheum* 39: 384–397.

Huguet N, Kaplan MS, Feeny D, *et al.* (2008). Socioeconomic status and health-related quality of life among elderly people: Results from the Joint Canada/United States Survey of Health. *Soc Sci Med* 66: 803–810.

Imai H, Fujii Y, Fukuda Y, *et al.* (2008). Health-related quality of life and beneficiaries of long-term care insurance in Japan. *Health Policy* 85: 349–355.

Kaboru BB, Muchimba M, Falkenbert T, *et al.* (2008). Quality of STIs and HIV/AIDS care as perceived by biomedical and traditional health care providers in Zambia: Are there common grounds for collaboration? *Complement Ther Med* 16: 155–162.

Konstam MA, Greenberg B (2009). Transforming health care through the medical home: the example of heart failure. *J Cardiac Failure* 15: 736–738.

Kramer RA, Dickinson KL, Anderson RM, *et al.* (2009). Using decision analysis to improve malaria control policy making. *Health Policy* 92: 133–140.

Lee GA (2008). Patients reported health-related quality of life five years post coronary artery bypass graft surgery: A methodological study. *Eur J Cardiovasc Nurs* 7: 67–72.

Lin V (2008). Evidence-based public health policy. In. Kris II (ed.) *International Encyclopedia of Public Health*. Oxford: Academic Press, pp. 527–536.

Makai P, Klazinga N, Wagner C, *et al.* (2009). Quality management and patient safety: Survey results from 102 Hungarian hospitals. *Health Policy* 90: 175–180.

Nakrem S, Vinsnes AG, Harkless GE, *et al.* (2009). Nursing sensitive quality indicators for nursing home care: International review of literature, policy and practice. *Int J Nurs Studies* 46: 848–857.

O'Mara AM, Denicoff AM (2010). Health related quality of life in NCI-sponsored cancer treatment trials. *Semin Oncol Nurs* 26: 68–78.

Pasman HR, Wolf JE, Hesselink BA, *et al.* (2009). Policy statements and practice guidelines for medical end-of-life decisions in Dutch health care institutions: Developments in the past decade. *Health Policy* 92: 79–88.

Paton C (2008). Health policy: overview. In: Kris H (ed.) *International Encyclopedia of Public Health*. Oxford: Academic Press, pp. 211–225.

Phillips C, Main C, Buck R, *et al.* (2008). Prioritising pain in policy making: The need for a whole systems perspective. *Health Policy* 88: 166–175.

Prinz L, Cramer M, Englund A. Telehealth: A policy analysis for quality, impact on patient outcomes, and political feasibility. *Nurs Outlook* 56: 152–158.

Purshouse RC, Meier PS, Brennan A, *et al.* (2010). Estimated effect of alcohol pricing policies on health and health economic outcomes in England: an epidemiological model. *Lancet* 375: 1355–1364.

Ramesh M, Wu X (2009). Health policy reform in China: Lessons from Asia. *Soc Sci Med* 68: 2256–2262.

Rosati RJ (2009). The history of quality measurement in home health care. *Clin Geriatr Med* 25: 121–134.

Rowett D, Ravenscroft PJ, Hardy J, *et al.* (2009). Using national health policies to improve access to palliative care medications in the community. *J Pain Symptom Manage* 37: 395–402.

Ryan JG (2009). Cost and policy implications from the increasing prevalence of obesity and diabetes mellitus. *Gender Med* 6: 86–108.

Ryashchenko SV, Gukalova IV (2010). Public health in the system of regional indicators of the quality of life in Russia and Ukraine. *Geogr Natural Resources* 31: 11–17.

Short NM (2008). Influencing health policy: Strategies for nursing education to partner with nursing practice. *J Prof Nurs* 24: 264–269.

Simpson LA, Fairbrother G (2009). How health policy influences quality of care in pediatrics. *Pediatr Clin North Am* 56: 1009–1021.

Unger J-P, Van Dessel P, Sen K, *et al.* (2009). International health policy and stagnating maternal mortality: is there a causal link? *Reproduct Health Matters* 17: 91–104.

Velasco Garrido M, Gerhardus A, Rottingen JA, *et al.* (2010). Developing health technology assessment to address health care system needs. *Health Policy* 94: 196–202.

Case Study

Electronic prescribing (e-prescribing)

E-prescribing has been touted as a method to increase the quality of the drug use process not only in the USA but also abroad. The drug use process is flawed, and e-prescribing is but one of numerous health information technologies (HITs) that have shown promise in furthering the ideal of enhanced drug use. Health policy support for e-prescribing has come from a multitude of encouraging entities, not least of which is the US federal government.

Many factors have been suggested to help stem the problem of drug misuse in the USA and elsewhere. Health professional interventions, calls for enhanced prescribing and dispensing processes, case management, medication therapy management services, and electronic mechanisms such as e-prescribing have all been suggested to be a potential means to impact the impreciseness of the drug use process.

Background on electronic prescribing from AHRQ

The AHRQ of the US HHS provides the following background on e-prescribing. Electronic prescription writing is defined by the eHealth Initiative as "the use of computing devices to enter, modify, review, and output or communicate drug prescriptions." Although the term "e-prescribing" implies the use of a computer for any type of prescribing action, a wide range of e-prescribing activities exist with varying levels of sophistication:

- level 1: electronic reference handbook
- level 2: standalone prescription writer
- level 3: patient-specific prescription creation or refilling
- level 4: medication management (access to medication history, warnings, and alerts)
- level 5: connectivity to dispensing site
- level 6: integration with an electronic medical record.

These levels and listing are adapted from *Electronic Prescribing: Towards Maximum Value and Rapid Adoption* (eHealth Initiative 2004). Materials in this case study have been adapted from Fincham (2009).

All levels of electronic prescription writing confer varying degrees of improvements in patient safety. Level 6, which is the most sophisticated, has been shown to confer the highest degree of patient safety and also provides the largest return on the investment. Over the last 10 years, national interest in e-prescribing has increased as the federal government has enacted legislation, including the Medicare Modernization Act of

2003 (MMA), aimed at increasing the adoption of e-prescribing. CMS released a report to Congress entitled *Pilot Testing of Initial Electronic Prescribing Standards* (Leavitt 2007). This report was mandated by the MMA, and it details the rigorous pilot testing of information standards by five leading e-prescribing organizations. AHRQ and the National Resource Center's evaluation report recommended that the medication history, formulary and benefits, and prescription fill status indicator standards were ready for implementation under Part D. Prior authorization, structured and codified signature (sig), and the RxNorm standards were not ready for implementation in their current state. (RxNorm is a standardized nomenclature for clinical drugs and drug delivery devices and is produced by the US National Library of Medicine.)

In addition, the pilot projects evaluated key issues in e-prescribing such as reduction of adverse drug events, provider uptake, and potential gains in efficiency and effectiveness. Use of the proposed standards advances interoperability in the US health care system and greatly enhances the ability of HIT to improve safety and quality. Such efforts are integral to AHRQ's mission to improve the quality, safety, efficiency, and effectiveness of health care for all Americans.

Areas of current e-prescribing applications

Existing e-prescribing tools have begun to consider a variety of new uses for a medication history. Those uses include knowing what medications a patient has received from a pharmacist using data from pharmacy benefit managers (PBMs). Services such as SureScripts provide this information to electronic prescription-writing systems, allowing providers to see a complete view of the patient's medication history. Another current trend is transmission of electronic prescriptions using a standard known as NCPDP-SCRIPT. This standard supports interfaces to pharmacy information systems and was adopted by the US HHS in 2005. A frequently used practice is to communicate via fax, which is often plagued by inaccurate fax numbers, poor management of faxes that are received by pharmacies, and poor systems to provide feedback about the status of fax delivery.

The MMA requires that Part D plans support an electronic prescription program, if any of their providers and pharmacies voluntarily choose to e-prescribe. This program is required to provide for the electronic transmittal of prescription orders; plan eligibility queries and responses; plan benefit information; drug interactions, warnings or cautions, and any dosage adjustments related to the drug being prescribed or dispensed; appropriate lower-cost alternatives, if any, for a drug being prescribed; and the patient's medical history related to a covered Part D drug being prescribed or dispensed. For each requirement, HHS released the final ruling on e-prescribing and the foundation standards in November 2005 in the Federal Register. These standards are compatible with existing ones, especially the transactions specified in the administrative simplification provisions of the Health Insurance Portability and Accountability Act of 1996. MMA also required pilot projects during 2006 to test any standards for which there is not adequate industry experience. AHRQ and CMS collaborated to issue grants and contracts for pilot-testing e-prescribing standards. Results of these pilot projects were released in April 2007 in the form of an evaluation report from the AHRQ National Resource Center for Health Information Technology. Final e-prescribing standards were released in the Federal Register on April 7, 2008, with implementation up to a year later. In the spring 2008 session of the US Congress, the Medicare Improvements for Patients and Providers Act of 2008 was passed, offering physicians financial incentives for e-prescribing. Under the new law, Medicare physicians who e-prescribe will receive a 2% payment bonus in 2009 and 2010, a 1% bonus in 2011 and 2012, and a 0.5% bonus in 2013. In addition, payments to Medicare physicians who do not e-prescribe will be reduced by 1% in 2012, 1.5% in 2013 and 2% in subsequent years.

In addition to the MMA, The Joint Commission for the Accreditation of Hospital Organizations (The Joint Commission) endorsed medication reconciliation in 2006. Hospitals that are accredited by The Joint Commission need to demonstrate methods to verify that medication histories are reconciled and up to date with medication lists after each care transition (e.g., from outpatient to inpatient status; from inpatient ward to inpatient intensive care unit; from outpatient hospital to nursing home facility). Medication reconciliation has been shown to be a time-intensive activity on the part of those people involved. E-prescribing tools may improve the process by providing more accurate and complete histories.

Specific information regarding e-prescribing

Using e-prescribing to impact quality of prescription prescribing

The enacted PPACA contains numerous items attempting to enhance the quality of medication prescribing and use in the USA. For example, from the bill the following is listed:

> The Secretary may incorporate reporting requirements and incentive payments related to the physician quality reporting initiative (PQRI), including such requirements and such payments related to electronic prescribing, electronic health records, and other similar initiatives.

Electronic transmission has been mandated to be used for all Medicare Part D prescription claims transmitted by pharmacies as a requirement for participation.

In 2009, and as an incentive for physicians to encourage adoption of e-prescribing systems, the Medicare Improvements for Patients and Providers Act of 2008 began a 5-year program of incentive payments to prescribing professionals when they e-prescribe for Medicare patients seen in ambulatory care offices. And as a disincentive, as previously noted, physicians eligible for the incentive payments but who fail to adopt e-prescribing will face penalties, beginning in 2012.

Historical aspects of e-prescribing

E-prescribing systems were first used in the mid to late 1970s; they became more significant when the US Institute of Medicine endorsed their use as a way to diminish the 98 000 hospitalized patients who die each year from a medication error. Often when we are presented with a new technology, or an upgrade to existing options, there is a sense that problems will be much easier to solve. With the case of drug use problems, there are many variables that impact medication errors, adverse effects, and problems with patient compliance. E-prescribing can help to ameliorate some of these vexing problems, but it will not solve them all. How can health policy decisions regarding e-prescribing impact the drug use process?

Limits of e-prescribing

Many of the many positive components of e-prescribing will be described here. It is important first to discuss what e-prescribing should not be expected to do. A number of problems within the prescribing, dispensing, and drug use process will not be influenced by e-prescribing. Some of these factors are drug-specific, patient-specific, or system-specific. Patient medication non-compliance and persistence, over-the-counter (OTC) drug misuse, occurrence of adverse drug reactions (ADRs), prescribing errors, and/or dispensing errors are commonplace. No systems yet devised or planned can totally eliminate these problems from negatively influencing appropriate drug use in the US health care system. Let's explore some of the problems related to drug use that cannot be remedied by e-prescribing.

Consideration of improper access to prescribing information and resultant impacts

Abuses have been noted when patients are unaware of accessed information, often for marketing purposes. Examples might be patient contacts identified through data mining, with the data subsequently sold, without the patient's knowledge or, most importantly, consent. Along with the many positive features and outcomes associated with e-prescribing, there are cautions. Abuses can occur if attendant safeguards relating to data collection are not in place. Wingfield *et al.* (2004) note that the access to electronic patient medication records allows for data mining to occur; sometimes for economic and not therapeutic endpoints. In both the UK NHS and the US PBM industry, collection of data will allow for population-level assessment of drug outcomes, both good and bad. However, the rights of an organization versus individual control over access to archived information will need to be clarified (O'Harrow 1998a, b). For example, there have been instances when a new drug has been promoted to patients who were unaware of how they were identified or singled out (Ohliger 1999).

Errors occurring with e-prescribing

Paradoxically, drug errors can occur with e-prescribing, which is widely touted to decrease drug errors. In an analysis of a serious drug error with intravenous potassium chloride ordered via computerized physician order entry (Horsky *et al.* 2005), the authors characterized errors in several converging aspects of the drug-ordering process: confusing on-screen laboratory results review, system usability difficulties, user training problems, and suboptimal clinical system safeguards contributed to a serious dosing error. As with any technology, new or old, all problems will not be solved by implementing e-prescribing. In a *Washington Post* column from 2005, Boodman (2005) noted:

> Computerized drug ordering systems have been regarded as essential in reducing medication errors, the most prevalent and preventable kind of mistake that experts say affects an estimated 770 000 hospitalized patients annually. A review of death certificates from 1993 found that drug errors killed nearly 7400 patients, according to the Institute of Medicine (IOM) (p. HE01).

Even with the positive features of e-prescribing, errors can still occur. Boodman (2005) points out that:

> among the potential or actual mistakes researchers found occurred weekly: incorrect doses prescribed for patients; patients who failed to get medication in a timely manner because of computer-related problems; and difficulty determining which patient was supposed to get a drug that had been prescribed (p. HE01).

Impact on formulary adherence and generic drug utilization

In one retrospective study the influence of e-prescribing on formulary compliance and generic drug utilization was analyzed (Ross *et al.* 2005). Ross *et al.* found that for paid pharmacy claims from a large, national managed care organization there were no differences found between predominantly e-prescribers and traditional prescribers in measures of formulary compliance or generic drug utilization. The key word in the previous sentence is predominantly: does "predominantly" mean 50% or 100% e-prescribing activity by the physicians? As a more widespread adoption of e-prescribing by physicians occurs, rates of both formulary compliance and generic drug utilization undoubtedly will be expected to increase.

Varying uptake by community pharmacy

It has been observed that, from current environment of e-prescribing, small independent pharmacies are slow to upgrade their pharmacy management systems to accept e-prescriptions because of large fees charged by software vendors; large chain pharmacies embrace e-prescribing at the corporate level, but local store support is low and there is inadequate training of pharmacy staff (Tcimpidis and Rosenblatt 2005).

Varying factors influencing e-prescribing

There have been impediments to incorporation of e-prescribing into practices, facilities, or third-party programs. For example, physician resistance to change regarding e-prescribing, system cost, and inadequate planning to incorporate e-prescribing into the existing care process have been blamed for failures in introducing e-prescribing in health systems (Morrissey 2004).

Positive aspects of e-prescribing

E-prescribing has at various points been suggested to reduce clinical risk management, provide operational efficiency, and provide access to electronic patient records. Enabling clinical risk management can include reducing the occurrence of adverse drug events. Adverse drug events can be due to prescribing errors, wrong interpretation of orders, and dispensing errors. E-prescribing can provide accurate prescriptions and records.

Reducing adverse drug events

E-prescribing provides decision support for the selection of prescription products, information about formularies, dosing and frequency of such, checking for allergies to particular medications, drug interactions, avoidance of therapeutic duplication, and maximum or minimum dose amounts.

Other benefits of e-prescribing

Various authors have noted that e-prescribing systems can provide computer-based support for: creation, transmission, dispensing, and monitoring of drug therapies. In various countries, these systems have been shown in certain circumstances to increase both the safety and quality of patient care (Bates *et al.* 1998; Chertow *et al.* 2001; Chrischilles *et al.* 2002; Potts *et al.* 2004; Miller *et al.* 2005). Clinical decision support and computerized physician order entry have made an impact on medication errors, and have been promoted as techniques to make huge inroads on medication errors (Teich *et al.* 2007). McMullin *et al.* (2005) found that e-prescribing that included a clinical decision support system (CDSS) was associated with significant drug cost savings and reduction in the proportion of high-cost drugs in eight therapeutic categories that were the target of CDSS messages to prescribers. Thus, an e-prescribing system with a CDSS can influence prescribing and produce drug cost savings (McMullin *et al.* 2005).

Potential aspects of reducing costs in the US health care system

Spending on drugs as a percentage of what was spent on health care in total increased slightly from 2006 to 2007, from 10.07% to 10.14% (Poisal *et al.* 2007). Drivers for the significant costs of medications include increased technologies available, increasing numbers of patients and prescriptions per patient, and the number of seniors taking advantage of the Medicare Part D Drug Benefit. Generic drug use accounts for over 63% of prescriptions filled in the USA, but as a percentage of expenditures on drugs in total remains 20% (Kaiser Family Foundation 2007). Brand-name drug purchases fuel the increase in spending on drugs, as evidenced by these data (Kaiser Family Foundation 2007).

One of the tangible benefits of e-prescribing in third-party programs is the potential to reduce excess spending on drugs that are not on plan formularies, to reduce spending on drugs for which generic substitutes are available, and for drugs prescribed inappropriately. Third-party plans include prescription drug plans, Medicare Advantage plans, and Medicaid plans that have formulary and generic option warnings that indicate to the prescriber and/or dispenser that a certain drug may not be appropriate.

Several segments of e-prescribing systems will enable drugs to be used more appropriately and thus less expensively. Physicians will have alerts about formulary acceptability or lack thereof when entering a specific drug for patients; in addition pharmacists will have computer prompts that will serve as "gatekeeper" warnings for non-formulary, expensive, and inappropriately prescribed drugs (drug interaction, drug disease, drug dosage, or drug dosage form warnings). These prompts will help stem some of the drug expenses in the system that have been rising so precipitously from year to year.

Quality-enhancing capabilities of e-prescribing

Bell and colleagues (2004) note that e-prescribing may substantially improve health care quality. Despite the complexity involved in evaluating systems, these authors (2004) suggest developing a conceptual framework when evaluating needs and possible e-prescribing solutions. They point to 14 options that e-prescribing can help address:

1 patient selection or identification
2 diagnosis selection and diagnosis-based reminders
3 medication selection menus
4 safety alerts
   a drug choice errors, including allergies
      i drug–drug interactions
      ii drug–disease interactions
      iii drug–lab (renal, hepatic function)
      iv body size, age
5 formulary alerts and formulary adherence
6 dosage calculation
   a dosage errors
7 data transmission to inpatient, retail, and/or mail-order pharmacy
8 physician in-office dispensing
   a drug choice errors
9 patient education materials, coordination of education activities
10 medication administration aids

11 refill and renewal reminders
    a   outpatient adherence
12 corollary orders (e.g., for monitoring tests)
13 automated patient questionnaires to detect adverse effects; other structured follow-up communication
14 alerts for patients' failure to refill (whether patients refill prescriptions in a timely fashion)
    a   patient adherence.

Ability to detect fraudulent patient activity

Another measure to improve quality is the ability to identify providers from whom patients seek care. This measure to enhance quality, and one that would be controlled through e-prescribing, is a fraud detection capability that would be built into every e-prescribing system. Patients could not "shop around" for numerous physicians to write prescriptions for them. This has been a problem for decades in the USA as some patients have attempted to see numerous physicians with the intent of obtaining many prescriptions from differing doctors. These abuses have resulted in multiple prescribing of drugs of abuse, antibiotics, antidepressants, and other drugs. E-prescribing will help to eliminate this problem. Interestingly, prior to e-prescribing, other attempts to diminish this serious problem have all fallen short. At various times people had tried to use duplicate or triplicate prescription pads (paper) to try to stem the abuse – none worked to the same extent that e-prescribing will. At present, tamperproof prescriptions are being required in Medicaid programs, as is the case in some states regardless of payer.

Inherent systems to enable e-prescribing for optimal effects

The electronic architecture necessary to enable e-prescribing are in place at present in the USA. Major systems that have been effective in transmitting information from physicians' software to pharmacies and from pharmacies to PBMs and insurers have been shown to provide all the benefits available from e-prescribing. Hale (2007) noted:

> The electronic prescribing process also requires intermediaries for data transfer to communicate the prescription information between the software system in the physician offices to the system in the pharmacies, and also for transmitting information to and from PBMs and health plans. Currently, SureScripts is the major provider of communication between physician office software and pharmacies and RxHub is the major provider of secure communication between the pharmacies and physician software with PBMs and health plans (p. 1).

Viewing e-prescribing with a systems approach

A systems approach or failsafe analysis has been advocated to view prescribing safety and avoidance of prescribing misadventures in a similar fashion to other high-risk activities in society (Hale 2007). Don Berwick, a noted scholar on medication errors and President Obama's 2010 nominee for the position of Director of CMS and who was named to the post, and coauthors have suggested that protecting patient safety can be adapted from other high-risk industries such as civil aviation and nuclear power (Amalberti *et al.* 2005). These authors provide a framework to guide quality improvement that includes five systemic barriers to safe patient care and three problems that are specific to health care.

Dr. Berwick previously served as President and CEO of the Institute for Healthcare Improvement, and is a professor at Harvard Medical School and the Harvard School of Public Health.

The systemic barriers arise from the discretion permitted for workers, worker autonomy, a craftsmanship mindset (that needs to transition to a mindset of equivalent actors), insufficient system-level (senior leadership) arbitration to optimize safety strategies, and the need for simplification.

Foreign experience with e-prescribing

E-prescribing has been used abroad with much success for an extended period of time. The foreign systems have utilized e-prescribing to reduce costs, monitor drug use in an enhanced fashion, and for the streamlining of payment and patient access to prescribed medications.

Sweden

Because of a one-payer system of health insurance, and other factors regarding health professionals, electronic medical records are widely available in Sweden. In addition, data and information are accessible. The Swedes have found that:

- E-prescribing increases security and quality of prescriptions because the chain of information between the physician or hospital and pharmacy is unbroken.
- The prescription the doctor writes in patients' medical record has exactly the same information that the pharmacist uses to dispense the drugs; this has led to a reduction in prescription error both of drugs delivered and suggested dosage by 15%.
- There are considerable savings of time for health providers; the time saved can be used more effectively for patient diagnosis and treatment, which allows more time for patient care.

- Health provider organizations, hospitals, general practitioner surgeries, and pharmacies benefit from:
  - avoidance of illegible prescriptions: the pharmacist does not have to call the physician to verify what is on the prescription
  - considerable time saving by doctors and nurses using e-prescribing
  - reduced risk of fraud and prescription falsification, which previously was problematic
  - avoidance of duplicate prescriptions, which were necessary to replace lost or misplaced prescriptions.

The UK

Barber and colleagues (2006) in the UK have conducted a thorough analysis of e-prescribing in several health care settings. When evaluating e-prescribing in multiple settings, the following were key lessons learned from their research:

- Electronic prescribing (EP) needs to be addressed as a "sociotechnical" innovation, not just a technical solution "there for the taking".
- An extended implementation period needs to be resourced to provide support and to help good new practices embed.
- Emergent change should be expected and be managed. This can be quite profound, for example, EP could lead to a reduction in interaction with patients and between other professionals.
- Technical systems are never perfect; they should continue to be developed both to improve performance and to embody new and changing understanding.
- Software should be specified so it is possible to adapt it locally, and so that the data held are easily accessible for multiple purposes.
- Decision support is not straightforward; the purpose and limitations of decision support need to be clear to all concerned (p. 11).

Barber *et al.* (2006) conclude:

> Our findings, taken overall, tentatively suggest that for every 100 prescriptions written in a hospital there will be around 10 errors; the introduction of an electronic prescribing system, at the current stage of development, would avoid two or three of them (p. 136).

Canada

The Canadian equivalent of the US FDA is Health Canada. In Canada, the regulatory equivalent of the US FDA has been involved in e-prescribing. The Canada Health Infoway has worked to develop standards to enable e-prescribing activities between prescribers and pharmacists. Canada Health Infoway is a Canadian government effort and approach to enable electronic medical records to be available in Canada. The standards are required to support amendments under the regulation-making authority of the Food and Drug Act, the Controlled Drug and Substance Act and possibly the Personal Information Protection and Electronic Documents Act. Health Canada has interacted with interested parties along the way. These key stakeholders, such as pharmacy and health practitioner regulatory bodies and federal/provincial/territorial government institutions, have worked together on such efforts.

Similar US FDA efforts
The US FDA has initiatives under way to encourage e-prescribing. In a speech before the Urban Institute on November 12, 2003, then FDA Commissioner Dr. Mark McClellan (2003) noted:

> For example, to ensure that up-to-date drug information will be available to clinicians at the point of care, FDA is developing its new structured medical product labels in conjunction with new standards to make this label fully electronic, through our DailyMed program. The goal is to give the kind of IT-based support systems for good prescribing access to FDA's full, up to date database on the evidence on approved medical product use.

> FDA has worked with the National Library of Medicine to maintain a comprehensive inventory of these "electronic drug labels" and will distribute this information free of charge to providers and IT vendors, possibly along with other useful information from medical studies. This will serve as the definitive source of drug information, since it will represent the body of evidence reviewed and approved by FDA.

DailyMed provides high-quality information about marketed drugs. This information includes FDA-approved labels (package inserts). This website provides health information providers and the public with a standard, comprehensive, up-to-date, look-up and download resource of medication content and labeling as found in medication package inserts.

Other information about prescription drugs may also be available. The National Library of Medicine regularly processes data files uploaded from the FDA system and provides and maintains this website for the public to access information. Additional information about medicines is available on the National Library of Medicine's MedlinePlus website (http://www.nlm.nih.gov/medlineplus/medicines.html).

Finland

E-prescribing has been implemented in Finland for several years; the problems identified in the USA as concerns were also prominent in the inauguration of the Finnish system in 2005.

Numerous factors have enabled e-prescribing to be implemented in foreign systems, such as the Finnish system:

- a one-payer health care insurance system
- electronic medical records
- enhanced communication between physicians and pharmacists
- seamless interactions between prescribers, dispensers, and health care institutions.

US implementation progress

A relative lack of any of these points will not preclude a gradual implementation of e-prescribing in the USA. In fact, these foreign systems can help those seeking e-prescribing implementation in the USA to avoid pitfalls and problem areas. The USA can learn much from these foreign examples of forays into e-prescribing.

Impact of existing technology on e-prescribing

The emergence of the enhanced sophistication of handheld and wireless transmission of data will stimulate the additional application of e-prescribing. This technology factor is important, as are the time, error, and economic savings that e-prescribing can provide (Curtiss 2005b). Curtiss notes:

> in the last year, Blackberry and other wireless communication devices have been breaking down barriers of resistance to change. The ubiquitous and low effort features of this technology will transfer to clinician prescribing, and rather than resisting e-prescribing, clinicians will be demanding it. Yet, it will remain necessary to spend money on new and upgraded system software to integrate e-prescribing with the electronic medical record to overcome electronic silos of data that reside in pharmacies, at pharmacy benefit managers, or in data warehouses and are not available to clinicians at the point of care. What will shorten the timeline between the reality of

today and the inevitability of tomorrow is studious examination of the work of pioneers in adapting and implementing IT solutions in health care settings (p. 420).

Gaps that inhibit e-prescribing uptake

Current physician use of e-prescribing is estimated to be between 3% and 18% depending on definition. Ridinger (2007) notes that an e-prescribing system would ensure optimization of safety, quality, and cost–benefit of therapeutics in clinical practice but is only one critical component of broader initiatives being implemented to optimize health care delivery.

Gaps also occur in many places in health care

Curtiss (2005b) has suggested:

> the gap between expectations and reality is large nearly everywhere one looks in health care. While there are success stories, more often, the truth is that success stories are limited to distinct subsets or compartments of the health care system; use of the IT solution is voluntary by clinicians, thereby undermining the value of digital information because it is not complete; the IT system is plagued with errors (Fernando *et al.* 2004), or a backlash occurs among clinicians who find the new IT system burdensome rather than helpful (Morrissey 2004). The solution to IT over promises is lower expectations for IT proposals to meet the need for safety, quality, and administrative efficiency in health care (p. 419).

Fundamental flaws in drug use process

There are fundamental flaws in the drug use process in the USA. Medication compliance hovers around 50%; prescription drug misuse is rampant. OTC medications are misused. Adverse drug events occur (many of which are preventable). Antibiotic misuse has led to drug-resistant strains of many bacteria. Despite recent changes to Medicare, many patients remained uninsured with respect to prescription medications. E-prescribing will not by itself impact these and other systemic medication-related error-producing system segments.

Increase in self-medication

Self-medication can be broadly defined as a decision made by a patient to consume a drug without the explicit approval or direction of a health professional. The self-medication activities of patients increased dramatically in the late 20th and on into the 21st century. Many contemporary developments have continued to fuel this increase. There are ever-increasing locations from which to purchase OTC medications. Many medications have been switched to OTC classification from prescription-only in the last 50 years. In addition, patients are increasingly becoming comfortable with self-diagnosis and self-selection of OTC remedies.

These important OTC therapeutic agents, that just happen to be sold and used without a prescription, will not be able to be captured in e-prescribing systems. They are purchased by consumers in some instances without their health professionals being aware of their use. Important impacts on disease states and deleterious effects on other drugs which are prescribed can cause problems. For example, if a patient is taking aspirin, which has blood-thinning properties, together with another drug that is prescribed, such as sodium warfarin, this can lead to dangerous bleeding episodes. Using non-prescription analgesics such as acetaminophen with prescription analgesics also containing acetaminophen can be problematic. These duplications will not be addressed or influenced by e-prescribing.

Direct-to-consumer advertising
Direct marketing of drugs by pharmaceutical manufacturers to consumers has also contributed to rising prescription costs. Direct-to-consumer advertising for prescription drugs doubled in the recent past, from $1.1 billion in 1997 to $2.7 billion in 2001 (Jeffords 2004). Estimates for 2006 spending on direct-to-consumer advertising have been estimated to be $4.2 billion. As drugs have been switched from prescription to OTC status, the advertising and promotion of these newly classified OTC drugs have increased as well. Self-medication in and of itself has many positive aspects with many benefits to patients when done appropriately.

Systems cannot indicate where consumers obtain medications
Although pharmacists are seen as the gatekeepers for patients to obtain prescription drugs, patients can also obtain prescription medications from other pharmacies and/or from dispensing physicians. Patients may also borrow from friends, relatives, or even casual acquaintances. In addition, patients obtain OTC medications from physicians through prescriptions, on advice from pharmacists, through self-selection, or through the recommendations of friends or acquaintances. Through all of this, it must be recognized that both formal (structural) and informal (pervasive) system components are at

play. Pharmacists or physicians may or may not be consulted regarding the use of medications. In some cases, health professionals are unaware of the drugs patients are taking. In addition, herbal remedies or health supplements may be taken without the knowledge of a health professional.

As an example, consider the patient medication profiling capability of most pharmacists currently in place and those that will continue to be enabled by e-prescribing. Computerization of patient medication records is commonplace in pharmacy. This computerization allows for:

- ease in billing third-party prescription programs
- maintenance of drug allergy information
- drug use review
- notification of drug interactions
- aid in meeting the Omnibus Budget Reconciliation Act of 1990 requirements for patient counseling, drug use review, and estimation of appropriateness of therapy.

This computerization permits drug-related information to be easily entered, retained, and retrieved. However, OTC medications are rarely entered into such records (one exception may be OTC drugs prescribed by physicians and dispensed through a prescription by pharmacists). This exclusion of a whole class of drugs from the monitoring programs of pharmacy may have a profound effect upon the ability of pharmacists to monitor the drug therapies of their patients. If the patient purchases the OTC medication in the pharmacy, the pharmacist may have an idea of the drugs consumed. However, if OTC drugs are purchased in a non-pharmacy outlet, the pharmacist is completely unaware of many drugs a patient may be taking. Another factor adding to the complexity of the problem is the fact that a patient may utilize numerous pharmacies for varying prescription products. Thus there is no one record repository for all medications a patient may be taking.

Lack of insurance coverage
External variables may greatly influence patients and their drug-taking behaviors. Coverage for prescribed drugs allows those with coverage to obtain medications with varying cost-sharing requirements. However, many do not have insurance coverage for drugs or other health-related needs. It has been estimated that, in 2006, 17% of Americans, approximately 47 million people, lacked health insurance for all or part of the year (Kaiser Family Foundation 2004). This will change with the full

impact of PPACA, but drug coverage gaps will continue to exist. Certainly, these considerations have huge ramifications for how and when consumers obtain prescribed and OTC medications.

Those who do have health insurance have seen premiums rise drastically in the recent past, by 8.4–11% (Miller 2001). Miller notes that in some cases employees are not just being asked to pay more for health insurance but to pay for it all. Until this fundamental inequality is remedied through health policy changes and a differing perspective on insurance coverage for those who are currently uninsured, no amount of sophisticated HIT implementations or e-prescribing enabling will impact this component of the health care delivery and access to care conundrum.

Adverse drug reactions

ADRs are sometimes frequent, sometimes sporadic, and more often than not unpredictable. E-prescribing can help to reduce ADRs if proper notation occurs in patients' records and is accessible electronically by prescribers and pharmacists. These notations, indicating previous reactions, sensitivities, and alerts for drugs, must be in place and not overridden by prescribers and pharmacists.

The incidence of ADRs is unknown. Even in health care system institutions (hospitals and long-term care facilities) with elaborate HIT systems, ADRs still occur despite sophisticated electronic systems. There is not at present a foolproof system to report their occurrence; it is hoped that e-prescribing and associated systems will enable a more cohesive method of reporting and sharing ADR experiences.

A consideration for both patients and providers is that ADRs should be reported, the process is anonymous and confidential, and either can report ADRs. There has been a reluctance to submit ADRs on the part of providers who may fear retribution, but the process is designed to be non-judgmental and is certainly not punitive. ADRs can be submitted to the US FDA through the MedWatch program (http://www.fda.gov/safetymedwatch/default.htm).

Compliance

All involved in the drug use process need to understand patient compliance behaviors. Interventions cannot be tailored to meet patient therapeutic needs if patient drug-taking behavior is unclear. Conversely, if patient drug-taking patterns are discernible, it is possible to help patients take medications as they should through varying types of compliance interventions. E-prescribing systems are unlikely to impact individual patient behavior so as to enhance patient compliance and/or persistence.

Interventions that have been shown to be effective in enhancing compliance have included:

- patient counseling (verbal or written)
- specialized packaging (unit of use, unit dose, blister packs, specialized containers, and/or packaging of medications to be taken at the same time in the same unit of use containers)
- varying refill reminders (letters mailed, e-mailed, telephone calls)
- other types of specialized contacts.

If we cannot measure how patients are taking medications, it is not possible to formulate specialized aids to help them take medications. Measurement of compliance can vary from mildly invasive (pill counts or questioning patients) to very invasive (blood level determination of compliance).

Providers can ask patients whether compliance is a problem with them, and the veracity of each of the responses is subject to verification. Blood levels can be measured, therapeutic outcomes can be measured, and indirect methods of estimating compliance (side-effects, certain outcomes of drug use examined) can all be undertaken with varying assurances of accuracy.

Ultimately the decision to comply or not with recommendations, including prescription drug therapies, is a patient-specific decision. E-prescribing may streamline the process of providing the patient with the right drug, the correct dose, the appropriate dosing mechanism, and proper instructions for use. However, the decision to comply or not, or to help a caregiver enable compliance behavior for those for whom they provide care, is in the hands of the patient and/or caregiver.

Frank errors

Despite elaborate and sophisticated HIT-enabled e-prescribing, errors will continue to be made as long as humans are involved in health care. Physicians have the potential to make errors in prescribing (wrong patient, right patient but wrong drug, wrong dose, and/or wrong duration of therapy). Pharmacists are also capable of making errors in dispensing, labeling, misreading orders, and/or dispensing to the wrong patient. Patients are also able to underdose, overdose, use the wrong drugs for the wrong length of time, and/or use the right drug for the wrong period of time.

Wrong diagnoses

A startling 15% of diagnoses are estimated to be made in error (Groopman 2007). Groopman further suggests that 80% of these errors are predictable based on how physicians go about diagnosing patients' maladies in such a compressed and hurried fashion. E-prescribing will not reverse this startling rate of inaccuracy. If the right drug is prescribed for the wrong diagnosis, the patient will always suffer.

Taking the place of face-to-face encounters?

There will always be a need for pharmacists to contact physicians via the telephone to deal with patient-related issues, including:

- clarification of orders transmitted by physicians or physicians' representatives
- following up on questionable orders from physicians
- determining if the patient is in fact the correct patient
- drug, dose, dosage form clarifications
- dealing with therapeutic duplications, drug interactions (drug, food, supplement)
- third-party insurance-related concerns
- clarifying refill instructions for repeating medication regimens
- emergency contact when a physician is not near a computer, and needs to phone in an order
- suggesting therapeutic alternatives when appropriate or required for some reason (insurance, patient needs, better choice of drug over what has been prescribed).

So, regardless of how well structured an e-prescribing system is, there will always be situations where health care professionals will need to converse via phone contact as well as interacting electronically.

Summary

E-prescribing has unlimited potential to enhance the drug use process from prescribing to the point of patient delivery of medications. Error reduction, precise dosing, help in choosing the appropriate drug, and enhancement of quality are but a few of the potential and very real consequences of the uptake of e-prescribing. As is the case with any improvement in any industry, including the health care industry, the recognition of the many potential benefits and a thorough assessment of the issues that e-prescribing cannot address will bode well for all involved in the drug use process.

E-prescribing will not solve all of the ills present in the US prescribing, dispensing, and utilization processes for prescription drugs. Varying legislative enactments favorable to implementation of e-prescribing are examples of how legislation can drive health policy from a regulatory point of view.

Discussion questions

1 What are the impediments to the use of e-prescribing by physicians?

2 Incentives are provided to physicians to incorporate e-prescribing into their practices. What could be done further to enhance their uptake of e-prescribing?

3 What can e-prescribing provide from a quality standpoint?

4 What are several downsides to e-prescribing in the US health care system?

5 You are a product manager for a new therapeutic treatment for rheumatoid arthritis, Dudamove. What segments of e-prescribing can you use on behalf of the new drug and your company to grow sales of the product?

6 How can pharmacies use e-prescribing as a competitive advantage enhancement in the marketplace?

7 How does e-prescribing alter marketing of pharmaceuticals in the channel of distribution for prescription drugs in the USA?

8 What are the impediments to the uptake of e-prescribing in the developing world?

9 Why would you assume that mail-order pharmacies are enthused by the prospects of widespread utilization of e-prescribing?

10 What can be done to ensure that e-prescribing is compatible with other HIT advances in the short and long term?

References

Amalberti R, Auroy Y, Berwick D, *et al*. (2005). Five system barriers to achieving ultrasafe health care. *Ann Intern Med* 142: 756–764.

Barber N, Franklin ED, Cornford T, *et al*. (2006). Safer, faster, better? Evaluating electronic prescribing report to the patient safety research programme. Policy Research Programme of the Department of Health. Available online at: http://eprints.pharmacy.ac.uk/763/1/ElectronicPrescribingBarberFranklin.pdf.

Bates DW, Leape LL, Cullen DJ (1998). Effect of computerized physician order entry and a team intervention on prevention of serious medication errors. *JAMA* 280: 1311–1316.

Bell DS, Cretin S, Marken RS, *et al.* (2004). A conceptual framework for evaluating outpatient electronic prescribing systems based on their functional capabilities. *J Am Med Inform Assoc* 11: 60–70.

Boodman SG (2005). Not quite fail-safe, computerizing isn't a panacea for dangerous drug errors. *Washington Post* March 22: HE01.

Chertow GM, Lee J, Kuperman GJ (2001). Guided medication dosing for inpatients with renal insufficiency. *JAMA* 286: 2839–2844.

Chrischilles EA, Fulda TR, Byrns PJ, *et al.* (2002). The role of pharmacy computer systems in preventing medication errors. *J Am Pharm Assoc* 42: 439–448.

Curtiss FR (2005a). Clinical, service, and cost outcomes of computerized prescription order entry. *J Manage Care Pharm* 11: 353–355.

Curtiss FR (2005b). Why e-prescribe and the future of transforming data into information. journal of managed care pharmacy. *J Manage Care Pharm* 11: 419–420.

eHealth Initiative (2004). *Electronic Prescribing: Toward Maximum Value and Rapid Adoption: Recommendations for Optimal Design and Implementation to Improve Care, Increase Efficiency and Reduce Costs in Ambulatory Care (eRx Report).* A report of the Electronic Prescribing Initiative, eHealth Initiative. Washington, DC: eHealth Initiative.

Fernando B, Savelyich BS, Avery AJ (2004). Prescribing safety features of general practice computer systems: evaluation using simulated test cases. *Br Med J* 328: 1171–1172.

Fincham JE (2009). *e-Prescribing: The Electronic Transformation of Medicine.* Sudbury, MA: Jones and Bartlett.

Groopman J (2007). *How Doctors Think.* New York: Houghton Mifflin, p. 24.

Hale P (2007). Electronic prescribing update. *HIMSS fact sheet.* Available online at: http://www.himss.org/content/files/CBO/Meeting7/ElectronicPrescribingUpdate.pdf (accessed 4 December 2007).

Horsky J, Kuperman GJ, Patel VL (2005). Comprehensive analysis of a medication dosing error related to CPOE. *J Am Med Inform Assoc* 12: 377–382.

Jeffords J (2004). Direct-to-consumer drug advertising: you get what you pay for. *Health Aff*, W4-253–W4-255.

Kaiser Family Foundation (2004). *The Uninsured and their Access to Health Care.* Fact sheet #1420-06. Washington, DC: Kaiser Family Foundation.

Kaiser Family Foundation (2007). Drug trends, 2007. Fact sheet #3057-06. Available online at: http://www.kff.org/rxdrugs/upload/3057_06.pdf.

Leavitt MA (2007). Pilot testing of initial electronic prescribing standards – cooperative agreements required under section 1860D-(4) (e) of the Social Security Act as amended by the Medicare Prescription Drug, Improvement, and Modernization Action (MMA) of 2003. Available online at: www.healthit.ahrq.gov/portal/server.pt/...0.../eRxReport_041607.pdf (accessed 17 December 2010).

McClellan MB (2003). Protecting and advancing America's health through 21st century patient safety. Speech before the Urban Institute, November 12, 2003. Available online at: http://www.fda.gov/oc/speeches/2003/urbaninstitute1112.html (accessed 7 March 2008).

McMullin ST, Lonergan TP, Rynearson CS (2005). 12-month drug cost savings related to use of an electronic prescribing system with integrated decision support in primary care. *J Manage Care Pharm* 11: 322–332.

Miller JL (2001). *A Perfect Storm: The Confluence of Forces Affecting Health Care Coverage.* Washington, DC: National Coalition on Health Care.

Miller RA, Gardner RM, Johnson KB, *et al.* (2005). Clinical decision support and electronic prescribing systems: A time for responsible thought and action. *J Am Med Inform Assoc* 12: 403–409.

Morrissey J (2004). Harmonic divergence – Cedars-Sinai joins others in holding off on CPOE. *Mod Healthcare* February 23: 16.

O'Harrow R (1998a). Prescription sales, privacy fears: CVS Giant share customer records with drug marketing firm. *Washington Post* February 15: A1.

O'Harrow R (1998b). Giant Food stops sharing customer data: Prescription-marketing plan drew complaints. *Washington Post* February 18: A1.

Ohliger PC (1999). Are your medication records confidential? *AIDS Read* 9: 282–283.

Poisal JA, Truffer C, Smith S, *et al.* (2007). Health spending projections through 2016: Modest changes obscure Part D's impact. *Health Aff* 26: w242–w253.

Potts AL, Barr FE, Gregory DF, *et al.* (2004). Computerized physician order entry and medication errors in a pediatric critical care unit. *Pediatrics* 113: 59–63.

Ridinger MHT (2007). The electronic prescription conundrum: Why "e-Rx" isn't so "e-Z". *Clin Pharmacol Ther* 81: 13–15.

Ross SM, Papshev D, Murphy EL, *et al.* (2005). Effects of electronic prescribing on formulary compliance and generic drug utilization in the ambulatory care setting: A retrospective analysis of administrative claims data. *J Manage Care Pharm* 11: 410–415.

Tcimpidis L, Rosenblatt M (2005). Readers' perspectives. *Health Data Manage* May: 88.

Teich JM, Osheroff JA, Pifer EA, *et al.* (2007). Clinical decision support. *J Am Med Inform Assoc* 14: 141–145.

Wingfield J, Bissell P, Anderson C (2004). The scope of pharmacy ethics – an evaluation of the international research literature, 1990–2002. *Soc Sci Med* 58: 2383–2396.

Further reading

Bell DS, Cretin S, Marken RS, *et al.* (2004). A conceptual framework for evaluating outpatient electronic prescribing systems based on their functional capabilities. *J Am Med Inform Assoc* 11: 60–70.

Cooper RJ, Anderson C, Avery T, *et al.* (2008). Nurse and pharmacist supplementary prescribing in the UK – A thematic review of the literature. *Health Policy* 85: 277–292.

Cooper-DeHoff RM, Handberg-Thurmond EM, Marks RG, *et al.* (2000). Control of blood pressure in a population of women with hypertension and CAD using an internet-based electronic prescribing system. *Am J Hypertens* 13(suppl. 1): S117–S118.

Cusack CM (2008). Electronic health records and electronic prescribing: Promise and pitfalls. *Obstet Gynecol Clin North Am* 35: 63–79.

De Salvia MA, Macchiarulo C, Lerro G, *et al.* (2002). Prescribing patterns for angiotensin II-receptor blockers in an Italian antihypertensive division: A retrospective chart review. *Curr Ther Res* 63: 789–802.

Hill DA, Cacciatore M, Lamvu GM (2010). Electronic prescribing influence on calcium supplementation: a randomized controlled trial. *Am J Obstet Gynecol* 202: 236. e231–236.e235.

Hollingworth W, Devine EB, Hansen RN, *et al.* The impact of e-prescribing on prescriber and staff time in ambulatory care clinics: A time–motion study. *J Am Med Inform Assoc* 14: 722–730.

Jani YH, Ghaleb MA, Marks SD, *et al.* (2008). Electronic prescribing reduced prescribing errors in a pediatric renal outpatient clinic. *J Pediatr* 152: 214–218.

Johnson KB, FitzHenry F (2006). Case report: Activity diagrams for integrating electronic prescribing tools into clinical workflow. *J Am Med Inform Assoc* 13: 391–395.

Judge J, Field TS, DeFlorio M, *et al.* (2006). Prescribers' responses to alerts during medication ordering in the long term care setting. *J Am Med Inform Assoc* 13: 385–390.

McNulty CAM (2001). Optimising antibiotic prescribing in primary care. *Int J Antimicrob Agents* 18: 329–333.

Pagán JA, Pratt WR, Sun J (2009). Which physicians have access to electronic prescribing and which ones end up using it? *Health Policy* 89: 288–294.

Rosenbloom ST (2006). Approaches to evaluating electronic prescribing. *J Am Med Inform Assoc* 13: 399–401.

Schedlbauer A, Prasad V, Mulvaney C, *et al*. What evidence supports the use of computerized alerts and prompts to improve clinicians' prescribing behavior? *J Am Med Inform Assoc* 16: 531–538.

Shah NR, Seger AC, Seger DL, *et al*. Improving acceptance of computerized prescribing alerts in ambulatory care. *J Am Med Inform Assoc* 13: 5–11.

Shannon T, Feied C, Smith M, *et al*. (2006). Wireless handheld computers and voluntary utilization of computerized prescribing systems in the emergency department. *J Emerg Med* 31: 309–315.

Simpson M, Sweeney MA (2009). Implementing electronic prescribing. *Osteopath Fam Phys* 1: 41–44.

Terrell KM, Heard K, Miller DK (2006). Prescribing to older ED patients. *Am J Emerg Med* 24: 468–478.

Wang CJ, Marken RS, Meili RC, *et al*. (2005). Functional characteristics of commercial ambulatory electronic prescribing systems: A field study. *J Am Med Inform Assoc* 12: 346–356.

Weingart SN, Massagli M, Cyrulik A, *et al*. (2009). Assessing the value of electronic prescribing in ambulatory care: A focus group study. *Int J Med Informatics* 78: 571–578.

4

Justice and access to care

Introduction

In a pluralistic society, decisions will vary about what services should be provided by social insurance programs and for whom. Different calls have emanated seeking the implementation of a universal one-payer system in the USA. Others have argued for a market-based and market-driven provision of health care insurance and health care services. Those without insurance or those who are underinsured often lack strong advocates to enhance what they have available to them. Many will talk about the need to reform Medicare: the program has become too expensive and will be more so as the number eligible for Medicare increases in the future. But the political will to change such a popular program would come with enormous political costs. Some suggest that means testing (adjusting benefits based upon personal income) for receipt of funded benefits would help eliminate some of the costs and allow the uninsured and underinsured to receive some care. Although it may seem altruistically appealing to look at this issue as a zero-sum game whereby costs are shifted from one social program to another, the reality is that what might really be necessary is a reduction in costs period and not a recasting of funds across other programs, regardless of how worthy they might be. The preceding discussion has pertinence for the USA, but could be duplicated in many other areas. Access to care and to services is a major issue, not only in the developed, but also in the developing, world.

Ethics and health policy

Emanuel (2002) notes that ethics in a society examines what values are important to us, and why they are important. Churchill (2002) suggests that "there are ethical assumptions and implications for all health policies" (p. 51) and ethical application to the processes of policy-making. He further suggests that a lack of ethics has led us to the health care system that we deserve, and that more infusion of ethics into health policy decisions may allow us to obtain the health care system that we may optimally want.

Social justice and health care

Many see the issue of access to care as an issue of social justice. Two prominent bioethicists, Powers and Faden (2006), suggest six essential dimensions must be considered when looking at social justice: health, personal security, reasoning, respect for others, attachment, and self-determination. Building upon the work of Rawls (1971), Powers and Faden (2006) suggest not examining one of these, e.g., health, in isolation as a solution. Instead they posit that a sufficient level of adequacy for each of the six dimensions needs to be accomplished to address social justice issues. They suggest that all in society need to have access to these six dimensions for a truly equitable society to exist. Finding instances of injustice and subsequently correcting them is suggested to be important to the design of the final forms of health policy and public health interventions (Powers and Faden 2006).

Justice and health policy

Daniels *et al.* (2002), discussing justice and health policy, noted: "Justice requires that we ask whether these social determinants of health are fairly distributed, and where they are not, that we take steps to address these sources of health inequality" (p. 20). They give several options to address issues of inequality, including early-life intervention, increasing the quality of a work environment, and income redistribution. These authors note that race and class dimensions are involved, and for example, when discussing increasing income, mention earned income tax credits, increasing child care credits, and increasing the minimum wage as options for solutions (Daniels *et al.* 2002). Early-life interventions would include prenatal and postnatal care, vaccinations, and well-child check-ups.

Allocation of resources for at-risk populations

Danis and Patrick (2002) suggest that macro issues of equity and justice have received scant attention from bioethicists, who have focused on health care and not health per se. The focus has been on delivery systems, access points, care availability, and health care personnel versus health status and preventive efforts.

Market forces versus government control and health care

Callahan and Wasunna (2006), when viewing medical progress, note that medical progress and scientific progress are open-ended and infinite in scope. At the outer fringes of infinite medical advances, and as costs increase with the new advances, progress blurs between good health and enhanced human health. They further argue that a finite as opposed to infinite model would emphasize quality of life over quantity of life-years (Callahan and Wasunna 2006). They suggest that the "medical necessity" view of health care is fraught with what they term a "twilight zone" of a mix of available money, cultural preferences, medical biases, and public information. Callahan and Wasunna (2006) note the influence of research, endless progress, ever-expanding patient choices, and the market as a means and glorification of it as an end.

Global status of market forces in health care

The USA stands alone as a country with a health care system that is predominantly market-oriented. Europe (especially western Europe) has a mixed model with market forces affecting health care delivery to a lesser extent and government regulation impacting systems to a greater extent. Europe, especially western Europe, relies on a system of solidarity whereby citizens are taken care of by society, e.g., governments. The USA relies much more on market competition and on individualism. Market competition in the USA is reliant upon competition to reduce or rein in health care costs.

The developing world relies upon market forces and Callahan and Wasunna (2006) suggests this is detrimental. With the presence of appalling morbidity and mortality statistics, the overwhelming burden of communicable diseases (malaria, acquired immunodeficiency syndrome (AIDS), tuberculosis (TB)) and maternal-related conditions affecting childbirth are far too burdensome in scope and occurrence for countries to try to maintain mixtures of market and governmental influences within health care systems in developing countries. Chronic conditions are much more prevalent in the western developed world. These authors posit five crucial criteria when considering the benefits of market practices (p. 254):

1   What is the state of the population health within a country? Can population health be positively influenced by market forces?
2   Is equity an issue?
3   Are regulations in place to monitor or control activities?
4   How have market mechanisms been used in the past? How effective has this been?
5   Are market experiments being evaluated?

Again, they note that market experiments have not helped developing countries due to the focus on health care systems and not on improving health. These are certainly not one and the same construct.

Special market case of pharmaceuticals

Callahan (2003) suggests there is nothing quite like the pharmaceutical industry, with escalating higher prices seeking to save lives and reduce suffering.

The drug industry works within the market economy in the USA with prices set and able to float at increasing levels within a framework of competition and little regulation. In western Europe, Canada, and the UK regulation and price controls affect the market price for pharmaceuticals. In the developing world, the market economy allows prices to remain high and unattainable for the majority of patients.

Callahan and Wasunna (2006) elsewhere indicate that the market "wild cards" are pharmaceuticals – they can have either a high or low value. The authors suggest that in developing countries, a mix of public and private systems is necessarily pertinent to pharmaceuticals. The public component is the ability of governments to interfere in the market for the sake of health, e.g., in the case of pharmaceuticals which may be priced too high and thus are out of reach for many.

Access to care and its importance

Enabled access to appropriate care is a necessity for the true benefits of a health care system to be fully realized. Numerous factors impinge on access to care, and negative factors adversely affecting access have been shown to lead to deleterious health outcomes. It has been estimated that, currently in the USA, 20 000 die annually simply because they do not have a physician from whom to seek care. Unaffordable and too high levels of insurance deductibles, no regular physician or caregiver, and inability to pay insurance co-payments can all lead to a lack of proper outcomes. Without question, health policy decisions can certainly negatively influence access to care.

So why examine access to care at this point? Even with the passage of the Patient Protection and Affordable Care Act (PPACA) in the USA, access to care will remain an issue. It always has and always will be an issue for concern. Additional individuals will be insured in health plans, more patients will be eligible for coverage under state Medicaid plans, and more employers will be required to cover employees with health insurance policies. Even with the hope that improvements in coverage and scope of benefits will be available for many, the reality is that some with coverage will struggle to pay for health care needs that are not covered or for services that individuals cannot afford, even with additional coverage that they currently do not have.

Burden of uninsurance

The health burdens accumulating due to uninsurance are significant. Ziller *et al.* (2008) found in a study examining rural and urban families and health insurance coverage that 33% of rural families have at least one uninsured member. There are subsidies planned within PPACA to account for low-income families; this is certainly necessary due to many low-income rural households lacking health insurance coverage and not being currently eligible due to inability to meet income requirements.

Underinsured

The number of underinsured is in reality unknown. The US government does not track the number of underinsured and hard data and/or reliable estimates are not available. Another dilemma when trying to examine numbers of the US underinsured groups is that the numbers are not static. Loss of jobs, part-time employment, changing jobs, changes in family structures for various reasons, including death, can all make measurement an imprecise process. Other uninsured may have health insurance coverage, but due to high deductable amounts, co-insurance, or co-payments, simply cannot afford to purchase care when needed because of an inability to meet the co-insurance requirements before coverage ensues.

Kriss *et al.* (2008), accessing the problems of young adults and lack of insurance, indicated that young adults, aged 19–29 years, are one of the largest segments of the US population without health insurance: 13.7 million lacked coverage in 2006. These individuals often lose coverage at age 19 or upon high-school or college graduation – almost two out of five (38%) high-school graduates who do not enroll in college and one-third of college graduates are uninsured for a time during their first year after graduation. The passage of PPACA contains components allowing young adults to remain covered under their parents' health insurance plans until age 27 (through the end of individuals' 26th year). This was implemented on September 23, 2010. However, in late April 2010 it was determined that federal employees' children, falling under federal employee insurance, would not be eligible for such coverage until 2011, past 2010, when most privately employed insurance plans for non-governmental employees with differing coverage will allow such coverage.

Schoen and fellow researchers (2008) estimate that in 2007, 25 million insured people ages 19–64 were underinsured – a 60% increase since 2003. These researchers note that the rate of increase was steepest among those with incomes above 200% of the federal poverty limit, where underinsurance rates nearly tripled. A final estimate was that 42% of US adults were underinsured or uninsured (Schoen *et al.* 2008).

Voorhees *et al.* (2008) in a study of underinsurance in a sample of patients seeking care in primary care clinics found that, of those with insurance for a full year, 36.3% were underinsured. Of those who were underinsured, 50.2% felt that their health suffered because they could not afford recommended care, a rate similar among those who were uninsured. Winkelman and Westall (2008) also noted the prevalence of underinsurance within patient subpopulations seeking primary care health services.

Halterman and colleagues (2008) have examined the influence of health insurance coverage gaps on children via a study using the National Survey of Children's Health. They identified children with continuous public or private insurance and defined three groups with gaps in insurance coverage: (1) those currently insured who had a lapse in coverage during the previous 12 months (gained insurance); (2) those currently uninsured who had been insured at some time during the previous 12 months (lost insurance); and (3) those with no health insurance at all during the previous 12 months (full-year uninsured). The results indicated that 13% of children had coverage gaps (7% gained insurance, 4% lost insurance, and 2% were full-year uninsured). Many children with gaps in coverage had unmet needs for care (7.4%, 12.8%, and 15.1% among the gained insurance, lost insurance, and full-year uninsured groups, respectively). The authors conclude that many children with asthma have unmet health care needs and poor access to consistent primary care, and lack of continuous health insurance coverage may play an important role (Halterman *et al.* 2008).

Medical technology as an impediment to improving access to care

Noted medical ethicist, Daniel Callahan (2009a), deftly places the access to care dilemma in the context of two irreconcilable forces: the need for better access to care for those without care and the unrelenting desire for more and better health care technology at the same time – in other words, stressing the "common good and not just the private good" (p. 3). Callahan (2009b) suggests that unless and until the health care technology albatross is controlled, the system could easily collapse. Callahan (2009b) notes a three-tier system of care in the USA: (1) one in which patients have coverage through employers or Medicare and can cover any additional necessary outlays (co-pays or deductibles); (2) one in which patients may have coverage but simply cannot afford high co-payment requirements or meet necessary deductibles; and (3) those with no coverage or inadequate coverage provided through Medicaid. Further, he calls for a radical relook at how health care is viewed, away from the premise that death is inherently a bad thing for those of advanced age, and toward one of acceptance of death as a normal physiological component of the life cycle (Callahan 2009c). Obviously, the further one is away from the data point Callahan (2009c) uses (80 years of age), the more dispassionate one may be. Rather than view disease treatments as an infinite exploration with ever-increasing expenses associated with the treatments, a more finite and realistic view would enable more who are currently without care options to receive care with more resources available for use elsewhere (Callahan 2009d).

Callahan's (2009e) premise is that, unless difficult choices are made in controlling costs, diminishing the need for constantly seeking the best technology available, and seeking a widespread basic care model for more in society and less focus on the best care available if one can afford it, the USA will not approach the level of coverage that is seen in continental European and UK systems pertaining to health care coverage of the population.

Emergency rooms as source of care

Individuals without regular access to points of care must rely upon emergency rooms for their source of care. Chronically ill patients without insurance are more likely to seek care from emergency rooms than similarly categorized patients with health insurance coverage (Wilper *et al.* 2008). In this study, after controlling for age, sex, and race or ethnicity, chronically ill patients without insurance were more likely than those with coverage not to have visited a health professional (22.6% versus 6.2%) and not to have a standard site for care (26.1% versus 6.2%) but more likely to identify their standard site for care as an emergency department (ED) (7.1% versus 1.1%) ($P < 0.001$ for all comparisons). However, Weber and colleagues (2008) found that the rise in ED visits between 1996 and 2003 could not be primarily attributed to the uninsured. In this study, major contributors to increasing ED utilization appear to be disproportionate increases in use by non-poor persons and by persons whose usual source of care is a physician's office. Owens and colleagues (2008) when examining ED use by pediatric patients across 14 states found that over 1.5 million or nearly one-third of ED visits were for pediatric injuries. The researchers found that injuries account for a significant portion of pediatric ED visits and that upwards of 47% were Medicaid-covered patients (Owens *et al.* 2008).

Hsia *et al.* (2008), when studying ED payments for 1996–2004, found the proportion of charges paid for outpatient ED visits from Medicaid, Medicare, and privately insured and uninsured patients persistently decreased from 1996 to 2004. These authors suggest that decreases may threaten the survival of EDs and their ability to continue to provide care as safety nets in the US health care system. This trend is doubly disconcerting when considering that the PPACA enables and focuses increases in Medicaid roles in the states.

In the USA, it has long been known that public hospitals serve as safety nets for many without health care coverage and who lack resources to pay for necessary health care services. Blesch (2008) notes that rules promulgated by the Centers for Medicare and Medicaid Services (CMS) have the potential to affect adversely public hospitals reliant upon Medicare and Medicaid funding for survival. Blesch writes:

> With a new CMS rule looming that will strip away some funding, public hospitals went on the offensive by filing a lawsuit in Washington. The safety net providers want an injunction against the rule, which would limit payments to the bare costs of Medicaid services (p. 1).

Again the prospects of additional coverage under governmental programs (e.g., Medicare and Medicaid) despite lower reimbursement will challenge safety-net providers, such as public hospitals. Robbins *et al.* (2008) note that safety-net health clinics have been shown to reduce hospitalizations for ambulatory care-sensitive conditions. Their findings, from a large-scale study of Philadelphia health care clinics on re-hospitalizations, suggest that access to primary care through the health care clinics may have a protective effect against the poor health outcomes typically associated with lower socioeconomic status. For diabetes patients, enrollment in publicly funded safety-net health clinics may have prevented re-hospitalizations for vulnerable diabetics (Robbins *et al.* 2008).

Medicaid Managed Care (MMC) and Managed Care

As increasing pressures from enrollment and financing have stretched Medicaid programs, various attempts at managing costs have been tried. Paramount among these has been MMC programs. Waitzkin *et al.* (2008) found, in a study examining MMC in New Mexico, that there were no consistent changes after MMC, relatively favorable experiences for Medicaid patients, and persisting access barriers for the uninsured. It was also found that safety-net institutions experienced increased workload and financial stress; mental health services declined sharply. Finally, in what the authors termed an important sentinel effect, immunization rates deteriorated. The authors conclude that MMC exerted greater effects on safety-net providers than on individuals and did not address the problems of the uninsured (Waitzkin *et al.* 2008). Hall and Schneider (2008), commenting on health policy and impacting costs, note:

> The persistent riddle of healthcare policy is how to control the costs while improving the quality of care. The riddle's once promising answer – managed care – has been politically ravaged, and consumerist solutions are now winning favor . . . that insurers bargain with some success for rates for the people they insure. The uninsured, however, must contract to pay whatever a provider charges and then are regularly charged prices that are several times insurers' prices and providers' actual costs. Perhaps because they do not understand the healthcare market, courts generally enforce these contracts (p. 643).

Single payer

In the health policy halcyon days of the 2008 election campaigns, the idea of a US single-payer health care plan was debated and ultimately rejected for the time being. DeGrazia (2008), writing about a single-payer alternative, suggested:

Common sense and empirical evidence suggest that single-payer health insurance, combined with competitive private delivery, would be the most cost-effective way of achieving the major, widely accepted goals of health care reform (p. 23).

Specific diseases or health states

Cancer

Ward and colleagues (2008) write that lack of insurance and effects upon patients' cancer and treatments and advances in the prevention, early detection, and treatment of cancer have resulted in an almost 14% decrease in the death rates from all cancers combined from 1991 to 2004 in the overall US population. Specific cancers with declines in mortality include breast and colorectal cancer in women, and lung, colorectal, and prostate cancer in men. They conclude:

> Evidence presented in this paper suggests that addressing insurance and cost-related barriers to care is a critical component of efforts to ensure that all Americans are able to share in the progress that can be achieved by access to high-quality cancer prevention, early detection, and treatment services (p. 30).

Halpern and Yabroff (2008) write that, each year, over 1.1 million individuals are estimated to receive chemotherapy or radiation therapy for cancer. They analyzed the 2000–2004 Medical Panel Expenditures Survey and found that cancer patients younger than 65 receiving treatment who were uninsured were less likely to receive chemotherapy or combined chemotherapy/radiation therapy than those with public or private insurance. In another study, Halpern and colleagues (2008) found that those without private medical insurance in the USA are less likely to have access to medical care or participate in cancer-screening programs than those with private medical insurance. In addition, patients from ethnic minorities with cancer are more likely to be uninsured or Medicaid-insured than non-Hispanic white people. They conclude:

> In this US-based analysis, uninsured and Medicaid-insured patients, and those from ethnic minorities, had substantially increased risks of presenting with advanced-stage cancers at diagnosis. Although many factors other than insurance status also affect the quality of care received, adequate insurance is a crucial factor for receiving appropriate cancer screening and timely access to medical care (p. 222).

Elsewhere, Coburn et al. (2008) found breast cancer in women with no insurance and Medicaid is significantly worse than in those with private insurance. They specifically point to the lower proportions of breast cancer survivors and reconstruction among patients who are uninsured or have Medicaid.

Even with availability of insurance, actions of insurance companies can impact patients negatively. In April 2010, WellPoint (a major insurance carrier) in the USA was alleged to have denied further coverage to women with breast cancer. These so-called insurance rescissions were eliminated in the health insurance reform legislation (PPACA) implemented in late fall 2010. In a letter copied below, Secretary Kathleen Sebelius chastised WellPoint for this alleged activity (Sebelius 2010):

April 22, 2010

[To: Angela Braly, WellPoint]

Dear Ms Braly

I was surprised and disappointed to read media accounts indicating that WellPoint routinely rescinds health insurance coverage from women recently diagnosed with breast cancer. Today's report from Reuters indicating that your company "has specifically targeted women with breast cancer for aggressive investigation with the intent to cancel their policies" is disturbing, and this practice is deplorable.

As you know, the practice described in this article will soon be illegal. The Affordable Care Act specifically prohibits insurance companies from rescinding policies, except in cases of fraud or intentional misrepresentation of material fact.

WellPoint should not wait to end the unconscionable practice of deliberately working to deny health insurance coverage to women diagnosed with breast cancer. I urge you to immediately cease these practices and abandon your efforts to rescind health insurance coverage from patients who need it most.

Breast cancer is the second-leading type of cancer among women, has touched millions of families, and will affect one in eight American women during their lifetime. This year alone, an estimated 192 000 American women will be diagnosed with breast cancer.

I hope you will consider these women and their families as you work to end this harmful practice.

Sincerely

Kathleen Sebelius

In communication back to Secretary Sebelius, Braly denied the alleged rescission of breast cancer patients' insurance coverage. Late in the week after the Sebelius letter was sent to WellPoint, and the denial from WellPoint, the insurer indicated that effective from May 1, 2010, the company would stop canceling coverage plans for patients who develop illnesses. This is an example of a news agency, in this case Reuters, highlighting findings from journalistic investigations, leading to a response from the chief care architect in the federal government (Secretary Kathleen Sebelius) communicating with a health insurer chief executive officer (WellPoint's Braly) in an open manner. The end-result is a health policy influence on a major insurer from a multi-pronged exposé and subsequent governmental response affecting an insurer.

Other health insurers have played a positive role in the treatment of breast cancer. For example, Blue Cross and Blue Shield of Georgia announced in late May 2010 that it will unilaterally implement key provisions of the Breast Cancer Patient Protection Act introduced by US Representative Rosa DeLauro (D-CT).

Cancer in the developing world
In 2008, an estimated 63% of cancer deaths occurred in the developing world – these data are from the United Nation's International Agency for Research on Cancer (IARC) (Kaiser Family Foundation 2010). The most common cancers resulting in death in 2008 were, in order, lung, breast, and colorectal (Kaiser Family Foundation 2010). The IARC predicts that by 2030 cancer deaths worldwide will double from 2010 (Kaiser Family Foundation 2010).

Tuberculosis

Wang *et al.* (2008a), when examining rural Chinese migrants around Beijing seeking care for TB, found similar impacts of lack of insurance or means for payment for care that might be seen elsewhere globally. Specifically, migrants delayed treatment by more than 2 weeks. The reasons given for the delay in seeking care were lack of money and lack of perceived need for care. Females, people without health insurance, those without sufficient knowledge of TB, without full-time employment and people with low incomes also experienced longer patient delay. Wang and colleagues (2008a) suggest that for optimum TB control, control efforts need to be more accessible to the economically and socially vulnerable.

Preventive health activities

In probably not surprising findings, screening and other preventive actions are significantly impacted by insurance coverage or lack thereof.

Chlamydia screening

Pourat *et al.* (2008), when examining rates of self-reported *Chlamydia trachomatis* (CT) screening among young women found in a large sample ($n = 1649$) of 18–25-year-olds that being older, an immigrant, or having one sexual partner reduced the likelihood of CT screening, while being a smoker, being single, or having had multiple doctor visits as well as a Pap test or clinical breast exam increased this likelihood. The uninsured had the lowest rate and public managed care enrollees had the highest rate of CT screening, but this insurance effect was superseded by other explanatory variables. The authors conclude that the results suggest that self-reported CT screening rates were low, particularly among the uninsured. However, these rates were primarily influenced by CT risk factors rather than insurance coverage.

Mammography screening

Pagan *et al.* (2008), in a study of the lack of community insurance and effects on mammography screening rates among insured and uninsured women, found that women living in communities with high uninsurance are substantially less likely to undergo mammography screening. The researchers posit that these results are consistent with the view that the negative impact of uninsurance extends to everyone in the community, regardless of individual health insurance status.

New initiatives

Numerous and varied care delivery models, in the USA and globally, have been recently tried as a health policy impact upon the lack of access to health care. Some have been driven by economic considerations, e.g., retail clinics, but they have been preliminarily shown to increase access to care.

New care delivery models

In a study analyzing the various factors impacting the Chinese New Cooperative Medical Scheme (NCMS), Wang and colleagues (2008b) found that gender, socioeconomic status, adequate knowledge about the policy, subjective premium contribution, subjective co-payment rates, and need are significantly associated with enrollment. They conclude that the sustainability of the NCMS program is only significantly related to knowledge about the policy and satisfaction with the overall performance of the program and that the NCMS program should be further promoted through different media avenues. They also recommend expanding the types of services to include basic medical care and other specialized services to meet the different needs of the rural population. It should be noted that 87% of health care costs in China are borne by individuals: governmental contributions are 13%. This figure is woefully inadequate and portends a difficult future for the Chinese state of health.

Retail clinics

In the USA, retail clinics have been seen as an option to enhance access to primary care services outside traditional physicians' office-based care. Retail clinics are a relatively new yet rapidly growing phenomenon in the USA offering a cheaper and convenient alternative to physician offices for certain minor illness and wellness care. In a study of retail clinics and consumer preference for such, Ahmed and Fincham (2010) found that respondents preferred to seek care for both urinary tract infections and upper respiratory tract infections; were less likely to seek care for urinary tract infections; preferred to seek care at a physician office; and received care on the same day. All else being equal, cost savings of $31.42 would be required for them to seek care at a retail clinic and $82.12 to wait 1 day or more. Ahmed and Fincham (2010) conclude:

> Patients find the time and cost savings offered by retail clinics attractive and are likely to choose those over physician offices given sufficient cost savings. Further studies with additional patient, provider, and market characteristics and disease scenarios are needed (p. 122).

State Children's Health Insurance Program (SCHIP)

SCHIP was enacted by the US Congress in 1997 to increase health insurance coverage for low-income children. At that time in the USA, in the late 1990s, more than 10 million children lacked health insurance. A significant portion of these uninsured children lived in families living below the federal poverty limit. Many of these children had one or both parents who worked and did have health insurance coverage, but the families could not afford the payments required over and above what the insurance might cover (Anonymous 2010).

Shields and colleagues (2008), when writing about SCHIP and other programs, suggest that meeting the health care needs of Americans and reducing health disparities requires both the provision of health coverage to all and sufficient comprehensiveness of benefits within private and public programs to meet enrollees' health care needs. DeVoe *et al.* (2008), in a study of Oregonians, noted that low-income parents at the higher end of the public insurance income threshold and those with private insurance had the most difficulty keeping their children insured. The authors suggest that when parents succeed in pulling themselves out of poverty and gain employment with private health insurance coverage, children may be left behind.

Impact of Medicaid expansion

The expansion of Medicaid will challenge providers, professions, insurers, and those who pay for Medicaid services. Because Medicaid is jointly financed by both state and federal government, the impacts of the PPACA will influence many. Those states that see the largest gains in Medicaid enrollment under health reform will likely see the greatest financial burden (Evan 2010).

Significant changes in Medicaid include that childless adults will be eligible for safety-net insurance starting in 2014, the year in which the income threshold to qualify for Medicaid will be raised to 133% of the federal poverty guideline (Evan 2010). It is of note that currently 39 states do not offer Medicaid to childless adults (Evan 2010). All the burden will not fall immediately upon states. From 2010 through the end of 2016, the federal government will cover the entire cost of newly eligible Medicaid enrollees, but will reduce aid to 90% of costs by 2020 (Evan 2010). This increase in costs to states is in addition to economically driven hardships in play both currently and in the future for state governments.

Bizarre consequences of lack of access and affordability in the USA for health care services

Medical tourism

The phenomenon of medical tourism has arisen due to inability to receive adequate insurance coverage for services in the USA. Whether this entails travel to foreign countries to receive care at a reduced price, seeking non-covered treatment for cancer in other countries for a price, or other iterations, medical tourism is seen as a last resort for many Americans to obtain services outside US borders.

York (2008) notes that the rising costs of medical treatment in the USA are fueling a movement to outsource medical treatment. Estimates of the number of Americans traveling overseas for treatment range from 50 000 to 500 000. To respond to the growth in medical travel, the Joint Commission (formerly the Joint Commission on Accreditation of Health Care Organizations) initiated the Joint Commission International to accredit hospitals worldwide (York 2008). The cable news network CNN has also highlighted individuals who seek care abroad and why (Rice 2010). CNN suggested that 878 000 Americans traveled internationally for a medical procedure in 2010, and projects that the number will double by 2012 (Rice 2010).

Self-prescription

Coffman et al. (2008) note that the use of self-prescriptions in immigrant populations is commonplace. They conclude that the data indicate that this population experiences significant barriers to accessing health care, forcing them to seek treatment alternatives, including the purchase of drugs manufactured in Mexico (Coffman et al. 2008).

Coverage expansion under PPACA

In an update report dated April 22, 2010 (Foster 2010), the Chief Actuary of CMS, in a memorandum summarizing the Office of the Actuary's estimates of the financial and coverage effects through fiscal year 2019, estimated the financial effects of the PPACA legislation:

The Office of the Actuary at CMS has estimated the effects of the non-tax provisions of the PPACA on federal outlays, overall national health expenditures, and health insurance coverage in the USA. Our estimates are based on available data sources and what we believe are reasonable assumptions regarding individual, employer, and health plan responses to the legislation, together with analyses of the likely changes in the unit cost and use of health care services. Our primary estimates for the PPACA are as follows:

1   The total federal cost of the national insurance coverage provisions would be about $828 billion during fiscal years 2010 through 2019.
2   By 2019, an additional 34 million US citizens and other legal residents would have health insurance coverage meeting the essential-benefit requirements.
3   Total net savings in 2010–2019 from Medicare provisions would offset about $575 billion of the federal costs for the national coverage provisions. The Medicaid and CHIP [Children's Health Insurance Program] provisions, excluding the expansion of Medicaid and increased CHIP funding, would raise costs by $28 billion. Additional federal revenues would further offset the coverage costs; however, the Office of the Actuary does not have the expertise necessary to estimate all such impacts. The Congressional Budget Office and the Joint Commission on Taxation have estimated an overall reduction in the federal budget deficit through 2019 under the PPACA.
4   The new Community Living Assistance Services and Supports (CLASS) insurance program would produce an estimated total net savings of $38 billion through fiscal year 2019. This effect, however, is due to the initial 5-year period during which no benefits would be paid. Over the longer term, expenditures would exceed premium receipts, and there is a very serious risk that the program would become unsustainable as a result of adverse selection by participants.
5   Total national health expenditures in the USA during 2010–2019 would increase by about 0.9%. The additional demand for health services could be difficult to meet initially with existing health provider resources and could lead to price increases, cost-shifting, and/or changes in providers' willingness to treat patients with low-reimbursement health coverage.
6   The mandated reductions in Medicare payment updates for providers, the actions of the Independent Payment Advisory Board, and the excise tax on high-cost employer-sponsored health insurance would have a downward impact on future health cost growth rates. During 2010–2019, however, these effects would be

outweighed by the increased costs associated with the expansion of health insurance coverage. Also, the longer-term viability of the Medicare update reductions is doubtful. Other provisions, such as comparative effectiveness research, are estimated to have a relatively small effect on expenditure growth rates (Foster 2010).

Summary

Much has been written in this chapter concerning access to care and the impact lack of access has upon health status. Hoffman and Paradise (2008) point to the fact that research connects being uninsured with adverse health outcomes, including declines in health and function, preventable health problems, severe disease at the time of diagnosis, and premature mortality.

Health policy will continue to be used to implement changes in the lack of access to care both in the USA and internationally. The success of these implementations will depend on how the policies are designed and implemented, and evaluation of these influences will continue.

Discussion questions

1 Discuss the factors affecting access to care. Why are these factors so significant for patients, providers, and society?
2 Describe the changes in health access that will be enabled through the passage of PPACA in the USA.
3 What influence do co-insurance, co-payments, and deductibles have upon health care utilization?
4 Do you feel that cost-sharing by patients is an ethical means of limiting access and costs within health care systems?
5 How successful do you feel the PPACA will be in impacting those currently without health care coverage? Do you feel PPACA will be altered in the future? If so, how will it be changed?
6 A component of PPACA is the expansion of Medicaid to those who currently are not eligible for coverage. How successful do you think this health policy change will be within cash-strapped states in the future (after all, Medicaid is jointly financed by state and federal government)?
7 Describe several health burdens that result from uninsurance.
8 The Canadian system of National Health Insurance still results in some remaining uninsured. Do you see this happening in the USA? Why or why not?
9 Why have EDs played such a role in the health insurance system in the USA? What health policy implementations could affect this utilization in the future?

10	Comment on insurance company policies affecting rescissions. Do you see PPACA totally eliminating this practice?
11	Why is the issue of the underinsured so critical in health policy decisions and health care system delivery enhancements?
12	What role has SCHIP played in expanding service to uninsured and underinsured children in the USA?

References

Ahmed A, Fincham JE (2010). Physician office vs retail clinic: patient preferences in care seeking for minor illnesses. *Ann Fam Med* 8: 117–123.

Anonymous (2010). Families USA. Available online at: www.familiesusa.org/issues/medicaid/medicaid-action/ (accessed 29 April 2010).

Blesch G (2008). A matter of life and death. Public hospitals sue to stop pending CMS rule that would block extra Medicaid dollars steered to safety net providers. *Mod Healthcare* 38: 6–7, 14.

Callahan D (2003). *What Price Better Health? Hazards of the Research Imperative.* Berkeley, CA: The University of California Press.

Callahan D (2009a). *Taming the Beloved Beast, How Medical Technology Costs are Destroying our Health Care System.* Introduction. Princeton, NJ: Princeton University Press, p. 3.

Callahan D (2009b). *Taming the Beloved Beast, How Medical Technology Costs are Destroying our Health Care System.* Introduction. Princeton, NJ: Princeton University Press, p. 4.

Callahan D (2009c). *Taming the Beloved Beast, How Medical Technology Costs are Destroying our Health Care System.* Introduction. Princeton, NJ: Princeton University Press, p. 7.

Callahan D (2009d). *Taming the Beloved Beast, How Medical Technology Costs are Destroying our Health Care System.* Chapter 2, Medical technology. Princeton, NJ: Princeton University Press, pp. 37–66.

Callahan D (2009e). *Taming the Beloved Beast, How Medical Technology Costs are Destroying our Health Care System.* Chapter 7, Redefining "medical necessity". Princeton, NJ: Princeton University Press, pp. 142–200.

Callahan D, Wasunna AA (2006). *Medicine and the Market: Equity v. Choice.* Baltimore, MD: The Johns Hopkins University Press.

Churchill LR (2002). What ethics can contribute to health policy. In: Danis M, Clancy C, Churchill L (eds) *Ethical Dimensions of Health Policy.* New York: Oxford University Press, Chapter 3.

Coburn N, Fulton J, Pearlman DN, *et al.* (2008). Treatment variation by insurance status for breast cancer patients. *Breast J* 14: 128–134.

Coffman MJ, Shobe MA, O'Connell B (2008). Self-prescription practices in recent Latino immigrants. *Public Health Nurs* 25: 203–211.

Daniels N, Kennedy BP, Kawachi I (2002). Justice, health, and health policy. In: Danis M, Clancy C, Churchill L (eds) *Ethical Dimensions of Health Policy.* New York: Oxford University Press, Chapter 2.

Danis M, Patrick DL (2002). Health policy, vulnerability, and vulnerable populations. In: Danis M, Clancy C, Churchill L (eds) *Ethical Dimensions of Health Policy.* New York: Oxford University Press, Chapter 15.

DeGrazia D (2008). Single payer meets managed competition: the case for public funding and private delivery. *Hastings Center Rep* 38: 23–33.

DeVoe JE, Graham A, Krois L, *et al.* (2008). "Mind the gap" in children's health insurance coverage: does the length of a child's coverage gap matter? *Ambul Pediatr* 8: 129–134.

Emanuel E (2002). Foreword. In: Danis M, Clancy C, Churchill L (eds) *Ethical Dimensions of Health Policy.* New York: Oxford University Press.

Evan M (2010). Medicaid expansion will sock states: Moody's. Available online at: www.modernhealthcare.com (accessed 28 April 2010).

Foster R (2010). Available online at: http://johanns.senate.gov/public/?a=Files.ServeandFile_id =1835930b-9e63-4300-89c7-9051c920d76a (accessed 26 April 2010).

Hall MA, Schneider CE (2008). Patients as consumers: courts, contracts, and the new medical marketplace. *Michigan Law Rev* 106: 643–689.

Halpern MT, Yabroff KR (2008). Prevalence of outpatient cancer treatment in the United States: estimates from the Medical Panel Expenditures Survey (MEPS). *Cancer Invest* 26: 647–651.

Halpern MT, Ward EM, Pavluck AL, *et al.* (2008). Association of insurance status and ethnicity with cancer stage at diagnosis for 12 cancer sites: a retrospective analysis. *Lancet Oncol* 9: 222–231.

Halterman JS, Montes G, Shone LP, *et al.* (2008). The impact of health insurance gaps on access to care among children with asthma in the United States. *Ambul Pediatr* 8: 43–49.

Hoffman C, Paradise J (2008). Health insurance and access to health care in the United States. *Ann N Y Acad Sci* 1136: 149–160.

Hsia RY, MacIsaac D, Baker LC (2008). Decreasing reimbursements for outpatient emergency department visits across payer groups from 1996 to 2004. *Ann Emerg Med* 51: 265–274.

Kaiser Family Foundation (2010). Kaiser daily global health policy report. Available online at: http://globalhealth.kff.org/Daily-Reports/2010/June/02/GH-060210-Cancer.aspx (accessed 2 June 2010).

Kriss JL, Collins SR, Mahato B, *et al.* (2008). Rite of passage? Why young adults become uninsured and how new policies can help, 2008 update *Issue Brief (Commonw Fund)* 38: 1–24.

Owens PL, Zodet MW, Berdahl T, *et al.* (2008). Annual report on health care for children and youth in the United States: focus on injury-related emergency department utilization and expenditures. *Ambul Pediatr* 8: 219–240.

Pagan JA, Asch DA, Brown CJ, *et al.* (2008). Lack of community insurance and mammography screening rates among insured and uninsured women. *J Clin Oncol* 26: 1865–1870.

Pourat N, Tao GA, Walsh CM (2008). Association of insurance coverage with chlamydia screening. *Am J Manage Care* 14: 197–204.

Powers M, Faden R (2006). *Social Justice, The Moral Foundations of Public Health and Health Policy*. New York: Oxford University Press.

Rawls J (1971). *A Theory of Justice*. Cambridge, MA: Harvard University Press.

Rice S (2010). 'I can't afford surgery in the US', says bargain shopper. Available online at: www.cnn.com/2010/HEALTH/4/26/cheaper.surgery (accessed 30 April 2010).

Robbins JM, Valdmanis VG, Webb DA (2008). Do public health clinics reduce rehospitalizations? The urban diabetes study. *J Health Care Poor Underserved* 19: 562–573.

Schoen C, Collins SR, Kriss JL, *et al.* (2008). How many are underinsured? Trends among U.S. adults, 2003 and 2007. *Health Affairs* 27: w298–w309.

Sebelius K (2010). Available online at: http://www.hhs.gov/news/press/2010pres/04/20100423a.html (accessed 24 April 2010).

Shields AE, McGinn-Shapiro M, Fronstin P (2008). Trends in private insurance, Medicaid/State Children's Health Insurance Program, and the Healthcare Safety Net: implications for vulnerable populations and health disparities. *Ann N Y Acad Sci* 1136: 137–148.

Voorhees K, Fernald DH, Emsermann C, *et al.* (2008). Underinsurance in primary care: a report from the State Networks of Colorado Ambulatory Practices and Partners (SNOCAP). *J Am Board Fam Med* 21: 309–316.

Waitzkin H, Schillaci M, Willging CE (2008). Multimethod evaluation of health policy change: an application to Medicaid managed care in a rural state. *Health Services Res* 43: 1325–1347.

Wang Y, Long Q, Liu Q, *et al.* (2008a). Treatment seeking for symptoms suggestive of TB: comparison between migrants and permanent urban residents in Chongqing, China. *Trop Med Int Health* 13: 927–933.

Wang H, Gu D, Dupre ME (2008b). Factors associated with enrollment, satisfaction, and sustainability of the New Cooperative Medical Scheme program in six study areas in rural Beijing. *Health Policy* 85: 32–44.

Ward E, Halpern M, Schrag N, *et al.* (2008). Association of insurance with cancer care utilization and outcomes. *CA: Cancer J Clinicians* 58: 9–31.

Weber EJ, Showstack JA, Hunt KA, *et al.* (2008). Are the uninsured responsible for the increase in emergency department visits in the United States? *Ann Emerg Med* 52: 108–115.

Wilper AP, Woolhandler S, Lasser KE, *et al.* (2008). A national study of chronic disease prevalence and access to care in uninsured U.S. adults. *Ann Intern Med* 149: 170–176.

Winkelman K, Westall J (2008). Underinsurance in primary care: a report from the State Networks of Colorado Ambulatory Practices and Partners (SNOCAP). *J Am Board Fam Med* 21: 309–316.

York D (2008). Medical tourism: the trend toward outsourcing medical procedures to foreign countries. *J Continuing Ed Health Prof* 28: 99–102.

Ziller EC, Coburn AF, Anderson NJ, *et al.* (2008). Uninsured rural families. *J Rural Health* 24: 1–11.

Further reading

Allin S, Grignon M, Le Grand J (2010). Subjective unmet need and utilization of health care services in Canada: What are the equity implications? *Soc Sci Med* 70: 465–472.

Amado CA, Santos SP (2009). Challenges for performance assessment and improvement in primary health care: The case of the Portuguese health centres. *Health Policy* 91: 43–56.

Bertoldi AD, de Barros AJD, Wagner A, *et al.* (2009). Medicine access and utilization in a population covered by primary health care in Brazil. *Health Policy* 89: 295–302.

Brunton M, Jordan C, Fouche C (2008). Managing public health care policy: Who's being forgotten? *Health Policy* 88: 348–358.

D'Avolio DA, Feldman J, Mitchell P, *et al.* Access to care and health-related quality of life among older adults with nonurgent emergency department visits. *Geriatr Nurs* 29: 240–246.

Gehshan S, Snyder A (2009). Why public policy matters in improving access to dental care. *Dent Clin North Am* 53: 573–589.

Gulley SP, Altman BM (2008). Disability in two health care systems: Access, quality, satisfaction, and physician contacts among working-age Canadians and Americans with disabilities. *Disabil Health J* 1: 196–208.

Halterman JS, Montes G, Shone LP, *et al.* (2008). The impact of health insurance gaps on access to care among children with asthma in the United States. *Ambulat Pediatr* 8: 43–49.

Himmelstein DU, Woolhandler S (2009). US health care: single-payer or market reform. *Urol Clin North Am* 36: 57–62.

Jatrana S, Crampton P (2009). Primary health care in New Zealand: Who has access? *Health Policy* 93: 1–10.

Laditka JN, Laditka SB, Probst JC (2009). Health care access in rural areas: Evidence that hospitalization for ambulatory care-sensitive conditions in the United States may increase with the level of rurality. *Health Place* 15: 761–770.

Lotstein DS, Inkelas M, Hays RD, *et al.* (2008). Access to care for youth with special health care needs in the transition to adulthood. *J Adolesc Health* 43: 23–29.

Loubiere S, Boyer S, Protopopescu C, *et al.* (2009). Decentralization of HIV care in Cameroon: Increased access to antiretroviral treatment and associated persistent barriers. *Health Policy* 92: 165–173.

Luo J, Zhang X, Jin C, *et al.* (2009). Inequality of access to health care among the urban elderly in northwestern China. *Health Policy* 93: 111–117.

Ma CT, Gee L, Kushei MB, *et al.* (2008). Associations between housing instability and food insecurity with health care access in low-income children. *Ambulat Pediatr* 8: 50–57.

Mladovsky P (2009). A framework for analysing migrant health policies in Europe. *Health Policy* 93: 55–63.

Mwabu G (2008). The demand for health care. In: Kris H (ed.) *International Encyclopedia of Public Health*. Oxford: Academic Press, pp. 84–89.

Ngoasong MZ (2009). The emergence of global health partnerships as facilitators of access to medication in Africa: A narrative policy analysis. *Soc Sci Med* 68: 949–956.

Pauly B (2008). Shifting moral values to enhance access to health care: Harm reduction as a context for ethical nursing practice. *Int J Drug Policy* 19: 195–204.

Phillippi JC (2009). Women's perceptions of access to prenatal care in the United States: A literature review. *J Midwifery Women's Health* 54: 219–225.

Ratcliffe J, Bekker HL, Dolan P, *et al.* (2009). Examining the attitudes and preferences of health care decision-makers in relation to access, equity and cost-effectiveness: A discrete choice experiment. *Health Policy* 90: 45–57.

Rowett D, Ravenscroft PJ, Hardy J, *et al.* (2009). Using national health policies to improve access to palliative care medications in the community. *J Pain Symptom Manage* 37: 395–402.

Schneiderman JU, McDaniel D, Xie B, *et al.* (2010). Child welfare caregivers: An evaluation of access to pediatric health care. *Children Youth Serv Rev* 32: 698–703.

Short NM (2008). Influencing health policy: strategies for nursing education to partner with nursing practice. *J Professional Nurs* 24: 264–269.

Smith DL (2008). Disparities in health care access for women with disabilities in the United States from the 2006 National Health Interview Survey. *Disabil Health J* 1: 79–88.

Solon O, Peabody JW, Woo K, *et al.* (2009). An evaluation of the cost-effectiveness of policy navigators to improve access to care for the poor in the Philippines. *Health Policy* 92: 89–95.

Van Doorslaer E, Clarke P, Savage E, *et al.* (2008). Horizontal inequities in Australia's mixed public/private health care system. *Health Policy* 86: 97–108.

Case Study

Patient compliance

Some of the materials in this case study have been adapted from *Patient Medication Compliance, Issues and Opportunities* (Fincham 2007).

Importance of patient compliance in health care and health policy planning and evaluation

Patient compliance is a significant issue in health care. It has been in the past, is in the present, and will be in the future. Cutler and Everett (2010) have noted the issues of non-compliance and its importance, relevance, and pertinence in the era of PPACA.

The consequences and ramifications of patient non-compliance with medication regimens pervade all aspects of the delivery of health care. Non-compliance is potentially deleterious to pharmaceutical manufacturers, prescribers, dispensers, patients, and to society as a whole.

Non-compliance may seem to some patients as a viable alternative to complying with drug therapy regimens, especially when a patient may have definite opposing viewpoints to those of a physician.

Weintraub (1976) referred to patients purposely not complying with medication regimens and stated that patients' reasons for not complying seem to be valid in some cases. Elsewhere, non-compliance with mood-altering drugs may be a response by patients asserting their independence from psychiatric treatment (Kaplan 1997). The late Ivan Illich (1976) perhaps stated it best when he suggested:

> To take a drug, no matter which and for what reason – is a last chance to assert control over himself, to interfere on his own with his own body rather than let others interfere (p. 70).

Access to pharmaceuticals and compliance in the future

The form, delivery, and intended site of action of pharmaceutical products in the future may be dramatically different from standard dosage forms that are currently used (Fincham 2007). Pharmacogenomically derived products will alter the landscape of pharmacotherapeutics (Patrinos and Ansorge 2010). The following extract is from the Human Genome Project Information (2008):

> Pharmacogenomics is the study of how an individual's genetic inheritance affects the body's response to drugs. The term comes from the words pharmacology and genomics and is thus the intersection of pharmaceuticals and genetics.

> Pharmacogenomics holds the promise that drugs might one day be tailor-made for individuals and adapted to each person's own genetic makeup. Environment, diet, age, lifestyle, and state of health all can influence a person's response to medicines, but understanding an individual's genetic makeup is thought to be the key to creating personalized drugs with greater efficacy and safety.

> Pharmacogenomics combines traditional pharmaceutical sciences such as biochemistry with annotated knowledge of genes, proteins, and single nucleotide polymorphisms.

Pharmacogenomically derived products will change the concept of drug delivery and methods of formulation of new, novel pharmacologically active medications.

Pharmacogenomics and compliance

Pharmacogenomics provides a tantalizing view of the future, both therapeutically and economically. The use of single pharmacogenomic agents to avoid the use of multiple therapies can provide significant, positive outcomes for both therapeutic and cost considerations (Ginsburg and Willard 2010). However, the costs of new therapies will not be inexpensive. The ability of patients to pay coupled with the potential for enhanced compliance with less challenging compliance regimens will be difficult decisions for patients, caregivers, providers, and payers to make (Winkelman and Westall 2008). Will these new therapies, with associated expenses, be covered under health insurance plans stretched to provide wider coverage levels to more individuals than ever before? Is it ethical potentially to exclude these therapies from governmental programs due to their increased costs over current, traditional therapies?

Shaffer (2004b), in analyzing beneficial aspects of new pharmacogenomically derived products for treatment of human immunodeficiency virus (HIV), points to several positive advantages of the new and emerging therapies. At present, the predominant treatment regime for HIV, called highly active antiretroviral therapy (HAART), is complex and challenging to comply with. A new agent, which is pharmacogenomically derived, bevirimat, targets the final step of viral infection, when the virus is released from the cell. Emerging therapy with one agent can remove the need to take multiple therapies at multiple times during the day. These new therapies may, however, be accompanied by exorbitant costs.

Terry (2004) notes the promise of pharmacogenomics in both reducing side-effects and diminishing problems with patient non-compliance. Terry notes that side-effects with oral administration of drugs may be substantially reduced and both acceptance and patient compliance improved for patients. However, intravenous or other parenteral drug therapy administration needs may also stress patient compliance and acceptance. The paradox is that the new agents may be less complex to comply with, but more challenging to administer due to parenteral, storage, and administration requirements. The less complex dosing intervals may be offset by the increasing complexity of administration requirements.

Terry (2004) presents transdermal delivery devices that provide access to complex proteins that are the product of pharmacogenomic research. Use of the transdermal approach to administer drugs would eliminate the hassles associated with patient self-administration of parenteral therapies.

Shaffer (2004a) notes that a highly selective protein for use in treating Alzheimer's disease and Parkinson's syndrome has selective properties. Shaffer optimistically points out that this new therapy in clinical trials at present bypasses current dilemmas related to compliance with currently available pharmacotherapies for neurological conditions. Patients with these conditions will no doubt continue to require caregiver assistance in order to achieve beneficial therapeutic and compliance outcomes. Parenteral drug administration requirements will add stress to patient ability to self-administer these drugs, and require caregiver assistance.

Class (2004) argues that the pharmacogenomically derived designer drugs are worth paying for for therapeutic and economic reasons. Targeted cures, enhanced compliance, and positive cost–benefit ratio assessments highlight the appropriateness of payment for pharmacogenomically derived pharmaceuticals. The ushering in of personalized medicine will help patients, providers, and certainly manufacturers seeking top-dollar reimbursement for research and development, and marketing costs. Counterbalancing the promise of these new therapies with the realization of administration concerns related to compliance will be a task necessary to complete for patients, providers, caregivers, and policy decision-makers.

Cubanski and colleagues (2005) wrote of the impact of increasing numbers of drugs, and variable payment mechanisms excluding coverage as having a negative influence on patient compliance. Regardless, the outcomes and behaviors (for both patient and provider) will be rich empirical areas for drug-related research in the future. Will these drugs be accessible under future health insurance policies, and what health policy ramifications will ensue revolving around the coverage for these therapies?

Discussion questions

1   Why should patient non-compliance with drug regimens be discussed within health policy considerations?

2   From an access standpoint, why is patient compliance an important consideration?

3   With therapies looming on the horizon which are in effect personalized medicine, what impact will compliance with these unparalleled therapies have on patients, providers, and payers within health care systems?

4   Why are pharmaceutical manufacturers interested in patient compliance?

5   If you were a product manager for a major pharmaceutical corporation, what health policy components would be important for you to implement and monitor?

6   From your perspective, would it be ethical to require patients to be compliant with psychotropic medications in order to receive a pharmacy benefit?

7   What role should health policy considerations play in discussions regarding pharmacogenomically based therapies in the future?

8   What health policy discussions should surround drug therapy considerations for HIV/AIDS therapies?

9   What health policy inputs should surround cost–benefit studies examining pharmacy benefit payment for new, expensive Alzheimer's disease therapies versus benefit payment for new, expensive HAART HIV/AIDS treatments?

10 Will limits be placed on formulary access within Medicaid programs for pharmacogenomic therapies? Is it ethical to limit their use and/or access?

References

Class S (2004). Personalised medicine: Quality not quantity. IMS Global Insights. Available online at: http://www.imshealth.com/web/content/0,3148,64576068_63872702_70515404_70684915,00.html (accessed 27 April 2010).

Cubanski J, Voris M, Kitchman M, *et al.* (2005). *Medicare Chartbook*, 3rd edn. Washington, DC: Henry J. Kaiser Family Foundation.

Cutler D, Everett D (2010). Thinking outside the pillbox – medication adherence as a priority for health care reform. *N Engl J Med* 362: 1553–1555.

Fincham JE (2007). Current and future considerations. In: Fincham JE (ed.) *Patient Medication Compliance, Issues and Opportunities*. Binghamton, NY: Pharmaceutical Products Press, pp. 195–207.

Ginsburg GS, Willard HF (2010). *Essentials of Genomic and Personalized Medicine*. San Diego: Academic Press.

Human Genome Project Information (2008). Pharmacogenomics. US Department of Energy Office of Science, Office of Biological and Environmental Research, Human Genome Program. Available online at: www.ornl.gov/hgmis (accessed 21 May 2009).

Illich I (1976). *Medical Nemesis*. New York: Bantam Books.

Kaplan EM (1997). Antidepressant noncompliance as a factor in the discontinuation syndrome. *J Clin Psychol* 58: 31.

Patrinos GP, Ansorge WJ (2010). *Molecular Diagnostics*, 2nd edn. San Diego: Academic Press.

Shaffer C (2004a). Chaperone protein dissolves amyloid plaques. Available online at: www.genpromag.com (accessed 9 August 2009).

Shaffer C (2004b). New anti-HIV compound inhibits virus maturation. Available online at: www.genpromag.com (accessed 9 August 2009).

Terry M (2004). Dermatrends announces patent for amine drug delivery system. Available online at: www.genpromag.com (accessed 9 August 2009).

Weintraub M (1976). Intelligent noncompliance and capricious compliance. In: Lasagna L (ed.) *Patient Compliance*. Mt. Kisco, NY: Futura.

Winkelman K, Westall J (2008). Underinsurance is primary care: a report from the State Networks of Colorado Ambulatory Practices and Partners (SNOCAP). *J Am Board Fam Med* 21: 309–316.

5

Social and cultural issues in health care

We all have heard the phrase "the world is an increasingly smaller place." Ease of travel, international commerce, families scattered in many places, and global acceptance of others have made the world appear to be a smaller place. Different types of medical care have been used for centuries at differing points in time and in different places. Health policy considerations need to consider place, population, methods of care, and outcomes.

Introduction to complementary and alternative medicine

According to a US government website (US National Center for Complementary and Alternative Medicine (NCCAM) 2008): "There are many terms used to describe approaches to health care that are outside the realm of conventional medicine as practiced in the United States." Conventional medicine is that which is practiced by holders of medical doctor (MD) or doctor of osteopathy (DO) degrees and by their allied health professionals such as physical therapists, psychologists, and registered nurses. NCCAM, a component of the National Institutes of Health, defines some of the key terms used in the field of complementary and alternative medicine (CAM) (NCCAM 2008). CAM is a group of diverse medical and health care systems, practices, and products that are not presently considered to be part of conventional medicine. Complementary medicine is used together with conventional medicine, and alternative medicine is used in place of conventional medicine. While some scientific evidence exists regarding some CAM therapies, for most there are key questions that are yet to be answered through well-designed scientific studies – questions such as whether these therapies are safe and whether they work for the diseases or medical conditions for which they are used (NCCAM 2008). The NCCAM website descriptor concludes: "The list of what is considered to be CAM changes continually, as those therapies that are proven to be safe and effective become adopted into conventional health care and as new approaches to health care emerge." Some health care providers practice both CAM and conventional medicine.

Insurance coverage for complementary and alternative medicine

One of the many factors impacting the use of CAM is insurance coverage for services. With a group of seniors, it was shown that the use of CAM is inversely proportional to the presence of insurance coverage (Ness *et al.* 2005). Ness and colleagues (2005) found that those who had health insurance were less likely to use herbal supplements or personal practices than those who had no insurance.

Acceptance of complementary and alternative medicine

Globally, CAM is used widely by varying percentages. In the USA, it is estimated that 36–62% of the population uses CAM (Ness *et al.* 2005). In Canada, the percentage of use is 70%, and in Germany, it is 71–75% (Bodeker and Burford 2007). Acceptance would no doubt be more widespread if there was more insurance coverage for CAM, but since so many have a lack of insurance or underinsurance, it would be a tough sell. The Medicare website (www.medicare.gov) gives descriptors of those services that are covered.

In the past century, Brazil has viewed public health issues in a much broader context than simply medical and technical measures: it was "fundamental to the process of nation building" (Lima 2007). According to Lima (2007), public health concepts in the developing world may have a greater impact when "they are intertwined with social thought and with the processes of nation building and construction of a modern society" (p. 1169). Different world views are necessary when examining health needs and options such as acceptance of CAM.

In the UK, a wider case mix of patients has been observed using acupuncture. MacPherson and colleagues (2006) found most commonly that:

> patients had self-referred (39%), had previously consulted their doctor about their problem or symptom (78%), were paying for their own treatment (95%), and had received acupuncture before (87%). The most common main problem or symptom reported by patients was musculoskeletal (38%), followed by psychological (11%), general (9%), neurological (8%) and gynaecological/obstetric (8%), while 5% of patients were seeking treatment for their general well-being (p. 28).

Noticeable in this study is the percentage of individuals paying for their own therapies as opposed to National Health Service payment.

In Tanzania, traditional health practitioners and CAM practitioners have become widely and increasingly used in addition to biomedical health practitioners (western medical practitioners) (Mbwambo *et al.* 2007). Gaps that exist between traditional health practitioners and scientists/biomedical health practitioners in health research have been addressed through recognition of traditional health practitioners among stakeholders in the country's health sector, as stipulated in Tanzania via the National Health Policy, the Policy and Act of TRM (traditional medicine) and CAM (Mbwambo *et al.* 2007).

In Canada, naturopathic physicians, traditional Chinese medicine (TCM) practitioners, homeopathic physicians, and western herbalists have been focused on how the new Canadian policy implemented in 2004 regulating natural health products would affect access to products they need to practice effectively. Moss *et al.* (2006) suggest that additional research will need to focus on what impacts occur as the regulations are implemented more fully.

Incorporation of complementary and alternative medicine

Without proper analysis, impact evaluation, and assessment of how best to incorporate traditional medicine into mainstream health care systems, problems can occur and limit the use of traditional medicine (Orwa 2007).

Evidence-based evaluative techniques have been called for to evaluate the evidence base necessary to incorporate CAM fully into traditional medical practices and health care systems (Pang 2007).

Integration of traditional medicine with western medicine or vice versa

Asia

Southeast Asia has the most integrated policy, health care system, and insurance coverage schemes of anywhere in the world. Taiwan, Vietnam, Thailand, China, and Korea all have pluralistic, integrated systems. These countries provide a model for how dual systems of care and theory can operate in parallel fashion, yet be incorporated into health policy systems. Shih and fellow researchers (2008) detail the integrated system in Taiwan for incorporation of CAM and western medicine into policy, health care delivery, and insurance systems in Taiwan. Taiwan has a pluralistic health care system and comprehensive insurance program covering western medicine and TCM and provides an interesting case to explore what forms of CAM people use, and why and how often they use them (Shih *et al.* 2008).

Despite a centuries'-long tradition of use of traditional medicine in China, altering health policies has been an inconsistent process. Much of the difficulty is due to the geographical complexity of China, as well as the interregional differences in traditional medicine practiced in differing regions of China. For example, Fan and Holliday (2006) have noted the regional differences between three autonomous regions of the People's Republic of China: Inner Mongolia, Tibet, and Xinjiang provinces. They argue that, because indigenous forms of medicine have been practiced successfully across many generations, they should be treated as different but equal within wider health care systems. They go on to urge Chinese policy-makers to increase their efforts to give all established traditional medicines different but equal status within regional health care systems (Fan and Holliday 2006).

UK

Green and colleagues (2006), in an interview, qualitative study of UK Chinese migrant women, found that these women try to straddle two disparate health care delivery options to meet their needs. Green *et al.* note that most of the women drew upon both medical systems. They point out:

> Women who are more connected with majority English culture are more successful in their consultations with western health service practitioners but do not necessarily discontinue using Chinese medicine. We find that recourse to two different systems helps to overcome barriers when accessing health care. The health policy implications of the findings would suggest that a system that acknowledges and embraces medical pluralism would assist the development of culturally appropriate health care provision (p. 1497).

This use of both systems of care predominates in countries where provision of traditional medicine alongside western medicine is commonplace.

Evidence for effectiveness

Bell (2007) has detailed the use of nutritional, herbal, and homeopathic CAM options for stroke prevention, treatment, and rehabilitation. Bell concludes that an evidence base is lacking to back up the effectiveness of these agents as stroke therapies. The conclusion regarding these agents as stroke therapy adjuncts is:

> the evidence does not favor recommendation of most of these treatments from a public health policy perspective ... However, a great deal of systematic research effort lies ahead before most of the options discussed would meet mainstream medical standards for introduction into routine treatment regimens (p. 38).

Elsewhere Meier and Rogers (2007) note that TCM has justified its practice based on empirical phenomenology, but questions linger regarding its effectiveness in the 21st century. As is the case with evidence-based evaluation of any type of program, standardizing terminology and data collection across settings will be a key step in the evaluative process (Meier and Rogers 2007; Pang 2007).

Ethical concerns

Marian (2007) suggests the increasing use and practice of CAM globally raises important ethical issues for health care providers, researchers, and policy-makers. Specifically, Marian points to five complementary therapies provided by general practitioners: homeopathy, anthroposophic medicine, TCM, neural therapy, and phytotherapy. An evaluation in Switzerland was commissioned to provide data to support or refute inclusion of coverage for these CAM in basic insurance coverage. Marian concludes that evaluations should be transparent and fair when considering insurance inclusion of CAM-related therapies in their evaluations and policy decisions regarding coverage.

Melhado (2006) argues for a return to inclusion of public-interest ideals and extramarket values in health policy discussions and actions. "Extramarket" refers to issues outside economic and health care, organizing and trying to improve efficiency. Issues of organization and efficiency are certainly important, but policy deliberations should also include concerns about coverage, equity, and inclusiveness. In the reforms of the early 1980s and since regarding diagnosis-related groups and payments based on managing care, Melhado argues that other important concerns have been minimized.

Assimilation

There are many issues surrounding the assimilation of CAM into western medicine-dominant health care systems. One of these crucial areas deals with western health profession training. Obviously, CAM segments have educational programs specific to the type of services provided, e.g., chiropractic or acupuncture. But there is a realization that health professionals must have exposure to the different CAM options. Barbato-Gaydos (2001) notes that nurse educators are considering the inclusion of CAM in nursing curricula. The affected curricula may include undergraduate, graduate, or perhaps continuing education programs.

The reverse is true when considering the inclusion of western medicine into developing-world countries where CAM is the dominant form of care. For example, TCM or traditional healers may view western medicine practices with disdain, distrust, or disbelief. The adoption of western medicine ideologies in the developing world may also lead to problems such as cultural unsuitability (Manima 2003). There are also differences in how western physicians view their practice roles, and these differences have geographic connotations as well. Hoffmaster *et al.* (1991) found differences between US physicians and Canadian and UK counterparts when examining divulging information to patients, and becoming involved in patients' lifestyles. American physicians were more likely to divulge information, but less likely to become involved in patients' lifestyles (Hoffmaster *et al.* 1991).

Rajput and Bekes (2002) note that, in this century, medical ethics will be fascinating and fast-moving in our pluralistic western societies. These ethical dilemmas at a micro level will concern individual provision of care by physicians to patients, and certainly at a macro level considering allocation of resources in a just and equitable manner (Rajput and Bekes 2002). Rajput and Bekes suggest the challenges of regulation, policy, and ethical issues concerning policy decisions and the type of care provided in the hospital setting and elsewhere will impact physicians greatly. Post *et al.* (1997) note the influence of pharmaceutical manufacturers in educational processes, and the inherent ethical problems with company-provided education.

Bioethics

Not surprisingly, when western medical bioethics is presented in Asian cultures, adaptation and/or acceptance is not easily accomplished. Tai and Lin (2001) suggest that overt and outright adaptation of western bioethics in Asia will undoubtedly encounter problems, if not rejection. They suggest that, if western bioethical principles are adopted, cultural norms require reinterpretation in light of Asian beliefs and customs.

Ypinazar and Margolis (2004) suggest in Middle Eastern physician-training programs that Arabic-speaking students studying medicine in an Arabic country can be introduced to some of the principles of western medical ethical reasoning and in fact retain knowledge of these principles. The caveat is that this incorporation ideally is accomplished in the early part of medical curricula with English as the language of choice.

Influence of migration and displacement

The influence of migration upon health morbidity is increasingly becoming a major concern. The influence of human migratory patterns and inability to obtain basic primary health care services occur in many places. This effect is not just present in the developing world. Rousseau *et al.* (2008), discussing the situation in Canada, note that "the number of people with either undocumented or with a precarious status is growing in Canada" (p. 292). Clinicians working in primary care are becoming more concerned (Rousseau *et al.* 2008). In the past two decades, migrants from all over have settled in Scandinavian countries (Lofvander and Dyhr 2002). Differing issues of health, illness, and treatment modalities that are culturally defined have surfaced, with health workers in Scandinavia treating many from faraway places with different health and world views. For example, treatments for psychiatric illnesses are viewed much differently from one part of the world to another. Similar situations are extant in the UK. Leishman (2006) notes that nurses will be well served to work to understand the mental health needs of immigrants while being cognizant of differing cultural views toward mental health and treatments for mental conditions. Others (Kreitler 2005) note the problems of providing health care without incorporating cultural diversity and trying to eliminate barriers to communication. In an Australian analysis (Klimidis *et al.* 2006), the most prevalent problems were lack of access to bilingual allied health (70%), access to translated materials (58%), and low patient compliance with mental health assessment and treatment (64%).

Forty years ago Muslim Turks came to Germany as industrial workers; in Turkey their value system had been shaped by traditional Islamic parameters (Ilkilic 2002). The use of the modern German health care system by devout Muslims could lead to an ethical conflict between the Islamic legal responses (fatwa) and the classical theories of biomedical ethics. Ilkilic describes the need for respect for autonomy in the concept of "principalism." Elsewhere, mental health research across cultural groups has been noted to be often criticized for using imprecise measures of cultural groups and for using universal outcome measures as if they have validity (Bhui and Bhugra 2001).

The experience of migration coupled with underlying depression related to preimmigration or postimmigration can lead to further deteriorating health status during resettlement. War, border conflicts, and other situations causing displacement challenge health workers to provide care (Fox *et al.* 1998).

Education and practice concerns

In the first of two articles, Jukes and O'Shea (1998a) discuss the "implications for practice surrounding diagnosis across cultures, classification of illness, and the status and influence of psychological assessments within the field of mental health and learning disability" (p. 905). They suggest community mental health and learning disability nurses need to make dynamic alliances with communities, through the individual, and thus redirect the power relationship inherent in health care provision. In the second article, Jukes and O'Shea (1998b) suggest that individual practitioners and employing organizations need to be responsive and committed to developing multicultural services. Campbell and Campbell (1996) discuss cultural issues related to specific childbearing-stage abuse interventions. They note that cultural competence, abuse and childbearing-stage specificity, and empowerment must be used with clinical interventions with abused women.

Kemp (2005) suggests that increased culture-specific knowledge will provide nurses with a basis for beginning exploration of others' individual or family beliefs. Hilgenberg and Schlickau (2002), when examining nursing education and providing culturally competent care, suggest that many nurses lack the skill and knowledge necessary to provide culturally competent care. They suggest collaboration via an internet-mediated sharing program among different nursing programs specifically addressing transcultural knowledge and skills (Hilgenberg and Schlickau 2002).

Glittenberg (2004) describes the efforts of the Transcultural Nursing Society over the past 30 years; they have been pioneers in generating knowledge about transcultural health issues. She suggests:

> that worldwide changes, demographic disparities, and new discoveries necessitate transitioning what has been a nursing discipline approach to that of a more inclusive transdisciplinary alliance ... also link with other disciplines such as anthropology, genetics, epidemiology, law, economics, and health policy to build cutting-edge research and theory for transcultural health care (p. 9).

de Leon Siantz (2008) describes the need for an expanded leadership role in schools of nursing which are becoming more global, and with the diverse population of the USA rapidly growing. A need exists for nurses to partner with multicultural communities locally, nationally, and globally.

Influence of disparities

Campinha-Bacote (2007) suggests that, because of the compellingly documented racial and ethnic disparities in mental health care related to issues of misdiagnosis, underuse, overrepresentation, and improper treatment, individuals are receiving suboptimal care. Calls for research examining psychopharmacology and the role of individual-specific responses to medications accounted for by factors related to race, ethnicity, age, gender, family history, public policy, or lifestyle are presented (Campinha-Bacote 2007).

Ballenger *et al.* (2001) support empiric research examining biological diversity across ethnic groups and subsequent influence upon the differential sensitivity of some groups to psychotropic medication.

Spenceley (2005) in a Canadian analysis has suggested that sociocultural factors must be considered when planning for primary health care. In addition, access to chronic disease services must include economic and cultural contexts (Anonymous 1983). Health planning must incorporate "a health-oriented process including promotive, preventive, curative and rehabilitative services" (p. 28). In the USA, in the 1970s, Mexican-Americans in Texas were suggested to be structurally alienated from mainstream Anglo-American society, and this alienation carried over to health care utilization (Quesada and Heller 1977). This alienation encompassed language, cultural, and folk medicine tenets. Barr and Wanat (2005) found similar results – that closer collaborations between health care organizations and ethnic minority communities in the recruitment and training of staff may be needed to improve cultural and linguistic access to care. And most recently, in 2008, DuBard and Gizlice in an analysis of US Hispanics concluded that:

> Spanish-language preference marks a particularly vulnerable subpopulation of US Hispanics who have less access to care and use of preventive services. Priority areas for Spanish-speaking adults include maintenance of healthy behaviors, promotion of physical activity and preventive health care, and increased access to care.

Sadly, few, if any, health policy changes or suggestions have altered the situation regarding Spanish-speaking populations in the USA.

Impediments to care

Impediments to care can include many factors. At the turn of the 21st century in Angola, a large poliomyelitis outbreak occurred. This was attributable to a mix of variables that included massive displacement of unvaccinated persons to urban areas, low levels of routine oral poliomyelitis vaccination, a large segment of the population being unavailable during national immunization days, and inadequate sanitation (Valente *et al.* 2007).

Ethnicity

Iliffe and Manthorpe (2004) point to ethnicity as a factor impeding health care access. Ethnicity "subsumes and conceals" the impact of migration, education, health beliefs and socioeconomic status on health, and can be a major concern if unrecognized. When considering the situation in Europe, Cooper (2001) notes that progress in health policy achieving adequate access to health care for large segments of populations is subject to constraints imposed by service infrastructures, reductions in state responsibility, changing public attitudes, and growth of relative poverty.

Gender-specific impediments

Access to birth control methods, either oral contraceptives or condoms, is a major impediment for many women to achieve rudimentary success in their life worldwide. Whether it is inability to achieve educational goals, family goals, or other personal goals, this lack of access has a negative impact upon women (Moreland and Talburd 2006). In some places, a woman cannot access birth control without the approval or presence of her husband in the care-seeking process (Moreland and Talburd 2006). Other religious-focused impediments prevent women from seeking birth control (Moreland and Talburd 2006). Cates (2010) has noted:

> Achieving universal access to family planning is within our grasp, but we need to increase investment in contraceptive technology research, develop more evidence-based policies, engage the public and private sectors, and expand the local commitment to family planning worldwide (p. 461).

Bunting and Seaton (1999), in an assessment of perinatal women with human immunodeficiency virus, point to stigma, uncertainty, and limited access to information and health care as detrimental to seeking and acquiring health services. Finally, Ames (2007) in a qualitative series of focus groups examined the role of communication patterns among children's health care providers as well as information on children's access to care and found derivatives of both to be barriers and/or impediments to care delivery.

Transcultural issues, ethics, and health policy

The above references and commentary make the case for inclusion of cultural concerns in health policy discussions. Many voices are heard in health policy debates; some are amplified due to their prominence in the health care system. Insurance companies, pharmaceutical manufacturers, durable goods manu-facturers, practitioner groups, health systems, and/or other third-party payers have voices in debates about policy and implementation. For decades, those who advocate for the less well represented, including those promoting trans-cultural issues, cultural awareness, or the need to have a global view when viewing health care policy issues have not been heard as they should be. From an ethical perspective, transcultural issues should be more prominently con-sidered in health policy debates.

Purnell and Paulanka (2003) argue that:

> As globalization grows and population diversity with nations increases, health-care providers are increasingly confronted with ethical issues related to cultural diversity (p. 5).

These authors state that organizations and providers who understand clients' cultural values, beliefs, and practices are in a better position to provide culturally acceptable care. This care is enhanced if providers have both gen-eral and specific cultural knowledge. Table 5.1 lists culturally and racially based diseases.

Table 5.1 Cultural and/or racially based diseases

Group	Disease	Cause
Navajo	Ear anomalies	Genetic
	Arthritis	Genetic
	Albinism	Genetic
Hopi	Tyrosinase + albinism	Genetic
Pueblo	Albinism	Genetic
Zuni	Tyrosinase + albinism	Genetic
Eskimo	Amyloidosis	Genetic
	Methemoglobinemia	Genetic
	Haemophilus influenzae type B	Genetic
Vietnamese	Lactase deficiency	Genetic
	Leprosy	Genetic
	Tuberculosis	Lifestyle, environment
Asian Indian	Sickle-cell disease	Genetic
Black populations	Sickle-cell disease	Genetic, environment
	Hypertension	Genetic, lifestyle
Puerto Rican	Breast cancer	Genetic, lifestyle
	Prostate cancer	Genetic, lifestyle, environment

Adapted from: Purnell LD, Paulanka BJ (2003) *Transcultural Health Care: A Culturally Competent Approach,* 2nd edn. Philadelphia: FA Davis, appendix.

Healthy People 2020

There is closure on the extensive planning process in the USA that culminated in the publication of the new *Healthy People 2020* issue. The *Healthy People* project is a collaborative effort of numerous state, federal, foundation, and organizations (http://www.healthypeople.gov/hp2020/default.asp). The following is an extract from the website:

> *Healthy People* provides science-based, 10-year national objectives for promoting health and preventing disease. Since 1979, *Healthy People* has set and monitored national health objectives to meet a broad range of health needs, encourage collaborations across sectors, guide

individuals toward making informed health decisions, and measure the impact of our prevention activity. Currently, *Healthy People 2010* is leading the way to achieve increased quality and years of healthy life and the elimination of health disparities.

Every 10 years, the US Department of Health and Human Services leverages scientific insights and lessons learned from the past decade, along with new knowledge of current data, trends, and innovations. *Healthy People 2020* reflects assessments of major risks to health and wellness, changing public health priorities, and emerging issues related to our nation's health preparedness and prevention. The following are the *Healthy People 2020* segments that deal with health care disparities and access to health services (AHS):

- AHS HP2020–1: Increase the proportion of persons with health insurance.
- AHS HP2020–2 (developmental): Increase the proportion of insured persons with coverage for clinical preventive services.
- AHS HP2020–3: Increase the proportion of persons with a usual primary care provider.
- AHS HP2020–4 (developmental): Increase the proportion of persons who have access to rapidly responding prehospital emergency medical services.
- AHS HP2020–5: Increase the number of states and the District of Columbia that have implemented guidelines for prehospital and hospital pediatric care.

Objectives retained but modified from Healthy People 2010

- AHS HP2020–6: Increase the proportion of persons who have a specific source of ongoing care.
- AHS HP2020–7: Reduce the proportion of individuals who experience difficulties or delays in obtaining necessary medical care, dental care, or prescription medicines.
- AHS HP2020–8: Reduce the proportion of hospital emergency department visits in which the wait time to see an emergency department physician exceeds the recommended timeframe.

Objectives new to Healthy People 2020

- AHS HP2020–9 (developmental): Increase the proportion of persons who receive appropriate evidence-based clinical preventive services.
- AHS HP2020–10 (developmental): Increase the proportion of practicing primary care providers.

Summary

Cultural and ethical issues in health care are significant, or should be significant, elements in the formation of health policy. The developed and developing world are affected when disadvantaged groups are denied access to care, or receive less than ideal provision of health care services. Governmental and non-governmental entities attempt to influence health policy through organized and often grassroots activism. Patients and societies who lack a voice in these deliberations rely on those with collective and powerful voices (governmental, economic, political, or other) to intercede and make positive influences.

Discussion questions

1   Do you feel that CAM and western medicine can be compatible?
2   From a health policy perspective, do you feel that the US health care system should expand coverage under governmental health programs such as Medicare and Medicaid to pay for services provided by CAM providers?
3   Can you explain why the use of CAM is greater in Canada and Germany than it is in the USA?
4   What health policy impacts could increase the use of CAM by the US population?
5   Why have health policy-makers in Vietnam, Thailand, China, and Korea allowed for a dual system of care for their populations, incorporating traditional and western medicine into coverage options?
6   What studies could be commissioned that would inform health policy-makers concerning CAM?
7   Explain extramarket conditions and how they impinge on health policy decisions.
8   Discuss the ethics involved in the evaluation of CAM options for patients to consider when seeking treatment.
9   What health policy decisions could be considered to allow for assimilation of CAM into mainstream health care options for patients? Upon what should these considerations be based?
10 Why are traditional western bioethical principles accepted or rejected by other non-western cultures?

References

Ames N (2007). Improving underserved children's access to health care: practitioners' views. *J Child Health Care* 11: 175–185.

Anonymous (1983). Toward tomorrow's world: Practicing health for all – How the Alma Ata declaration can become a reality. *Nurs Times* 79: 28–29.

Ballenger JC, Davidson JR, Lecrubier Y, *et al*. (2001). Consensus statement on transcultural issues in depression and anxiety from the International Consensus Group on Depression and Anxiety. *J Clin Psychiatry* 62(suppl. 13): 47–55.

Barbato-Gaydos HL (2001). Complementary and alternative therapies in nursing education: trends and issues. *Online J Issues Nurs* 6: 5.

Barr DA, Wanat SF (2005). Listening to patients: cultural and linguistic barriers to health care access. *Fam Med* 37: 199–204.

Bell IR (2007). Adjunctive care with nutritional, herbal, and homeopathic complementary and alternative medicine modalities in stroke treatment and rehabilitation. *Top Stroke Rehabil* 14: 30–39.

Bhui K, Bhugra D (2001). Transcultural psychiatry: some social and epidemiological research issues. *Int J Soc Psychiatry* 47: 1–9.

Bodeker G, Burford G (2007). *Traditional, Complementary and Alternative Medicine – Policy and Public Health Perspectives*. London: Imperial College Press.

Bunting SM, Seaton R (1999). Health care participation of perinatal women with HIV: what helps and what gets in the way? *Health Care Women Int* 20: 563–578.

Campbell JC, Campbell DW (1996). Cultural competence in the care of abused women. *J Nurse-Midwifery* 41: 457–462.

Campinha-Bacote J (2007). Becoming culturally competent in ethnic psychopharmacology. *J Psychosoc Nurs Ment Health Serv* 45: 27–33.

Cates W (2010). Family planning: the essential link to achieving all eight millennium development goals. *Contraception* 81: 460–461.

Cooper B (2001). Public-health psychiatry in today's Europe: scope and limitations. *Soc Psychiatry Psychiatr Epidemiol* 36: 169–176.

de Leon Siantz ML (2008). Leading change in diversity and cultural competence. *J Prof Nurs* 24: 167–171.

DuBard CA, Gizlice Z (2008). Language spoken and differences in health status, access to care, and receipt of preventive services among US Hispanics. *Am J Publ Health* 98: 2021–2028.

Fan R, Holliday I (2006). Policies for traditional medicine in peripheral China. *J Altern Complement Med* 12: 483–487.

Fox PG, Cowell JM, Montgomery AC, *et al*. (1998). Southeast Asian refugee women and depression: a nursing intervention. *Int J Psychiatr Nurs Res* 4: 423–432.

Glittenberg J (2004). A transdisciplinary, transcultural model for health care. *J Transcult Nurs* 15: 6–10.

Green G, Bradby H, Chan A, *et al*. (2006). "We are not completely Westernised": dual medical systems and pathways to health care among Chinese migrant women in England. *Soc Sci Med* 62: 1498–1509.

Hilgenberg C, Schlickau J (2002). Building transcultural knowledge through intercollegiate collaboration. *J Transcult Nurs* 13: 241–247.

Hoffmaster CB, Stewart MA, Christie RJ (1991). Ethical decision making by family doctors in Canada, Britain and the United States. *Soc Sci Med* 33: 647–653.

Iliffe S, Manthorpe J (2004). The debate on ethnicity and dementia: from category fallacy to person-centred care? *Aging Ment Health* 8: 283–292.

Ilkilic I (2002). Bioethical conflicts between Muslim patients and German physicians and the principles of biomedical ethics. *Medicine Law* 21: 243–256.

Jukes M, O'Shea K (1998a). Transcultural therapy. 1: Mental health and learning disabilities. *Br J Nurs* 7: 901–906.

Jukes M, O'Shea K (1998b). Transcultural therapy. 2: Mental health and learning disabilities. *Br J Nurs* 7: 1268–1272.

Kemp C (2005). Cultural issues in palliative care. *Semin Oncol Nurs* 21: 44–52.

Klimidis S, Minas H, Kokanovic R (2006). Ethnic minority community patients and the Better Outcomes in Mental Health Care initiative. *Australas Psychiatry* 14: 212–215.

Kreitler S (2005). The effects of cultural diversity on providing health services. *EDTNA/ERCA J* 31: 93–98.

Leishman JL (2006). Culturally sensitive mental health care: a module for 21st century education and practice. *Int J Psychiatr Nurs Res* 11: 1310–1321.

Lima NT (2007). Public health and social ideas in modern Brazil year. *Am J Public Health* 97: 1168–1177.

Lofvander M, Dyhr L (2002). Transcultural general practice in Scandinavia. *Scand J Prim Health Care* 20: 6–9.

MacPherson H, Sinclair-Lian N, Thomas K (2006). Patients seeking care from acupuncture practitioners in the UK: a national survey. *Complement Ther Med* 14: 20–30.

Manima A (2003). Ethical issues in palliative care: considerations. *J Pain Palliat Care Pharmacother* 17: 141–149.

Marian F (2007). Complementary medicine: equity issues in evaluation and policy-making. *Forsch Komplementmed* 14 (suppl. 2): 2–9.

Mbwambo ZH, Mahunnah RL, Kayombo EJ (2007). Traditional health practitioner and the scientist: bridging the gap in contemporary health research in Tanzania. *Tanzan Health Res Bull* 9: 115–120.

Meier PC, Rogers C (2007). The need for traditional Chinese medicine morbidity research. *Complement Ther Med* 15: 284–288.

Melhado EM (2006). Health planning in the United States and the decline of public-interest policymaking. *Milbank Q* 84: 359–440.

Moreland RS, Talbird S (2006). *Achieving the Millennium Development Goals: The Contribution of Fulfilling the Unmet Need for Family Planning*. Washington, DC: USAID.

Moss K, Boon H, Ballantyne P, *et al.* (2006). New Canadian natural health product regulations: a qualitative study of how CAM practitioners perceive they will be impacted. *BMC Complement Altern Med* 6: 18.

Ness J, Cirillo DJ, Weir DR, *et al.* (2005). Use of complementary medicine in older Americans: results from the Health and Retirement Study. *Gerontologist* 45: 516–524.

Orwa JA (2007). Mainstreaming traditional medicine into national healthcare system: potential and limitations. *East Afr Med J* 84: 49–50.

Pang T (2007). Evidence to action in the developing world: what evidence is needed? *Bull World Health Organ* 85: 247.

Post SG, Beerman B, Brodaty H, *et al.* (1997). Ethical issues in dementia drug development. Position paper from the International Working Group on Harmonization of Dementia Drug Guidelines. *Alzheimer Dis Assoc Disord* 11 (suppl. 3): 26–28.

Purnell LD, Paulanka BJ (2003). *Transcultural Health Care: A Culturally Competent Approach*, 2nd edn. Philadelphia: FA Davis.

Quesada GM, Heller PL (1977). Sociocultural barriers to medical care among Mexican Americans in Texas: a summary report of research conducted by the Southwest Medical Sociology Ad Hoc Committee. *Med Care* 15: 93–101.

Rajput V, Bekes CE (2002). Ethical issues in hospital medicine. *Med Clin North Am* 86: 869–886.

Rousseau C, ter Kuile S, Munoz M, *et al.* (2008). Health care access for refugees and immigrants with precarious status: public health and human right challenges. *Can J Public Health* 99: 290–292.

Shih SF, Lew-Ting CY, Chang HY, *et al.* (2008). Insurance covered and non-covered complementary and alternative medicine utilisation among adults in Taiwan. *Soc Sci Med* 67: 1183–1189.

Spenceley SM (2005). Access to health services by Canadians who are chronically ill. *West J Nurs Res* 27: 465–486.

Tai MC, Lin CS (2001). Developing a culturally relevant bioethics for Asian people. *J Med Ethics* 27: 51–54.

US National Center for Complementary and Alternative Medicine (NCCAM) (2008). CAMBASICS. Available online at: http://nccam.nih.gov/health/whatiscam/ (accessed 13 September 2008).

Valente F, Otten M, Balbina F, *et al.* (2007). Improving underserved children's access to health care: practitioners' views. *J Child Health Care* 11: 175–185.

Ypinazar VA, Margolis SA (2004). Western medical ethics taught to junior medical students can cross cultural and linguistic boundaries. *BMC Med Ethics* 5:E4.

Further reading

Adams J, Hollenberg D, Lui CW, *et al.* (2009). Contextualizing integration: a critical social science approach to integrative health care. *J Manip Physiol Ther* 32: 792–798.

Ben-Arye E, Karkabi K, Karkabi S, *et al.* (2009). Attitudes of Arab and Jewish patients toward integration of complementary medicine in primary care clinics in Israel: A cross-cultural study. *Soc Sci Med* 68: 177–182.

Boon HS, Mior SA, Barnsley J, *et al.* The difference between integration and collaboration in patient care: Results from key informant interviews working in multiprofessional health care teams. *J Manip Physiol Ther* 32: 715–722.

Broom A, Doron A, Tovey P, *et al.* (2009). The inequalities of medical pluralism: Hierarchies of health, the politics of tradition and the economies of care in Indian oncology. *Soc Sci Med* 69: 698–706.

Broom A, Wijewardena K, Sibritt D, *et al.* (2010). The use of traditional, complementary and alternative medicine in Sri Lankan cancer care: Results from a survey of 500 cancer patients. *Public Health* 124: 232–237.

Chen W-T, Shiu C-S, Simoni J, *et al.* Attitudes toward antiretroviral therapy and complementary and alternative medicine in Chinese patients infected with HIV. *J Assoc Nurses AIDS Care* 20: 203–217.

Duarte RA, Argoff CE (2009). *Complementary and Alternative Medicine. Pain Management Secrets*, 3rd edn. Philadelphia: Mosby, pp. 364–369.

Engler RJM, With CM, Gregory PJ, *et al.* (2009). Complementary and alternative medicine for the allergist-immunologist: Where do I start? *J Allergy Clin Immunol* 123: 309–316.

Flesch H (2010). Balancing act: Women and the study of complementary and alternative medicine. *Complement Ther Clin Pract* 16: 20–25.

Gaboury I, Bujold M, Boon H, *et al.* (2009). Interprofessional collaboration within Canadian integrative healthcare clinics: Key components. *Soc Sci Med* 69: 707–715.

Gage H, Storey L, McDowell C, *et al.* (2009). Integrated care: Utilisation of complementary and alternative medicine within a conventional cancer treatment centre. *Complement Ther Med* 17: 84–91.

Handel MJ (2010). Integrative primary care and the internet: opportunities and challenges. *Primary Care: Clinics Office Pract* 37: 181–200.

Hsu M-C, Moyle W, Creedy D, *et al.* (2009). Use of antidepressants and complementary and alternative medicine among outpatients with depression in Taiwan. *Arch Psychiatr Nurs* 23: 75–85.

Jacobson IG, White MR, Smith TC, *et al.* (2009). Self-reported health symptoms and conditions among complementary and alternative medicine users in a large military cohort. *Ann Epidemiol* 19: 613–622.

Jones L, Sciamanna C, Lehman E (2010). Are those who use specific complementary and alternative medicine therapies less likely to be immunized? *Prevent Med* 50: 148–154.

Kantor M (2009). The role of rigorous scientific evaluation in the use and practice of complementary and alternative medicine. *J Am Coll Radiol* 6: 254–262.

Li X-M, Brown L (2009). Efficacy and mechanisms of action of traditional Chinese medicines for treating asthma and allergy. *J Allergy Clin Immunol* 123: 297–306.

Lorenc A, Blair M, Robinson N (2010). Parents' and practitioners' differing perspectives on traditional and complementary health approaches (TCAs) for children. *Eur J Integr Med* 2: 9–14.

Mitchell M (2010). Risk, pregnancy and complementary and alternative medicine. *Complement Ther Clin Pract* 16: 109–113.

Movaffaghi Z, Farsi M (2009). Biofield therapies: Biophysical basis and biological regulations? *Complement Ther Clin Pract* 15: 35–37.

Norris MC (2009). Interacting with complementary/alternative medical providers. *Osteopathic Fam Phys* 1: 57–63.

Pelletier KR, Herman PM, Metz RD, *et al.* (2010). Health and medical economics applied to integrative medicine. *EXPLORE: J Sci Healing* 6: 86–99.

Porzsolt F, Eisemann M, Habs M (2010). Complementary alternative medicine and conventional medicine should use identical rules to complete clinical trials. *Eur J Integr Med* 2: 3–7.

Robinson N, Lorenc A, Blair M (2009). Developing a decision-making model on traditional and complementary medicine use for children. *Eur J Integr Med* 1: 43–50.

Shorofi SA, Arbon P (2010). Complementary and alternative medicine (CAM) among hospitalised patients: An Australian study. *Complement Ther Clin Pract* 16: 86–91.

Siti ZM, Tahir A, Farah AI, *et al.* Use of traditional and complementary medicine in Malaysia: a baseline study. *Complement Ther Clin Pract* 17: 292–299.

Tom Xu K (2009). Socioeconomic aspects of the use of complementary and alternative medicine. In: Ross WR (ed.) *Complementary and Alternative Therapies and the Aging Population*. San Diego: Academic Press, pp. 275–298.

Xu J, Yang Y (2009). Traditional Chinese medicine in the Chinese health care system. *Health Policy* 90: 133–139.

Yates KM, Armour MJ, Pena A (2009). Complementary therapy use amongst emergency med icine patients. *Complement Ther Med* 17: 224–228.

Case Study

The occurrence of deltoid muscle fibrosis after antibiotic injections: public health pharmacy considerations in Vietnam

Introduction

Materials utilized in this section are partially from Fincham (2008).

A damaging muscle disease, deltoid muscle fibrosis (DMF), is commonplace affecting children in Vietnam. DMF usually results in the contraction of the deltoid muscle in the shoulders, causing deformities such as drooping shoulders or hunchback. Most Vietnamese victims have been children between the ages of 10 and 20 years. Estimates place the number of children with the disorder at close to 16 000 (Ngoc 2007). Treatment modalities include only surgery, after which 90% of patients remain scarred. Physical therapy may be of some help postsurgery, but access to allied health professionals (physiotherapists) has been limited in Vietnam.

The cause of the disorder is intramuscular injection of antibiotics into immature deltoid muscles which then predisposes toward fibrosis (Ko *et al.* 1998). The effects of DMF include children not being able to hold their arms close to their trunk. Initially, it was thought that DMF was caused by vaccinations (Trangle *et al.* 2004). However, epidemiological analyses indicate that the injection of large amounts of antibiotics into developing muscles is the causative pathway. Penicillin, gentamicin, lincomycin, and streptomycin have been identified as the most commonly used and causative antibiotics. These antibiotics dissolve slowly in muscle tissue, and the exposure and quantities of the injected drugs involved are problematic. Alternative antibiotics, orally administered, are suggested to be used in place of the intramuscularly administered drugs.

Why this situation occurs and historical antecedents

Broderson (2010) has noted that "reports of deltoid fibrosis began in the early 1960s." Before this time, there had been reports in non-English journals. Post World War II and before widespread availability of other antibiotic dosage forms, the intramuscular injection of antibiotics, antipyretics, and other drugs led to the occurrence of deltoid fibrosis, fractures, and other muscle maladies (Broderson 2010). The occurrence of DMF in the USA and elsewhere in the developed world has been infrequent. Broderson noted that a prevalence rate of 10% was common in some areas of Taiwan. Because of the rarity of the disorder in the USA, manufacturers of injectable drugs do not list DMF as a potential reaction postinjection in professional package inserts. For example, there is no mention whatsoever of DMF in the professional package insert for Lincocin, manufactured by Pfizer (Lincocin package insert 2010). In fact, there is no mention of any cautions pertaining to muscle damage anywhere in the professional package insert. Professional package inserts are country-specific; products packaged for sale in the USA must comply with US Food and Drug Administration requirements.

Vietnam precipitators

Vietnam is a rapidly advancing country with a resilient population. Per capita spending on health care is much lower than elsewhere; the per capita spending on health from 2001 to 2006 is given in Table 5.2 (Euromonitor 2007). Access to adequate antibiotics for use in younger children may be limited due to:

Table 5.2 Per capita health spending in Vietnam, in US dollars

Year	Dollar amount
2001	$21.00
2002	$23.00
2003	$22.00
2004	$26.00
2005	$27.11
2006	$45.00 ($15.00 from government sources)

Source: Euromonitor (2007) World Health Organization, health financing. Available online at: http://www.wpro.who.int/vietnam/sites/dhs/health_financing/.

- poorly structured channels of distribution for pharmaceuticals
- excessive rate of poverty
- lack of access to new antibiotics, including oral dosage forms, both tablet and liquid. Furthermore, liquid formulations needing refrigeration may not be able to be refrigerated due to lack of storage options in refrigerators
- the US-imposed economic embargo for Vietnam until the late 1990s, when the embargo was lifted by then President William Clinton
- lack of education regarding infectious disease pharmacotherapy, including that pertinent to newer antibiotics
- poorly structured pharmacy distribution system in institutional or ambulatory clinics
- spending necessary for other medical care items
  - hospital care
  - physician services
  - other necessary services such as trauma care.

Although there is universal coverage for health needs in Vietnam, the resources for maintaining this access to care through insurance are not sufficient to meet needs. The burgeoning private practice market for medical care services may also divert appropriately administered anti-biotics to those who can afford to pay out of pocket.

Oral antibiotics in solid dosage forms, antibiotic powders for sus-pension, antibiotic liquid suspensions, or refrigerated antibiotics appro-priate for administration for children are not readily available throughout Vietnam in rural and some urban locations. Refrigeration may be a problem in rural, isolated areas and pose stability risks for antibiotic suspensions or reconstituted suspensions that require refrig-eration. The access to suitable sterile, safe water to use in such suspen-sions may also be scarce. Physicians may feel that they have no choice but to administer intramuscular antibiotics normally reserved for older patients often in institutional settings elsewhere.

Literature regarding DMF

Postinjection skeletal muscle fibrosis has been discussed in the literature. Shanmugasundaram (1980) presents a profile of numerous cases of the condition affecting various skeletal muscle segments. The presentation highlights a series of 169 cases of postinjection fibrosis of skeletal muscle consisting of 78 cases of deltoid fibrosis, 84 cases of quadriceps fibrosis, six cases of gluteal fibrosis, and one case of triceps fibrosis. These cases follow antibiotic injections in the affected skeletal muscle areas. This paper includes a discussion and an extensive review of the literature. Shanmugasundaram (1980) makes a plea for prevention of the condition.

Discussion of health policy needs

Patient package inserts and professional inserts are regulatory agency-specific and do not always express the experiences of patients and physicians elsewhere. This process should be changed to reflect contemporary experiences and adverse reactions that might be occurring elsewhere and should be instructive for use of these products in other countries. Much has been made of the harmonization process for the reporting of adverse drug reactions. International standards for adverse drug reaction reporting have been in place since the late 1980s (Waller 2006). The sponsoring group for such congregate reporting is the International Organization of Medical Sciences (www.cioms.ch) (Waller 2006). The French pharmacovigilance centers are perhaps the most sophisticated in the world, and certainly have been successful in stimulating the reporting of significant adverse drug reactions (Thiessard *et al.* 2005). A similar international compilation of significant new reactions with older drugs due to inappropriate prescribing could be achieved as well. There is no reason why a harmonization process could not be instituted for a "universal" package insert that could list reactions that occur, such as DMF, in varying countries. Prevention of DMF is the key to solving this problem. Avoiding intramuscular injections in young children will require education not only of patients and families, but also of caregivers. It must be noted that just because an adverse effect does not appear to be significantly impacting patients in developed countries, this does not absolve companies that market their products globally from a developed country from providing education, regulatory input, and promulgation of appropriate practice guidelines for various products, including intramuscular injections of antibiotics.

Discussion questions

1   What ethical responsibilities do pharmaceutical companies have when marketing and selling their products and product lines in a global economy?
2   What other causative factors might lead to the development of DMF?

3 Why did the US government and allies have in place an embargo for medicines and other goods until the late 1990s?

4 This embargo had health policy ramifications for the Vietnamese population. What were these ramifications? Would you support this health policy (foreign policy) decision between 1975 and 1995?

5 What options would you recommend from a health policy standpoint apart from the use of injectable antibiotics as first-line therapy against infections?

6 A discussion of the etiology and causation of DMF was presented in this case study. Was this the first time you have heard of this condition? Why is that?

7 Should the US Food and Drug Administration (FDA) require differing professional package inserts when an American drug with FDA approval is used elsewhere in the world? Would you support this health policy decision?

8 If DMF occurred as a result of antibiotic injections in the US population, what do you think would be the result from a health policy standpoint in America?

9 When health care resources are scarce, what ethical decisions are involved in health policy deliberations?

10 From a health policy perspective, do you think that foreign patients experiencing adverse reactions, such as DMF, should have legal recourse to obtain resources from US pharmaceutical manufacturers whose products are felt to be the causative agent?

References

Broderson M (2010). Deltoid fibrosis. Available online at: http://www.emedicine.com/orthoped/topic481.htm (accessed 12 April 2010).

Euromonitor (2007). *Total Health Expenditure: Euromonitor International from OECD/WHO National Statistics*. London: Euromonitor International.

Fincham JE (2008). Deltoid muscle fibrosis after antibiotic injections: public health considerations. *J Publ Health Pharm* 1: 51–56.

Ko J, An K, Yamamoto R (1998). Contracture of the deltoid muscle, results of distal release. *J Bone Joint Surg* 80-A: 229–238.

Lincocin (Lincomycin for injection, USP) (2006). Package insert, Lab-0138-3.0. Pfizer, Inc. New York, NY: Pharmacia and Upjohn.

Ngoc HN (2007). Fibrous deltoid muscle in Vietnamese children. *J Pediatr Orthop B* 16: 337–344.

Shanmugasundaram TK (1980). Post-injection fibrosis of skeletal muscle: A clinical problem. *Int Orthop* 4: 31–37.

Thiessard F, Roux E, Miremont-Salamé G, *et al.* (2005). Trends in spontaneous adverse drug reaction reports to the French pharmacovigilance system (1986–2001). *Drug Safety* 28: 731–740.

Trangle KL, Fallon LF, Awosika-Olumo A (2004). Deltoid muscle atrophy secondary to hepatitis B injection? A case report *J Controvers Med Claims* 11: 9–12.

Waller PC (2006). Making the most of spontaneous adverse drug reaction reporting. *Basic Clin Pharmacol Toxicol* 98: 320–323.

Further reading

Ali M, Thiem VD, Park JK, *et al.* (2007). Geographic analysis of vaccine uptake in a cluster-randomized controlled trial in Hue, Vietnam. *Health Place* 13: 577–587.

Chaudhuri A, Roy K (2008). Changes in out-of-pocket payments for healthcare in Vietnam and its impact on equity in payments, 1992–2002. *Health Policy* 88: 38–48.

Dao HT, Waters H, Le QV (2008). User fees and health service utilization in Vietnam: How to protect the poor? *Public Health* 122: 1068–1078.

Glassman A, Buse K (2008). Politics, and public health policy reform. In: Kris H (ed.) *International Encyclopedia of Public Health*. Oxford: Academic Press, pp. 163–170.

Granlund D, Chuc NT, Phuc HD, *et al.* (2010). Inequality in mortality in Vietnam during a period of rapid transition. *Soc Sci Med* 70: 232–239.

Hill PS, Ngo AD, Khuong TA, *et al.* (2009). Mandatory helmet legislation and the print media in Viet Nam. *Accident Anal Prevent* 41: 789–797.

Hoa NQ, Öhman A, Lundborg CS, *et al.* (2007). Drug use and health-seeking behavior for childhood illness in Vietnam – a qualitative study. *Health Policy* 82: 320–329.

Hoa NP, Chuc NT, Thorson A (2009). Knowledge, attitudes, and practices about tuberculosis and choice of communication channels in a rural community in Vietnam. *Health Policy* 90: 8–12.

Krakauer EL, Ngoc NTM, Green K, *et al.* (2007). Vietnam: integrating palliative care into HIV/AIDS and cancer care. *J Pain Symptom Manage* 33: 578–583.

Lan PT, Faxelid E, Chuc NT, *et al.* (2008). Perceptions and attitudes in relation to reproductive tract infections including sexually transmitted infections in rural Vietnam: A qualitative study. *Health Policy* 86: 308–317.

Murakami H, Van Cuong N, Huynh L, *et al.* (2008). Implementation of and costs associated with providing a birth-dose of hepatitis B vaccine in Viet Nam. *Vaccine* 26: 1411–1419.

Ngo AD, Schmich L, Higgs P, *et al.* (2009). Qualitative evaluation of a peer-based needle syringe programme in Vietnam. *Int J Drug Policy* 20: 179–182.

Oosterhoff P, Anh NT, Yen PN, *et al.* (2008). HIV-positive mothers in Viet Nam: using their status to build support groups and access essential services. *Reprod Health Matters* 16: 162–170.

Sepehri A, Sarma S, Simpson W, *et al.* (2008). How important are individual, household and commune characteristics in explaining utilization of maternal health services in Vietnam? *Soc Sci Med* 67: 1009–1017.

Son NT, Thu NH, Tu NT, *et al.* (2007). Assessment of the status of resources for essential trauma care in Hanoi and Khanh Hoa. *Vietnam Injury* 38: 1014–1022.

Teerawichitchainan B, Phillips JF (2008). Ethnic differentials in parental health seeking for childhood illness in Vietnam. *Soc Sci Med* 66: 1118–1130.

Tsu VD, Luu HTT, Mai TT (2009). Does a novel prefilled injection device make postpartum oxytocin easier to administer? Results from midwives in Vietnam. *Midwifery* 25: 461–465.

6

Varying organizational roles

Introduction

The funding of international public health efforts is a multifaceted process. Financing can come from any number of sources, with countries, specific disease advocacy groups, and/or global health organizations all competing for scarce and limited funds. Significant groups include: government agencies, individuals, local communities, multilateral organizations, and non-governmental organizations (NGOs). Membership in these differing categories is not mutually exclusive as it is possible for entities to be classified in multiple ways.

Government agencies

The main governments involved in supporting financially global health concerns include those belonging to the Group of Eight (G8) countries (Canada, France, Germany, Italy, Japan, Russia, UK, and the USA). Of these G8 members, the USA is and has been the largest contributor. These donated US funds are funneled through varying US governmental agencies for targeted efforts abroad.

Individuals

When considering the contributors to global health-funding projects, the predominant names that come to mind are the Bill and Melinda Gates Foundation and the William J. Clinton Foundation. The Gates Foundation is primarily funded through the private donations of Bill and Melinda Gates. In fact, the Bill and Melinda Gates Foundation prefers that donors contribute directly to the agencies that the Gates Foundation supports rather than to the foundation itself! The Clinton Foundation solicits funding from external entities and applies these funds globally to address numerous health issues and problems. Predominant African initiatives have been the treatment of malaria and human immunodeficiency virus (HIV)/acquired immunodeficiency syndrome (AIDS). The Clinton Foundation has also been active in Asia with a focus on similar diseases. The Clinton Foundation, through the intercession of former President

Clinton, has been a proactive force stimulating the availability of generic drugs within the focal countries, as well as pressurizing brand-name pharmaceutical companies to lower prices for enhanced access.

From the What We Do (2010) section on the Clinton Foundation website, the following can be found:

> The Clinton Health Access Initiative (CHAI)* is a global health organization committed to strengthening integrated health systems in the developing world and expanding access to care and treatment for HIV/AIDS, malaria and tuberculosis. CHAI's solution-oriented approach focuses on improving market dynamics for medicines and diagnostics; lowering prices for treatment; accelerating access to life-saving technologies; and helping governments build the capacity required for high-quality care and treatment programs.
>
> Established in 2002 by President Clinton as the Clinton HIV/AIDS Initiative, CHAI initially focused on addressing the limited access to HIV/AIDS treatment faced by developing countries, where more than 90% of individuals living with HIV/AIDS reside. By working in collaboration with governments and NGO partners, CHAI has been able to expand treatment access and save lives.
>
> Since its inception, CHAI has helped more than 2 million people access the medicines needed for treatment, which represents nearly half of all the people living with HIV and on treatment in developing countries.
>
> Building on its model, CHAI has expanded its scope to include efforts to strengthen healthcare delivery systems and to combat malaria and tuberculosis.
>
> *Note: As of January 1, 2010, the Clinton HIV/AIDS Initiative became a separate nonprofit organization called the Clinton Health Access Initiative (CHAI).

One of the significant components of the CHAI in combination with other groups such as the Bill and Melinda Gates Foundation has been a dramatic lowering of the cost of antiretroviral (ARV) drug therapy from $35 per day in the late 1990s to 40 cents or less daily today. This is a result of health policy effects brought to bear on the issue from eclectic sources including foundations, governmental entities and agencies, and pharmaceutical industry deliberations and agreements.

Local communities

Local community health policy supports may come from local public health departments or perhaps from groups soliciting funds for use in a local or regional disaster relief effort. An example might be the efforts to raise funds emanating from New Orleans and/or the Mississippi Gulf Coast for Hurricane Katrina disaster relief. A significant portion of these efforts was directed to health-specific relief efforts. One component of health policy-related interventions in New Orleans post-Katrina was an enabling of health information technology sharing of information about patients and patient needs in a heretofore unseen capacity. These efforts, cutting across state and federal regulatory boundaries, were sterling examples of how health policy must be proactive rather than reactive in times of crisis, whether natural disaster or otherwise.

Multilateral organizations

Health policy at the international level requires collaboration and cooperation, and a central organizing entity. Multilateral organizations such the World Health Organization (WHO) play a major role in financing global health care efforts. Through the oversight of the United Nations (UN), health care-impacting efforts are financed throughout the world. Other agencies within the UN fund health care efforts, including the Joint UN Programme on HIV/AIDS (UNAIDS) and UN Children's Fund (UNICEF). Other multilateral examples include the Global Fund to Fight AIDS, Tuberculosis and Malaria and the Global Alliance for Vaccines and Immunization (GAVI). Recently GAVI and the Global Fund to Fight AIDS pressed nations to help raise $24 billion to fight infectious diseases (Guth 2010). Guth writes:

> The groups now are trying to coax money out of a broader group of nations that either don't contribute today or that give relatively little – including Japan, South Korea, China and Germany. But governments now also face competing global demands.

These groups have been successful in the past decade in making steady progress towards reducing infant mortality, and according to Guth (2010), "mitigating the impact of some deadly diseases."

Waning and colleagues (2010) have analyzed global initiatives for access to ARV therapies. They point to the positive influence exerted by Global Fund. They also found the creation of fairly efficient markets for older ARVs, but markets for newer ARVs are less competitive (from a pricing standpoint) and slower to evolve. They point out that large-scale procurement policies may decrease the numbers of buyers and sellers, paradoxically rendering the market less competitive in the longer term. Waning *et al.* (2010) suggest that global policies must be developed with consideration for their short- and long-term impact on market dynamics.

In date 2010 and early 2011 controversy erupted as fraud was found in diversion of Global Fund funding endpoints (Zarocostas 2011). This report, published by the Global fund, detailed cases of fraud and abuse of grants by various ministries of health, national bodies, and civil society organizations (Zarocostas 2011). Countries described in the report included Djibouti, Mali, Mauritania, Zambia, Cameroon, Ivory Coast, Haite, the Philippines, and Papua New Guinea. As a result the Global find sought the return of $34 million from a total of $13 billion in provided founds (Zarocostas 2011).

International collaborative efforts are in place to address the problem of drug-resistant tuberculosis (TB); much of this effort is focused on Africa. In late May 2010, an announcement was made concerning the Expanding Access to New Diagnostics for TB (EXPAND-TB) project (Stop TB Partnership 2010). Countries covered in the initial project were: Azerbaijan, Bangladesh, Côte d'Ivoire, the Democratic Republic of the Congo, Ethiopia, Georgia, Indonesia, Kazakhstan, the Kyrgyz Republic, Lesotho, Myanmar, the Republic of Moldova, Tajikistan, Ukraine, Uzbekistan, and Vietnam. The May 2010 agreement also includes Cameroon, Djibouti, Haiti, India, Kenya, Peru, Senegal, Swaziland, Uganda, the United Republic of Tanzania, and Zambia (Stop TB Partnership 2010). The EXPAND-TB goal is to accelerate access to diagnosis for patients at risk of multidrug-resistant TB. The project is funded by UNITAID, a collaborative effort between WHO, the Global Laboratory Initiative, the Foundation for Innovative New Diagnostics, and the Stop TB Partnership's Global Drug Facility (Stop TB partnership 2010).

Non-governmental organizations

Numerous NGOs provide global health relief efforts. One such NGO is the Bill and Melinda Gates Foundation (see above). Other groups, such as faith-based initiatives, are also NGOs: one such group is the Catholic Church. It has been estimated that the Catholic Church provides care for one-third of the HIV/AIDS patients in the world (Ferris 2005). Other groups provide relief through any number of advocacy actions, which include providing services, research, specific advocacy activities, economic and social development, education, and/or emergency relief.

The United States President's Emergency Plan for AIDS Relief – a case study of success

In his January 2003 State of the Union Address (The United States President's Emergency Plan for AIDS Relief 2010), then President George W. Bush announced the President's Emergency Plan for AIDS Relief (PEPFAR) – the largest international health initiative ever initiated by a single government to address one disease – HIV/AIDS. In the first 5 years of the program (First Annual Report to Congress on PEPFAR Program Results 2005; Second Annual

Report to Congress on PEPFAR Program Results 2006; Third Annual Report to Congress on PEPFAR Program Results 2007; Fourth Annual Report to Congress on PEPFAR Program Results 2008; Fifth Annual Report to Congress on PEPFAR Program Results 2009), PEPFAR focused on establishing and scaling up prevention, care, and treatment programs. It achieved success in expanding access to HIV prevention, care, and treatment in low-resource settings. During its first phase, PEPFAR supported the provision of treatment to more than 2 million people, care to more than 10 million people, including more than 4 million orphans and vulnerable children, and prevention of mother-to-child treatment services during nearly 16 million pregnancies (The United States President's Emergency Plan for AIDS Relief 2010).

Much of the following text is in the public domain and available through the PEPFAR website (www.pepfar.gov). This emergency plan, as required by Section 305 of P.L. 108-25, the United States Leadership Against HIV/AIDS, Tuberculosis, and Malaria Act of 2003, was initiated to help turn the tide against the global pandemic of HIV/AIDS. On January 23, 2004, US Congress approved the first funds to put the President's vision into motion. The goals of this unprecedented effort included a special focus on 15 nations that account for more than 50% of the world's infections, where support for treatment will impact the lives of 2 million people infected with HIV/AIDS, hopefully prevent 7 million new HIV infections, and support care for 10 million people infected and affected by HIV/AIDS. This program continues under the administration of President Barack H. Obama. Nations with PEPFAR-supported research projects through the US Agency for International Development in 2003 and in 2010 can be found in Table 6.1.

Numerous US federal government agencies are charged to play roles in the PEPFAR program (Table 6.2). This integrated effort works across agency-delineating lines to promote a unified US effort toward supporting PEPFAR. This level of interagency cooperation and collaboration is a unique reason for the success of the PEPFAR program.

On July 30, 2008, H.R. 5501, the Tom Lantos and Henry J. Hyde United States Global Leadership Against HIV/AIDS, Tuberculosis, and Malaria Reauthorization Act of 2008, was signed into law, authorizing up to $48 billion over the following 5 years to combat global HIV/AIDS, TB, and malaria (Fact Sheet 2010).

This global epidemic requires a comprehensive, multisectoral approach that expands access to prevention, care, and treatment. As PEPFAR works to build upon its successes, it will focus on transitioning from an emergency response to promoting sustainable country programs:

- Sustainable programs must be country-owned and country-driven. Given that the AIDS epidemic represents a shared global burden among nations, the next phase of PEPFAR represents an opportunity for the USA to

Table 6.1 PEPFAR research studies in affected countries in 2003 and 2010

Initial countries with PEPFAR-supported studies (2003) (USAID)	Current countries with PEPFAR-supported studies (2010) (USAID)
Botswana	Angola
Côte d'Ivoire	Botswana
Guyana	Caribbean region
Haiti	China
Kenya	Côte d'Ivoire
Mozambique	Democratic Republic of Congo
Namibia	Dominican Republic
Nigeria	Ethiopia
Rwanda	Ghana
South Africa	Guyana
Tanzania	Haiti
Uganda	India
Vietnam	Indonesia
Zambia	Kenya
	Lesotho
	Malawi
	Mozambique
	Namibia
	Nigeria
	Russia
	Rwanda
	South Africa
	Sudan
	Swaziland
	Tanzania
	Thailand

(continued overleaf)

Initial countries with PEPFAR-supported studies (2003) (USAID)	Current countries with PEPFAR-supported studies (2010) (USAID)
	Uganda
	Ukraine
	Vietnam
	Zambia
	Zimbabwe

Source: http://www.pepfar.gov/countries/index.htm.
PEPFAR, President's Emergency Plan For AIDS Relief; USAID, US Agency for International Development.

support shared responsibility with partner countries. To seize this opportunity, PEPFAR is supporting countries in taking leadership of the responses to their epidemics. In addition, to support an expanded collective impact at the country level, PEPFAR is increasing collaboration with multilateral organizations.

- Sustainable programs must address HIV/AIDS within a broader health and development context. PEPFAR must be responsive to the overall health needs faced by people living with HIV/AIDS, their families, and their communities, linking the HIV response to a diverse array of global health challenges. As a component of the Global Health Initiative, PEPFAR will be carefully and purposefully integrated with other health and development programs.

- Integration expands country capacity to address a broader array of health demands and to respond to new and emerging challenges presented by HIV. Strategic coordination furthers the reach of bilateral assistance, leverages the work of multilateral organizations, promotes country ownership, and increases the sustainability of national health programs.

- Sustainable programs must build upon our strengths and increase efficiencies. PEPFAR is renewing its emphasis on a "whole of government" response, ensuring that agencies focus on core competencies and better coordination to maximize the effectiveness of US government assistance. It is also identifying and implementing efficiencies in its work at both field and headquarter levels to ensure value for money. To build upon the strengths of proven programs, PEPFAR is scaling up effective interventions, particularly in prevention. Finally, it is working to ensure that increased access to coverage is accompanied by an emphasis on quality of services.

Table 6.2 US departments and subdepartments with involvement in PEPFAR

US Agency for International Development (USAID)

Child survival HIV/AIDS

Other accounts HIV/AIDS, TB, and malaria

Child survival TB and malaria

Child Survival Global Fund

Department of Health and Human Services (HHS)

CDC HIV/AIDS

NIH HIV/AIDS research

CDC TB and malaria

Mother and child HIV/AIDS prevention initiative

NIH global fund

Department of Labor (DOL)

Department of Defense (DOD)

State department

Foreign military finance

US Global AIDS Coordinator's Fund

Departments are listed in **bold**; subdepartments follow beneath the departments.
Source: www.pepfar.gov.
PEPFAR, President's Emergency Plan For AIDS Relief; HIV, human immunodeficiency virus; AIDS, acquired immunodeficiency syndrome; TB, tuberculosis; CDC, Centers for Disease Control and Prevention; NIH, National Institutes of Health.

PEPFAR's goals

PEPFAR goals include:

- Transition from an emergency response to promotion of sustainable country programs.
- Strengthen partner government capacity to lead the response to this epidemic and other health demands.
- Expand prevention, care, and treatment in both concentrated and generalized epidemics.
- Integrate and coordinate HIV/AIDS programs with broader global health and development programs to maximize impact on health systems.
- Invest in innovation and operations research to evaluate impact, improve service delivery, and maximize outcomes.

Programmatic strategy

In this second phase of PEPFAR, a new program strategy is under way that supports the administration's overall emphasis on improving health outcomes, increasing program sustainability and integration, and strengthening health systems. Some of these changes were beginning to be implemented with planning and programming for fiscal year 2010. During 2010 and 2011, PEPFAR worked closely with country teams in order to translate, prioritize, and implement this strategy in a manner appropriate to the country context. More information on the broader strategic framework for PEPFAR activities can be found at www.pepfar.gov/strategy.

PEPFAR's targets for fiscal years 2010–2014

Prevention

- Support the prevention of more than 12 million new HIV infections.
- Ensure that every partner country with a generalized epidemic has both 80% coverage of testing for pregnant women at the national level, and 85% coverage of ARV prophylaxis and treatment, as indicated, of women found to be HIV-infected.
- Double the number of at-risk babies born HIV-free, from the 240 000 babies of HIV-positive mothers who were born HIV-negative during the first 5 years of PEPFAR.
- In every partner country with a generalized epidemic, provide 100% of youth in PEPFAR prevention programs with comprehensive and correct knowledge of the ways HIV/AIDS is transmitted and ways to protect themselves, consistent with Millennium Development Goal indicators in this area.

Care, support, and treatment

- Provide direct support for more than 4 million people on treatment, more than doubling the number of people directly supported on treatment during the first 5 years of PEPFAR.
- Support care for more than 12 million people, including 5 million orphans and vulnerable children.
- Ensure that every partner country with a generalized epidemic reaches a threshold of 65% coverage for early infant diagnosis at the national level, and testing of 80% of older children of HIV-positive mothers, with increased referrals and linkages to care and treatment.

Sustainability

- Support training and retention of more than 140 000 new health care workers to strengthen health systems.

- In order to support country ownership, ensure that in each country with a major PEPFAR investment (greater than $5 million), the partner government leads efforts to evaluate and define needs and roles in the national response.
- Ensure that in every partner country with a Partnership Framework, each country will change policies to address the larger structural conditions, such as gender-based violence, stigma, or low male partner involvement, which contribute to the spread of the epidemic.

Prevention

Prevention remains the paramount challenge of the HIV epidemic, and the major priority for the next 5 years of PEPFAR. Successful prevention programs require a combination of evidence-based, mutually reinforcing biomedical, behavioral, and structural interventions. PEPFAR is expanding its prevention activities with an emphasis on the following:

- working with countries to track and reassess the epidemiology of the epidemic, in order to fashion a prevention response based on best available and most recent data
- emphasizing prevention strategies that have been proven effective and targeting interventions to most at-risk populations with high incidence rates
- increasing emphasis on supporting and evaluating innovative and promising prevention methods.

Progress achieved through September 30, 2009

- Through its partnerships with more than 30 countries, as of September 30, 2009, PEPFAR directly supported life-saving ARV treatment for over 2.4 million men, women, and children. They represent more than half of the estimated 4 million individuals in low- and middle-income countries on treatment.
- In fiscal year 2009, PEPFAR directly supported prevention of mother-to-child transmission programs that allowed nearly 100 000 babies of HIV-positive mothers to be born HIV-free, adding to the nearly 240 000 babies born without HIV due to PEPFAR support during fiscal years 2004–2008.
- In fiscal year 2009, PEPFAR also directly supported HIV counseling and testing for nearly 29 million people, providing a critical entry point to prevention, treatment, and care.

Linking HIV/AIDS to women's and children's health

According to the WHO, AIDS is the leading cause of death among women aged 15–44 years worldwide. Nearly 60% of those living with

HIV in sub-Saharan Africa are women. UNICEF estimates that nearly 12 million children in sub-Saharan Africa have lost one or both parents to HIV/AIDS. Women and children living with HIV also face other conditions, ranging from inadequate access to family planning to lack of antenatal care to the need for food and nutrition support. As part of its overall prevention, care and support, and treatment efforts, PEPFAR is leveraging and linking HIV services to broader delivery mechanisms that improve health outcomes for women and children. Some of these activities include:

- increasing investment in prevention of mother-to-child transmission to meet 80% coverage levels in HIV testing and counseling of pregnant women and 85% coverage levels of ARV prophylaxis for those women who test positive
- increasing the proportion of HIV-infected infants and children who receive treatment commensurate with their representation in a country's overall epidemic, helping countries to meet national coverage levels of 65% for early infant diagnosis, and doubling the number of at-risk babies born HIV-free
- expanding integration of HIV prevention, care and support, and treatment services with family planning and reproductive health services, so that women living with HIV can access necessary care, and so that all women know how to protect themselves from HIV infection
- strengthening the ability of families and communities to provide supportive services, such as food, nutrition, education, livelihood, and vocational training to orphans and vulnerable children
- expanding PEPFAR's commitment to cross-cutting integration of gender equity in its programs and policies, with a new focus on addressing and reducing gender-based violence.

Treatment

PEPFAR's treatment programs provide essential medications to more than 2 million people. PEPFAR also contributes to the strengthening of the health systems needed to deliver these drugs in low-resource settings. In addition, PEPFAR serves populations with special treatment needs, like children. Together, all global efforts support approximately 4 million people on ARV treatment, but at least 5 million more are still in need of ARV drugs. This figure will likely double with the recent revision of WHO and other recommendations for treatment initiation (Thompson *et al.* 2010). As part of its reauthorization, PEPFAR was charged with supporting increased treatment commensurate with increased appropriations and efficiencies realized. PEPFAR's treatment strategy over the next 5 years emphasizes the following activities:

- directly supporting more than 4 million people on treatment, more than doubling the number of patients directly supported by PEPFAR in its first 5 years
- scaling up treatment with a particular focus on serving the sickest individuals, pregnant women, and those with HIV/TB co-infection
- increasing support for country-level treatment capacity by strengthening health systems and expanding the number of trained health workers
- working with countries and international organizations to develop a shared global response to the burden of treatment costs in the developing world, and assisting countries in achieving their defined treatment targets.

Health system strengthening

PEPFAR has had a positive impact on the capacity of country health systems to address the WHO's six building blocks of health systems functions ((1) service delivery; (2) health workforce; (3) health information; (4) medical products, e.g., vaccines and treatments for conditions such as tuberculosis; (5) financing; and (6) leadership/governance: World Health Organization 2008). However, the program to date has not placed a deliberate focus on the strategic strengthening of health systems. In its next phase, PEPFAR is working to enhance the ability of governments to manage their epidemics, respond to broader health needs impacting affected communities, and address new and emerging health concerns. PEPFAR now emphasizes the incorporation of health systems-strengthening goals into its prevention, care, and treatment portfolios. Doing so will help to reduce the burden of HIV/AIDS on the overall health system. Planned activities include:

- training and retention of health care workers, managers, administrators, health economists, and other civil service employees critical to all functions of a health system
- implementing a new health systems framework to assist country teams in targeting and leveraging PEPFAR activities in support of a stronger country health system
- supporting efforts to identify and implement harmonized health systems measurement tools
- coordinating US government activities across multilateral partners to leverage and enhance broader health system-strengthening activities.

Country ownership

PEPFAR's commitment to the principles of country ownership highlights a new focus on engaging in true partnership with countries. These partnerships pave the way for new approaches to foreign assistance based upon principles and directions common to partner country plans and US government objectives. Over the next 5 years, PEPFAR's emphasis on country ownership will include:

- continuing bilateral engagement through its Partnership Frameworks and other efforts to promote and develop a more sustainable response to the local epidemic, whether concentrated or generalized
- ensuring that the services PEPFAR supports are aligned with the national plans of partner governments and integrated with existing health care delivery systems
- strengthening engagement with diplomatic efforts at all levels of government to raise the profile and dialogue around the AIDS epidemic and its linkages with broader health and development issues
- expanding technical assistance and mentoring to country governments, in order to support a capable cadre of professionals to carry out the tasks necessary for a functioning health system
- partnering with governments through bilateral regional and multilateral mechanisms to support and facilitate South-to-South (geographical section of globe sectioning) technical assistance.

Integration

As the largest component of President Obama's Global Health Initiative, PEPFAR is actively working to enhance the integration of quality interventions with the broader health and development programs of the US government, country partners, multilateral organizations, and other donors. Through activities like co-location of services and expanded training of health care workers, PEPFAR can expand access to overall care and support for infected and affected individuals. As noted earlier, a particular focus of PEPFAR's integration is to expand access to care for women and children. PEPFAR is also emphasizing engagement with broader health and development programs. Examples include:

- expanding HIV/TB integration by ensuring that people living with HIV/AIDS are routinely screened and treated for TB, and that people with TB are tested for HIV and referred, with follow-up, for appropriate prophylaxis and treatment
- linking PEPFAR food and nutrition programs with the new US government Global Hunger and Food Security Initiative
- expanding partnerships with education, economic strengthening, microfinance, and vocational training programs
- promoting accountable and responsive governance through increased bilateral engagement and capacity building with partner governments.

Multilateral engagement

PEPFAR is part of a shared global responsibility to address global health needs. Its success has been closely linked to the success of newer multilateral initiatives such as the Global Fund for AIDS, Tuberculosis and Malaria (Global Fund), and long-standing multilateral organizations, including UNAIDS and WHO. PEPFAR is expanding its multilateral engagement with the goal of strengthening these institutions and leveraging their work to maximize the impact of PEPFAR. PEPFAR's multilateral engagement includes a new emphasis on the following:

* supporting the Global Fund's efforts to improve oversight, grant performance, and its overall grant architecture in order to position it as a key partner for PEPFAR
* supporting UNAIDS efforts to mobilize global action and facilitate adoption of country-level changes that allow for rapid scale-up of key interventions
* negotiating a strategic framework for greater PEPFAR–WHO engagement
* increasing coordination with multilateral development banks to improve the performance of health systems investments and better integrate with their broader economic development efforts.

Funding crisis

In May 2010, Médecins Sans Frontières (Doctors Without Borders) issued a report highlighting the funding crisis for AIDS programs in Africa. Specifically the report (Médecins Sans Frontières 2010) presents the following assessment of the funding shortfall and resultant effects:

> One key donor, **PEPFAR,** has flatlined its funding for 2009–2014 and as of 2008–9, further decreased its annual budget allocations for the coming years by extending the period to be covered with the same amount of money. The funding for purchase of ARVs will also be reduced in the next few years. All this translates into a reduction in the number of people starting on ART, as we have seen in South Africa and Uganda.

> The **World Bank** currently prioritises investment in health system strengthening and capacity building in planning and management over HIV-dedicated funding. However, without funding for ARV [antiretroviral therapy] drugs and related costs, the impact of such capacity to support HIV/AIDS care will remain very limited.

> **UNITAID** is phasing out its funding. By 2012, the drug and other medical commodity procurement organised by the Clinton

Foundation for HIV/AIDS and funded by UNITAID for second-line ARVs and paediatric commodities should end in Zimbabwe, Mozambique, DRC [Democratic Republic of Congo] and Malawi.

The **Global Fund** is currently facing a serious funding shortfall. In October 2010, a donor replenishment conference is planned with the aim of mobilizing more resources, but donors have already requested the Global Fund to lower its financial ambitions. All current funding scenarios are inadequately reflecting demand, as none includes the additional resources required to implement the new WHO guidelines on earlier treatment and improved drug regimens (p. 5).

Monitoring, metric, and research

PEPFAR's work can and should be systematically studied and analyzed to help inform public health and clinical practice. PEPFAR is not a research organization, but is expanding its current partnerships with implementers, researchers, and academic organizations to improve the science that guides this work. As PEPFAR transitions to support sustainable, country-led systems, it will improve efforts to contribute to the evidence base around HIV interventions, as well as broader health systems strengthening and integration. Over its next phase, PEPFAR will support the following new initiatives:

- building the country capacity necessary to implement and maintain a fully comprehensive data use strategy
- reducing the reporting burden on partner countries and supporting transition to a single, streamlined national monitoring and evaluation system
- working to expand publicly available data.

PEPFAR has not been initiated and continued without controversy. The percentage distribution of expenditures can be found in Figure 6.1; these percentages are for fiscal year 2009. Preventive expenditures account for 30.5% of dollars spent. And within the preventive segment, 6.3% is slotted for the category of "abstinence, be faithful". PEPFAR's "Abstinence, Be faithful, and, as appropriate, correct and consistent use of Condoms" (ABC) approach was criticized at the start of PEPFAR due to the limitation on numbers of condoms that could be purchased with PEPFAR funding. The issue took on added importance when considering the efficacy of condom use in HIV/AIDS prevention with the population of men having sex with men.

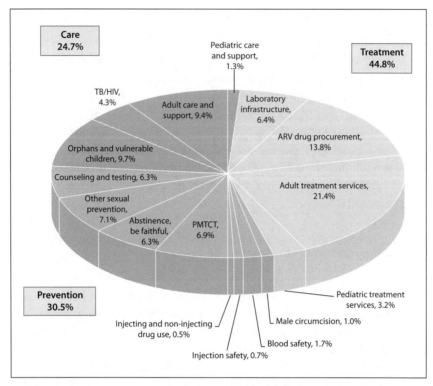

Figure 6.1 Breakdown of fiscal year 2009 President's Emergency Plan for AIDS Relief (PEPFAR) funding categories. TB, tuberculosis; HIV, human immunodeficiency virus; ARV, antiretroviral; PMTCT, prevention of mother-to-child transmission. Source: Sixth Annual Report to Congress on PEPFAR Program Results (2010), available online at: www.pepfar.gov/press/sixth_annual_report/ (accessed 3 February 2010).

Recently the successes of PEPFAR in Uganda have been highlighted (Parkhurst 2010). Within the successes attributed to PEPFAR, the importance of ABC has been extolled. However, the actual use of ABC for successful outcomes, or the suggested use of ABC to reach successful outcomes as well as maintain PEPFAR funding levels has been brought into the equation (Parkhurst 2010).

Summary

In summary, PEPFAR has been the most aggressive and expensive effort from one country to many differing countries to impact a devastating disease epidemic. This example of health policy from one country to many is a classic example for health policy debate and consideration.

Discussion questions

1 PEPFAR is an international aid program with noble intentions. How could this program be used for political purposes as well?

2 How could PEPFAR funding be diverted for non-program use by recipient countries?

3 How does the Global Fund for AIDS intersect with other international-based efforts?

4 How has ABC evolved over time and changes in US presidential administrations?

5 What have been the major accomplishments of PEPFAR after initiation during the presidency of George W. Bush?

6 From a health policy perspective, do you feel that prevention or treatment efforts are the best treatment approach to address the HIV/AIDS crisis globally?

7 Considering malaria, TB, and HIV/AIDS, which has the most importance for the future of global health issues and health policy?

8 How can NGOs with differing missions and advocacy objectives best interact with governmental international health policy initiatives?

9 When considering the spending categories and percentages associated with each segment, would you allocate funding in a different fashion? If yes, how would your funding be allocated?

10 How can the drug component of PEPFAR expenditures be best managed with so many different countries, health systems, distribution schemes, and procurement policies in place internationally?

References

Fact Sheet, The US President's Emergency Plan for AIDS Relief (PEPFAR) (2010). US Global Health Policy, The Henry J. Kaiser Family Foundation. Available online at: http://www.kff.org/globalhealth/upload/8002-02.pdf (accessed 9 April 2010).

Ferris E (2005). Faith-based and secular humanitarian organizations. *Int Rev Red Cross* 87: 311–325.

Fifth Annual Report to Congress on PEPFAR Program Results (2009). Available online at: http://2006-2009.pepfar.gov/press/fifth_annual_report/index.htm (accessed 3 February 2010).

First Annual Report to Congress on PEPFAR Program Results (2005). Available online at: http://2001-2009.state.gov/s/gac/rl/c14961.htm (accessed 3 February 2010).

Fourth Annual Report to Congress on PEPFAR Program Results (2008). Available online at: http://2006-2009.pepfar.gov/press/fourth_annual_report/index.htm (accessed 3 February 2010).

Guth RA (2010). Two groups push for health funds. *Wall Street Journal*, March 29, 2010. Available online at: http://online.wsj.com/article/SB10001424052702304434404575149690099745482.html (accessed 5 April 2010).

Médecins Sans Frontières (2010). *No Time to Quit: HIV/AIDS Treatment Gap Widening in Africa*. Brussels Operational Centre: Médecins Sans Frontières, p. 5.

Parkhurst JO (2010). Evidence, politics and Uganda's HIV success: Moving forward with ABC and HIV prevention. *J Int Dev*. Available online at: www.interscience.wiley.com (accessed 22 February 2010).

Second Annual Report to Congress on PEPFAR Program Results (2006). Available online at: http://2001-2009.state.gov/s/gac/rl/c16742.htm (accessed 3 February 2010).

Stop TB Partnership (2010). Boosted EXPAND-TB agreement will broaden access to MDR-TB diagnosis. Available online at: http://www.stoptb.org/news/stories/2010/ns10_033.asp (accessed 31 May 2010).

The United States President's Emergency Plan for AIDS Relief (2010). Available online at: www.pepfar.gov (accessed 3 January 2010).

Third Annual Report to Congress on PEPFAR Program Results (2007). Available online at: http://2006-2009.pepfar.gov/press/c21604.htm (accessed 3 February 2010).

Thompson MA, Aberg JA, Cahn P, *et al.* (2010). Antiretroviral treatment of adult HIV infection 2010. Recommendations of the International AIDS Society–USA Panel. *JAMA* 304: 321–333.

Waning B, Kyle M, Diedrichsen E, *et al.* (2010). Intervening in global markets to improve access to HIV/AIDS treatment: an analysis of international policies and the dynamics of global antiretroviral medicines markets. *Globaliz Health* 6: 9.

What We Do (2010). W.J. Clinton Foundation. Available online at: http://www.clintonfoundation.org/what-we-do/clinton-health-access-initiative (accessed 17 May 2010).

World Health Organization (2008). Measuring health systems strengthening and trends: a toolkit for countries. Available online at: www.who.int/healthinfo/statistics/toolkit_hss/EN_PDF_Toolkit_HSS_Introduction.pdf (accessed 20 December 2010).

Zarocostas J (2011). Donor countries have responsibility to root out corruption in aid flows. *Br Med J* 342: d714.

Further reading

Andrus JK, Sherris J, Fitzsimmons JW, *et al.* (2008). Introduction of human papillomavirus vaccines into developing countries – international strategies for funding and procurement. *Vaccine* 26 (suppl 10): K87–K92.

Atun R, Kazatchkine M (2010). The Global Fund's leadership on harm reduction: 2002–2009. *Int J Drug Policy* 21: 103–106.

Brugha R (2008). Global health initiatives and public health policy. In: Kris H (ed.) *International Encyclopedia of Public Health*. Oxford: Academic Press, pp. 72–81.

Claeson M, Folger P (2008). Health issues of the UN millennium development goals. In: Kris H (ed.) *International Encyclopedia of Public Health*. Oxford: Academic Press, pp. 197–204.

Doyle C, Patel P (2008). Civil society organisations and global health initiatives: Problems of legitimacy. *Soc Sci Med* 66: 1928–1938.

Eckhouse S, Lewison G, Sullivan R (2008). Trends in the global funding and activity of cancer research. *Mol Oncol* 2: 20–32.

England R (2009). The GAVI, Global Fund, and World Bank joint funding platform. *Lancet* 374: 1595–1596.

Fryatt R, Mills A, Nordstrom A (2010). Financing of health systems to achieve the health millennium development goals in low-income countries. *Lancet* 375: 419–426.

Horton R (2009). Global science and social movements: towards a rational politics of global health. *Int Health* 1: 26–30.

Jayaraman SP, Ayzengart AL, Goetz LH (2009). Global health in general surgery residency: a national survey. *J Am Coll Surg* 208: 426–433.

Kelly PJ, Geller SE (2008). Unintended consequences of US policies on international women's health. *J Midwifery Women's Health* 53: e35–e39.

Lu C, Schneider MT, Gubbins P, *et al.* (2010). Public financing of health in developing countries: a cross-national systematic analysis. *Lancet* 375: 1375–1387.

Magnusson RS (2009). Rethinking global health challenges: Towards a 'global compact' for reducing the burden of chronic disease. *Public Health* 123: 265–274.

McCoy D, Kembhavi G, Patel J, *et al.* (2009). The Bill and Melinda Gates Foundation's grant-making programme for global health. *Lancet* 373: 1645–1653.

Ngoasong MZ (2009). The emergence of global health partnerships as facilitators of access to medication in Africa: A narrative policy analysis. *Soc Sci Med* 68: 949–956.

Ooms G, Decoster K, Miti K, *et al.* (2010). Crowding out: are relations between international health aid and government health funding too complex to be captured in averages only? *Lancet* 375: 1403–1405.

Primarolo D, Malloch-Brown M, Lewis I, *et al.* (2009). Health is global: a UK government strategy for 2008–13. *Lancet* 373: 443–445.

Ranson K, Law TJ, Bennett S (2010). Establishing health systems financing research priorities in developing countries using a participatory methodology. *Soc Sci Med* 70: 1933–1942.

Ravishankar N, Gubbins P, Cooley RJ, *et al.* (2009). Financing of global health: tracking development assistance for health from 1990 to 2007. *Lancet* 373: 2113–2124.

Sridhar D, Woods N (2010). Are there simple conclusions on how to channel health funding? *Lancet* 375: 1326–1328.

Sridhar D, Batniji R (2008). Misfinancing global health: a case for transparency in disbursements and decision making. *Lancet* 372: 1185–1191.

van Oranje M (2008). International funding mechanisms for AIDS care and prevention. In: Volberding PA, Sande MA, Lange J, *et al.* (eds) *Global HIV/AIDS Medicine*. Edinburgh, WB Saunders, pp. 793–800.

World Health Organization Maximizing Positive Synergies Collaborative Group (2009). An assessment of interactions between global health initiatives and country health systems. *Lancet* 373: 2137–2169.

Wright A, Zignol M, Van Deun A, *et al.* (2009). Epidemiology of antituberculosis drug resistance 2002–07: an updated analysis of the Global Project on Anti-Tuberculosis Drug Resistance Surveillance. *Lancet* 373: 1861–1873.

7

Reimbursement issues

Introduction

Health policy guides reimbursement issues for health care commodities. These items may include services provided by physicians, hospitals, laboratory panels, pharmaceuticals, long-term care for seniors, home health care, and/or hospice care. Each of the services listed in the previous sentence has groups, professional organizations, or governmental entities that may be advocating for more payment for such services, more access at a lower cost, or trying to limit total amounts that are paid.

Having such disparate goals from many interested parties ensures, if nothing else, that health policy formulations, deliberations, and outcomes can hardly be predicted. Despite this, oftentimes the outcomes across countries are strikingly similar. The construct of comparative effectiveness research is one such type of outcome that has similar effects in the UK, in Canada, and perhaps in the USA with the passage of the Patient Protection and Affordable Care Act and its tenets stressing comparative effectiveness research.

The balance of this chapter will focus on three systems of care, in the UK, Canada, and the USA, and discuss programs implemented in each of these countries that have their formative roots in health policy components. For the UK, discussion will focus upon primary care trusts (PCTs) and the National Institute for Health and Clinical Excellence (NICE). For Canada, it will be on the Canadian process of evaluating and recommending reimbursement for pharmaceuticals. And for the USA, a discussion of diagnosis (diagnostic)-related groups (DRGs) and drug pricing will be presented.

The UK

The UK is a prime example of a true system of a publicly financed, one-payer national health system – the National Health Service (NHS). Physicians are salaried employees of the NHS, hospitals and domiciliary homes (nursing homes) are owned, and care provided within is financed, by the NHS. Pharmacies are privately owned, but reimbursed directly by the NHS. There are prescription co-pays, around $10.00 for prescriptions, but pensioners, veterans, and young children are exempt from the co-pay (United Kingdom Department of Health 2002).

Recent changes in the UK system include the institution of PCTs. Care trusts were introduced in 2002 to provide a better system of integrating health and social care. By combining both NHS and local authority health responsibilities, care trusts conceivably can increase continuity of care and simplify administration of health and social services. Fundamentally this health policy change was in response to the notion that if patients are to receive the best possible care, then the old divisions between health and social care need to be overcome. A total of three-fourths of funding for health is funneled through the PCTs in the UK (United Kingdom Department of Health 2002). (Current plans (2011) are to abolish PCTs in 2013 with general practitioner (GP) consortiums projected to allocate about 80% of NHS resources.)

The NHS and local councils are currently using existing Health Act flexibilities covering over 230 schemes and involving £2 billion in funding. This basic health policy change is an example of the devolution process in the UK health care system. Each of the components of the UK (England, Northern Ireland, Scotland, and Wales) sets specific priorities for the delivery of health care on a country-specific basis.

PCTs are also providing a unique opportunity to foster closer working between the NHS and local government, particularly social services. As the next stage in this evolution, the NHS Plan announced a new kind of organization, called care trusts. Care trusts will enable the even closer integration of health and social care services. The necessary legal framework is set out in the Health and Social Care Act. Care trusts will build on existing joint working and enable local authorities to fulfill their community leadership role (United Kingdom Department of Health 2002).

Regarding prescription medications, in the UK there are few direct drug pricing controls, and the reimbursement mechanism is different to many other European countries (Mossialos *et al.* 2002). The branded drug price is set using the Pharmaceutical Price Regulation Scheme and the drug is then reimbursed by the NHS according to the manufacturer's list price. There is a profitability cap for pharmaceuticals in the UK, roughly 23%. If this percentage is exceeded for company profits, the companies are fined or prohibited from participating within the UK NHS.

The UK National Institute for Health and Clinical Excellence

In the UK, NICE (www.nice.org.uk) is the independent organization responsible for providing national guidance on the promotion of good health and the prevention and treatment of ill health. In order to spend NHS funds in the most cost-effective way, NICE was instituted to provide guidance on the most appropriate utilization of health funds in the UK. NICE was begun in 1999 and the first item to be analyzed was the product zanamivir, a treatment for influenza. Subsequent NICE evaluations have evaluated treatments, drugs, and screenings, all in a health economics framework. This NHS-driven process enacts health policy decision-making throughout the UK. NICE traditionally has provided health policy decisions in three areas of health: public health (health promotion and disease prevention), technologies, and clinical practice guidelines.

NICE guidance is developed using the expertise of the NHS staff, consultants, and formal health economic evaluation units, e.g., at the University of Aberdeen and Oxford University.

For the sake of discussion, quality of life (QOL) will be used as an example of a health economic measure.

How can NICE use quality of life quantitatively?

Over the past decades, QOL has been used in an applied fashion in numerous places. The 1980s saw the initial development and applied use of QOL via the "quality-adjusted life-year" (QALY) approach to valuing outcomes. QALYs take into account the QOL of the additional years of life in a particular health state. For example, individuals may prefer to be in a healthy state x for 8 years as opposed to being in non-healthy state y for 10 years. By examining individuals' willingness to trade off the quantity of life for QOL, a QALY weight or utility weight can be identified, from 0 to 1. The length of time in life-years is multiplied by the utility weight (a QOL adjustment) to calculate the number of QALYs. Just as is the case with QOL, there are generic and condition-specific QALYs (Auld *et al.* 2002). To develop condition-specific QALYs, one can use existing health outcome profile measures or develop specific health state descriptions for a particular condition (Salkeld *et al.* 2000; Medical Research Council 2001).

QALYs have been used in the UK within NICE when assessing formulary additions of new medications. The UK NICE uses QALYs to determine which drugs are added to the NHS formulary or not approved for use. NICE recognizes that social value judgments via QOL determinations are an important and necessary component of the evaluative processes for high-cost therapies and formulary inclusion. This process is not without controversy (Auld *et al.* 2002), but places the decision for formulary acceptance in the range of $30 000–50 000 for derived QALYs. Using QALYs to determine formulary acceptance places a quantitative focus around qualitatively derived measures. Until recently in the UK, statins and Alzheimer's drugs were rejected for formulary acceptance with challenges and criticism (Getsios *et al.* 2007; Steinbrook 2008). However, since these papers were published, the NHS (in 2010) has reversed the strict formulary exclusion regarding Alzheimer's drugs and softened the prohibition against statin use. A perhaps tangible measure of the impact of these types of QOL-driven QALY analyses may be that elimination of expensive drugs from formulary consideration will require these drugs to become more competitively priced. In the USA, a standard figure of $50 000 for a QALY has been suggested to be the norm for drug acceptance (Haycox 2007).

Currently the UK applies QOL in QALYs to assess the worthiness of adding specific drugs to the NHS formulary. Similar applications of QALYs will no doubt be applied elsewhere, including the USA, as scarce resources are further reduced, yet additionally requested for expenditures for drug therapies.

Canada

Pricing and reimbursement for medications in Canada are regulated at three levels:

1   the federal Patented Medicine Prices Review Board (PMPRB)
2   the 17 federal, provincial, and territorial public drug plans
3   the Common Drug Review (CDR).

Health Canada

In Canada, drugs are federally regulated under the Food and Drugs Act, and the Food and Drug Regulations administered by the health products and food branch within Health Canada, the equivalent of the US Food and Drug Administration. Health Canada reviews new drug submissions for assurances regarding the safety, efficacy, and quality of manufactured products. A notice of compliance is issued on approval and this in turn allows for marketing authorizations. Health Canada does not become involved in issues pertaining to the pricing of drugs in Canada.

Patented Medicine Prices Review Board

The PMPRB was created in 1987 under the federal Patent Act. The PMPRB is responsible for ensuring that patented medicines sold in Canada are not excessively priced. This includes biologics, prescription and over-the-counter drugs, and veterinary drugs.

Patentees are concerned that the PMPRB is continually expanding its jurisdiction. It had found that patent dedication ousted its jurisdiction, but the PMPRB has now reversed this position. The PMPRB regulates the price at which patented medicines are sold to wholesalers, hospitals, or pharmacies. It does not regulate the prices of patented medicines throughout the distribution chain or those prices negotiated on behalf of the federal, provincial, or territorial drug plans.

Provincial Public Drug Plans

Canada's publicly funded universal health care system (named Medicare; the Australian health care system is also termed Medicare) does not contain a

universal publicly funded prescription drug plan. However, drugs administered in hospitals are fully funded by the Medicare system. There is some
coverage for outpatient prescriptions at certain federal and provincial levels.
Public outpatient drug coverage is offered at both federal and provincial or
territorial levels. Provincial health plans offer drug coverage for those 65 years
and older, for those receiving social insurance or disability-related benefits,
and for those classified as needing extraordinary help due to high drug
expenditures in relation to their income. Co-payments, co-insurance, and
deductibles are also required of each of the provincial plans. Employers do
provide a private drug insurance option for employees and their families.

Common Drug Review

In 2003, the CDR was implemented to assess centrally all publicly funded
drug plans in Canada, with the exception of those administered by the province of Quebec (which continues to maintain an independent review process).
According to the CDR, it conducts objective, rigorous reviews of the clinical
and cost-effectiveness of drugs, and provides formulary listing recommendations to the publicly funded drug plans in Canada (except Quebec).

When evaluating a drug, CDR is charged to evaluate the following:

- How does it compare with alternatives?
- Which patients will it benefit?
- Will it deliver value for money?

In this manner, the Canadian CDR is similar to NICE in the UK. Both are
examples of comparative effectiveness reviews. Each of the public drug plans
considers the CDR recommendations for possible formulary listing of agents
and reimbursement recommendations. Not surprisingly, the CDR process has
been criticized by patients, providers, and manufacturers.

US reimbursement issues

Materials utilized in following sections are partially from Fincham
(2006, 2007).

One unique (at the time) element of the US health care system was the
implementation of diagnosis-related reimbursement for health care services.
The development of the concept of DRGs began in the late 1960s at Yale
University in the USA (Averill *et al.* 2003). The impetus for development came
from the need for US federal government mandates to assess quality and
resource allocation in the Medicare program in the USA (Averill *et al.*
2003). To obtain quality and cost comparisons across disparate medical
diagnoses it was necessary to incorporate a case-based system of determining
average costs, including severity of illness, risk of mortality, prognosis, treatment difficulty, need for intervention, and resource intensity (Averill *et al.*

2003). In a seminal paper by Arrow (1963), the concept of market failure pertaining to medical care is presented – the use of prospective payment based on DRGs is a societal response to the lack of competitive preconditions, and as Arrow noted, an "attempt to bridge it" (p. 142). Achieving horizontal equity (Donaldson and Gerard 2005), equal length of stay for equal conditions, and equal pay for equal need by equitably distributing resources for all, and yet achieving vertical equity (Donaldson and Gerard 2005) by ensuring adequate distribution of resources for diagnoses that command higher levels of resource assignment and utilization can both be addressed by prospective pricing (DRGs or HRGs – the UK acronym for health care resource groups). Etheredge (2001), in a perspective on the historical roots of prospective reimbursement, noted that instituting payment prospectively via DRGs was motivated by "the need for utilization review, mandated by the 1965 Medicare legislation" (p. 18) paying for hospital services for the elderly.

According to the US Centers for Medicare and Medicaid Services (CMS), prospective reimbursement works as follows (http://www.cms.gov/ProspMedicareFeeSvcPmtGen/). A Prospective Payment System (PPS) is a method of reimbursement in which Medicare payment is made based on a predetermined, fixed amount. The payment amount for a particular service is derived based on the classification system of that service (for example, DRGs for inpatient hospital services). CMS uses separate PPSs for reimbursement to acute inpatient hospitals, home health agencies, hospices, hospital outpatients, inpatient psychiatric facilities, inpatient rehabilitation facilities, long-term care hospitals, and skilled nursing facilities.

First applications of prospective reimbursement

Initially begun as a component of Medicare in 1983 (the US social insurance program started in 1965), DRG payment prospectively for hospital inpatient services has now been incorporated in concept in private insurance programs in the USA and beyond. As the paradigm of payment for services changed, hospital departments and units that had traditionally been seen as profit centers in retrospective reimbursement (laboratory, pharmacy, central stores, or central supply) were now viewed, and have continued to be viewed over the succeeding decades, as cost centers. Expenditures from these cost centers added to the total costs of care, and thus affected the total charge for care provided. The pharmacy administration segments of our collective curricula have necessarily adapted to the shift in how pharmacy services have been subsequently perceived and reimbursed.

Positive results from governmental regulation in the USA through prospective reimbursement have included: improvements in access to care in rural areas through mandated increased payment rates to hospitals relative to urban areas, financial support to medical schools through Medicare (a response to the realization that care provided from academic medical centers was inherently more costly due to their education and training components, and expanded financial support for hospitals serving poor or disadvantaged patients) (Etheredge 2001).

The continuing failure of the US system health reforms to provide more coverage for more individuals (horizontal equity) is a reflection of the difficulty of the US combined system of public and private insurance components merging to attempt to provide coverage for those without insurance.

International comparisons

The pitfalls of comparison between countries and associated systems, as noted by Culyer *et al.* (1991), should not diminish the need to look at foreign systems for experience in new programs such as prospective reimbursement and how educational demands have needed to adapt. It might be best to begin a system knowing that refinement is a necessary component for evolving success. Vertrees and Manton (1993) note that: "it is better to start with a simple but imperfect system than to wait for some possibly unattainable level of perfection" (p. 172). The allocative efficiency in differing systems of payment for preventive or acute services, and technical efficiency of effective bundling of purchases to reduce costs, will vary both within countries and between countries (Mossialos *et al.* 2002). This will make comparative data examination tenuous as well.

Patient diagnoses can be complex and, as more patient categories, even those with multiple conditions and attendant increases in severity, are included in DRG-type classifications, the need to address increasing costs with outliers comes into play regardless of the country studied. All patient refined DRGs encompass differing levels of severity of illness and risks of mortality.

Differing methods for analyzing such patients have been an issue in Belgium as well as other countries (Pirson *et al.* 2006). Swedish researchers have noted that improving overall health quality is also a component of DRG systems (Leister and Stausberg 2005); thus the issue of equity becomes important in any system of prospective payment for institutional care.

Palmer *et al.* (1991) note that the Australian DRG scheme was incorporated with cost modeling using the US experience to institute the process in Australia. Duckett (2000) has indicated that, since 1992, the Australian refined DRG (AR-DRG) classification is now in use and allows for ongoing refinement and adjustment, with specific differences in Australian health care service delivery incorporated into the scheme. Australian researchers (Jackson *et al.* 1999) have outlined the issues in "costing" differing patient levels: the process of costing in the DRG framework is not unlike the "costing" that needs expressing in cost–benefit and cost-effectiveness analyses. In effect, costs are identified for direct and indirect items and included in a thorough process considering the expenditures involved in a diagnostic category (e.g., cardiology), a specific condition (e.g., myocardial infarction), and the costs associated with its treatment.

The AR-DRG has now also been used in New Zealand and Singapore (Duckett 2000). Ashton and Press (1997) point to the New Zealand experience of separating purchaser from provider as a mechanism for stimulating competition between providers; in such systems DRGs have been used as a mechanism to keep prices from rising beyond norms and to allow purchasing units (governmental entities) to help control rising costs.

Heavens (1999) noted that "the principles underlying the development of DRG or HRG type groupings are that they should be: clinically meaningful, resource homogeneous, limited to a manageable number of groups, and derived from routinely collected data" (p. 7). Here, "resource homogeneous" means keeping similar diagnoses and associated costs separate from other diagnoses that have differing associated costs (e.g., costs pertaining to treatment of myocardial infarction versus hip replacement surgery).

In France, in 1982 le Programme de Médicalisation du Système d'Information (PMSI) (the French version of DRG or HRG) was instituted (Rodrigues 1993). One tangible result of the French PMSI has been a reallocation of resources throughout France. For example, hospitals with costs above the regional mean have lost 1% of their budget with the amount distributed to facilities with a cost ranking that is below the cost outlier facilities (Rodrigues *et al.* 1998).

The Portuguese experience with DRGs began in the 1990s after health care reform legislation was enacted (Lima and Whynes 2003). Lima and Whynes, when discussing the Portuguese experience with DRGs, noted that costs per admission decreased over a decade, principally due to associated cost decreases accompanying decreased average length of stay per admission. As the per-admission length of stay decreased in Portugal, the actual number of admissions increased owing to a more equitable distribution of resources.

Common and probable effects of DRG use worldwide have led to predictable results. There has been an initial slowing in the rate of increase in payments for hospital services. Length of stay has on average decreased as specific limits are in place for average length of stay for certain diagnoses. The additional revenue freed up from the institution of prospective reimbursement has allowed for payment for increased admissions with shorter length of stay.

Refinement of the classification of diagnoses has necessarily evolved to incorporate severity indices for complex patients. In any case, there are instances of patients being dismissed too soon not based on sound medical rationale, but because of economic ramifications of extending length of stays and subsequent increased costs over and above reimbursement levels. More pressure has been brought to bear on the use of resource utilization during hospital stays. The needs of academia to respond to these dramatic changes have been met, but continue to need addressing.

As prospective reimbursement has evolved, it has become more important to use more refined definitions of DRG classification. Initially begun as a Medicare payment mechanism for elderly inpatient hospital care, DRG classifications have necessarily been used for patient diagnoses for non-elderly patients, e.g. pediatric, adolescent, middle age, and/or females of child-bearing ages.

The average length of stay in the USA for inpatient hospital patients has decreased from an average of 9.9 days per admission in the 1980s to 6.6 days per admission in 2007 (National Center for Health Statistics 2009). A part of this reduction is surely due to DRG reimbursement for hospital services; other factors may include increasing levels of medical technology and provider skills in treatment of patients (National Center for Health Statistics 2009). This would be expected to occur elsewhere as well. Bodenheimer (2002) notes that governmental efforts such as prospective pricing have helped to reduce costs; annual increases in Medicare spending per capita dropped from 11.2% from 1975–1980 to 1.8% for 1995–1999 (Bodenheimer 2002). Such decreases would be expected to be seen in managed care applications in other countries.

Summary of international considerations

Determining which, if any, of the above prospective payment options is preferred in comparison with the other systems is tenuous but necessary. The paper by Culyer *et al.* (1991) points out that the context of the system (social, political, and economic milieu in which it operates) and the relevant data collected make such comparisons difficult, if not impractical. Thus, it makes sense to apply segments that would seem to aid in the implementation of DRG reimbursement elsewhere with the realization that alterations will be necessary. Specific examination of aspects of systems that have been unworkable or disappointing can aid in avoiding similar pitfalls in implementing such systems worldwide.

Drug pricing in the USA

In the USA at present, roughly 26% of health insurance coverage and 45% of all health care payments are made by government programs (state and federal). Much of the discussion surrounding the Medicare Part D drug program has centered on the profits derived from increased drug coverage, which has proven to be a windfall for the major US pharmaceutical manufacturers and insurers participating in plans offered by the program.

Writing about the Medicare Modernization Act of 2003 (P.L. 108-173), Hogan (2005) noted:

> The Medicare Modernization Act (MMA) included three policies to limit the financial risks that Medicare Part D prescription drug plans (PDPs) must bear. These were:

- risk adjustment of the payments to plans, based on the demographics and health status of each plan's enrollees, resulting in higher payments for more costly enrollees;
- reinsurance for catastrophic costs, with the federal government directly paying most of the cost when an enrollee's total drug spending exceeds $5100; and
- risk corridors that limit the bottom-line profits and losses for PDPs, regardless of the reason for the profit or loss (p. 7).

In effect, participating insurers were thus assured profitability regardless of what happened from a risk standpoint with their proffered plans.

The "cost to dispense" study prepared for the Coalition for Community Pharmacy Action has noted an average cost of dispensing per prescription of $10.50 for a sample of 832 million prescriptions, and a cost of dispensing per pharmacy of $12.10 (reflecting the differential in high- and low-volume prescription pharmacies) (Grant Thornton 2007). Every third-party program, whether managed care provided by private insurers or governmental Medicaid and Medicare programs, is moving in an economic, diametrically opposed vector from this payment need for pharmacy viability to providing and pushing for lower prescription costs, including ratcheting down dispensing fees.

Drug reimbursement (historical perspective)

The average wholesale price (AWP) concept was created in 1969 by Dr. George Pennebaker, State of California Pharmaceutical Program Coordinator (Pennebaker 1969). It was designed to provide a reference price for adjudicating claims for California's Medicaid (Medi-Cal) drug program.

Before 2003, Medi-Cal typically reimbursed drugs at the lower of AWP – 5% or the direct price for a handful of selected manufacturers, or federal upper limit (FUL) price or California maximum allowable ingredient cost (MAIC). The FUL is a federally established maximum price for a drug product if there are three (or more) generic versions of the product rated therapeutically equivalent (A-rated) and at least three suppliers. Effective from 2003, the legislature changed Medi-Cal's reimbursement formula to the lower of AWP – 10%, or FUL or MAIC. Direct price is no longer used. Effective from October 1, 2004, the California legislature reduced Medi-Cal's reimbursement to the lower of AWP – 17%, or FUL or MAIC.

Other states have relied on similar AWP or wholesale acquisition cost (WAC) pricing formulas since the 1960s to reimburse for prescription drugs within the Medicaid programs. As Medicaid came into play, private health insurance companies since the 1970s have offered a drug benefit that was also based on an AWP plus dispensing fee framework. Since the initiation of a drug benefit provided by health insurance companies, the reimbursement for prescriptions has seen an eroding payment platform for the cost of the drug (to a now approximate AWP – 12% or WAC +15%, whichever is less) plus a dispensing fee that has decreased in most cases over time. However, Medicaid dispensing fees are higher than other managed care prescription dispensing fees on average.

Table 7.1 gives an example of how pricing levels differ dramatically in the USA. Generic drug costs are projected to be based on an average manufacturer price of 175% above FUL. This was a price that had been targeted to be only 150% over FUL until heavy lobbying occurred during the Patient Protection and Affordable Care Act deliberation and its ultimate passage. Because of the tiered pricing in place in the USA there are numerous pricing levels based on volume purchased, type of pharmacy (mail-order pharmacies receive the most preferential price), and perhaps warehouse pricing (chains and major wholesalers).

The use of pharmacy benefit managers (PBMs), companies, that manage the drug benefit for major insurers, has also revised how drugs are reimbursed. Formularies are used to control the drugs used within specific health plans. Formularies are listings of drugs that are paid for in a particular plan. These listings contain all the drugs that are eligible to be supplied on prescriptions covered by the Part D plan. Table 7.2 provides a comparison of what a three-tiered drug formulary might look like. The first tier, for generic drugs, requires the patient to pay a $5.00 per-prescription co-payment. The second tier, preferred drugs, may require a $25.00 per-prescription co-payment, and the third tier allows for drugs to be covered that are brand-name, but not pre-ferred, at a higher cost – in this depiction $60.00. The tiered reimbursement and co-payment scheme is intended to drive the higher utilization of generic drugs. Also, the higher-priced drugs that are eligible or not eligible for cov-erage require higher payments on the part of the prescriber. These prescrip-tion co-payments are most often for a 30-day supply of a maintenance medication only. Patients may also use a mail-order pharmacy, obtain a 90-day supply, and pay a lower co-payment on the drug prescribed and dispensed to them via mail order. More often than not, the PBM also owns a mail-order pharmacy, and thus funnels prescriptions through their mail-order operation, bypassing other pharmacy outlets.

Health policy decisions have ramifications that last generations and take turns into unforeseen tangents over time. A social health insurance program in the 1960s, Medicaid, that had as an optional benefit coverage for prescription drugs, has evolved dramatically over time. Although still an optional benefit within Medicaid programs, the drug benefit has been shown to be an effective health system variable that reduces hospital admissions and downstream costs that are more expensive, and allows individuals to manage complex health conditions and disease states. This drug benefit under Medicaid has also been structured into private health insurance plans. Although different in design

Table 7.1 Pricing level fluctuations in the USA

Pricing level	Amount
Drug pricing for a hypothetical drug product	
Average wholesale price (AWP)	$100.00
Discounted pharmacy price (price paid to pharmacy by pharmacy benefit manager, Medicaid, etc.)	$88.00
Wholesale acquisition cost (WAC)	$80.00
Average manufacturer price (AMP)	$79.00
Best price available	$70.00
Federal supply schedule price	$67.00
Pricing terms	
Average wholesale price (AWP)	A national average of prices charged by wholesalers to pharmacies, calculated by pricing services. This is a fictitious price used for pharmacy reimbursement
Pharmacy discount price	The price paid to the pharmacy by a program (Medicaid, Medicare part D) for drugs
Wholesale acquisition cost (WAC)	Sometimes called "list price." WAC is the price set by manufacturers, and often has been manipulated for sales and marketing purposes
Average manufacturer price (AMP)	The average price paid to a manufacturer by wholesalers for drugs distributed to retail pharmacies. A confidential price
Best price	The lowest price paid to a manufacturer for a brand-name drug, taking into account rebates, chargebacks, discounts, or other pricing adjustments. Chargebacks are amounts reimbursed to wholesalers or pharmacy buying groups by manufacturers for selling product below a WAC or acquisition cost for preferential contract buyers (chains, chains with warehouses, etc.)
Federal supply schedule price	The maximum price that manufacturers can charge covered entities participating in the various federal governmental programs (Veterans Affairs system, US Department of Defense, etc.)
Wholesaler discount	Discount offered by wholesalers to direct purchasers for large volume and prompt payment, usually within 10 days of receipt of the product and billing for such
Federal upper limit (FUL) price	Federally established maximum price for a drug product if there are three (or more) generic versions of the product rated therapeutically equivalent (A-rated) and at least three suppliers
Acquisition cost (AC)	The net cost of a drug paid by a pharmacy, including discounts, rebates, chargebacks, and other adjustments

Table 7.2 An example of a tiered arrangement for a type of drug

Tier	Drugs covered	Amount to pay
First tier	A generically available drug (generic)	$500
Second tier	A preferred brand-name drug	$2500
Third tier	A non-preferred brand drug	$60.00

This is a hypothetical example and is for illustrative purposes only.

and scope than Medicaid counterpart drug plans, private health insurance drug plans have been shown to reduce other costs in the health care system in an analogous fashion. Both Medicaid and managed care plans utilized formularies. Medicaid formularies are by design open: physicians for the most part can prescribe any therapy for a Medicaid patient. Private health insurance or managed care drug benefits use a closed formulary structure and rely upon the exclusion of certain available drug therapies, or use a tiered formulary and co-payment mechanism to reduce costs.

Discussion questions

1 The concept of managed care originated in the USA. Does this effort to manage health care costs and the growth in expenditures have applicability for health care systems in other countries?

2 Has managed care been a successful health policy initiative in the USA? If yes why, and if no, why not?

3 How does Health Canada differ from the US Food and Drug Administration?

4 In the UK, the PCTs exert local control of some health and social expenditures (roughly 75%). Could this model of local control and input into health care policy determination be exported elsewhere?

5 Would a prescription drug pricing scheme such as the UK Pharmaceutical Price Regulation Scheme work in the USA to the same degree?

6 Explain how the Canadian CDR benefits Canadian consumers.

7 How do the provincial health care plans, including provincial public drug plans, work in Canada?

8 Discuss the similarities and differences between the UK NICE and the Canadian CDR.

9 Compare and contrast allocative and technical efficiency in relation to health policy considerations.

10 Do you feel the French PMSI is a fair, equitable, and ethical system of allocation of health resources?

References

Arrow KJ (1963). Uncertainty and the welfare economics of medical care. *Am Econ Rev* LIII: 141–149.

Ashton T, Press D (1997). Market concentration in secondary health services under a purchaser–provider split: the New Zealand experience. *Health Econ* 6: 43–56.

Auld C, Donaldson C, Mitton C, *et al.* (2002). Health economics and public health. In: Detels R, Beagehole R, Lansing MA, *et al.* (eds) *Oxford Textbook of Public Health.* Oxford: Oxford University Press, pp. 877–901.

Averill R, Goldfiels N, Hughes J, *et al.* (2003). All patient refined diagnosis related groups (APR-DRGs). In: Averill R, Goldfiels N, Hughes J, *et al.* (eds) *Methodology Overview,* Version 20.0. Wallingford, CT: 3M Health Information Systems.

Bodenheimer T (2002). The not-so-sad history of Medicare cost containment as told in one chart. *Health Affairs* Jul–Dec: Suppl Web Exclusives: W88–W90.

Culyer AJ, Maynard AK, Williams AG (1991). Alternative systems of health care provision: an essay on motes and beams. In: Culyer AJ (ed.) *The Economics of Health Care,* vol. II. Camberley, Surrey: Edward Elgar, pp. 321–340.

Donaldson C, Gerard K (2005). Economic objectives of health care. In: Donaldson C, Gerard K (eds) *Economics of Health Care Financing, The Visible Hand.* Basingstoke, Hampshire: Palgrave Macmillan, pp. 73–88.

Duckett SJ (2000). The development of Australian refined diagnosis related groups: the Australian inpatient casemix classification. *Casemix* 2: 115–120.

Etheredge L (2001). On the archaeology of health care policy, periods and paradigms 1975–2000. *The Robert Wood Johnson Health Policy Fellowships Program, Special Report, Institute of Medicine, Shaping the Future for Health.* New York: Robert Wood Johnson Foundation.

Fincham JE (2006). A global perspective on managed care and pharmacy education. *Am J Pharm Educ* 70: 86.

Fincham JE (2007). The need to invest in community pharmacy practice. *Am J Pharm Educ* 71: 26.

Getsios D, Migliaccio-Walle K, Caro JJ (2007). NICE cost-effectiveness appraisal of cholinesterase inhibitors: was the right question posed? Were the best tools used? *Pharmacoeconomics* 25: 997–1006.

Grant Thornton LLP (2007). *National Study to Determine the Cost of Dispensing Prescriptions in Community Retail Pharmacies.* Washington, DC: The Coalition for Community Pharmacy Action.

Haycox A (2007). When NICE says no! *Pharmacoeconomics* 25: 995–996.

Heavens J (1999). Casemix – the missing link in South African healthcare management. *An Overview of Casemix Groupings such as DRGs and HRGs, Their Use for Improved Clinical and Administrative Healthcare Management, and Recommendations for a Way Forward in South Africa.* Tygerberg, South Africa: The Health Informatics RandD Coordination Programme of the Informatics and Communications Group.

Hogan C (2005). Impact of policies to limit drug plan's financial risk. Available online at: http://aspe.hhs.gov/health/reports/06/drug06/index.htm#TOC (accessed 6 February 2010).

Jackson T, Watts J, Lane L, *et al.* (1999). Data compatibility in patient level clinical costing. Available online at: http://www.casemix.org/pubbl/pdf/1_1_5.pdf (accessed 5 June 2010).

Leister J, Stausberg J (2005). Comparison of cost accounting methods from different DRG systems and their effect on health care quality. *Health Policy* 74: 46–55.

Lima E, Whynes D (2003). *Finance and Performance of Portuguese Hospitals.* Working paper series no. 20. Núcleo de Investigação em Microeconomia Aplicada. Braga, Portugal: Universidade do Minho.

Medical Research Council Laparoscopic Groin Hernia Trial Group (2001). Cost–utility analysis of open versus laproscopic groin hernia repair: results from a multicentre randomised clinical trial. *Br J Surg* 88: 653–881.

Mossialos E, Dixon A, Figueras J, *et al.* (2002). Funding health care in Europe: weighing up the options. In: Mossialos E, Dixon A, Figueras J, *et al.* (eds) *Funding Health Care:*

Options for Europe. Copenhagen, Denmark: European Observatory on Health Care Systems Series, pp. 1–17.

National Center for Health Statistics (2009). Health, United States, 2009 with chartbook on trends in the health of Americans. Hyattsville, MD: National Center for Health Statistics.

Palmer G, Aisbett C, Fetter R, *et al.* (1991). Estimates of costs by DRG in Sydney teaching hospitals: an application of the Yale cost model. *Aust Health Rev* 14: 314–334.

Pennebaker G (1969). Available online at: http://averagewholesaleprice.com (accessed 29 June 2009).

Pirson M, Dramaix M, Leclercq P, *et al.* (2006). Analysis of cost outliers within APR-DRGs in a Belgian general hospital: two complementary approaches. *Health Policy* 76: 13–25.

Rodrigues J-M (1993). Origin and dissemination throughout Europe. In: Casas M, Wiley M (eds) *Diagnosis Related Groups in Europe.* London: Springer-Verlag, pp. 17–29.

Rodrigues J, Coca E, Tombert-Paviot B, *et al.* (1998). How to use casemix to reduce inequities and efficiencies among French hospitals. Available online at: http://www.casemix.org/pubbl/art. asp?articoloID=4 (accessed 6 May 2006).

Salkeld G, Cameron ID, Cumming RG, *et al.* (2000). Quality of life related to fear of falling and hip fracture in older women: a TTO study. *Br Med J* 320: 341–364.

Steinbrook R (2008). Saying no isn't NICE – the travails of Britain's National Institute for Health and Clinical Excellence. *N Engl J Med* 359: 1977–1981.

United Kingdom Department of Health (2002). Care trusts in the United Kingdom National Health Service (NHS). Available online at: http://www.dh.gov.uk/prod_consum_dh/groups/ dh_digitalassets/@dh/@en/documents/digitalasset/dh_4074326.pdf (accessed 3 May 2010).

Vertrees J, Manton K (1993). Using case mix for resource allocation. In: Casas M, Wiley M (eds) *Diagnosis Related Groups in Europe.* London: Springer-Verlag, pp. 155–172.

Further reading

Aalto-Setälä V, Alaranta A (2008). Effect of deregulation on the prices of nicotine replacement therapy products in Finland. *Health Policy* 86: 355–362.

Almarsdóttir AB, Traulsen JM (2009). Multimethod research into policy changes in the pharmacy sector – the Nordic case. *Res Soc Admin Pharm* 5: 82–90.

Babar ZD, Izham MIM (2009). Effect of privatization of the drug distribution system on drug prices in Malaysia. *Public Health* 123: 523–533.

Barozzi N, Tett SE (2009). Gastroprotective drugs in Australia: Utilization patterns between 1997 and 2006 in relation to NSAID prescribing. *Clin Ther* 31: 849–861.

Cameron A, Ewen M, Ross-Degnen D, *et al.* (2009). Medicine prices, availability, and affordability in 36 developing and middle-income countries: a secondary analysis. *Lancet* 373: 240–249.

Garattini L, Motterlini N, Cornago D (2008). Prices and distribution margins of in-patent drugs in pharmacy: A comparison in seven European countries. *Health Policy* 85: 305–313.

García-Alonso MDC, García-Mariñoso B (2008). The strategic interaction between firms and formulary committees: Effects on the prices of new drugs. *J Health Econ* 27: 377–404.

Håkonsen H, Horn AM, Toverud EL (2009). Price control as a strategy for pharmaceutical cost containment – What has been achieved in Norway in the period 1994–2004? *Health Policy* 90: 277–285.

Harrington JE, Jr Hsu EB (2010). Stockpiling anti-viral drugs for a pandemic: The role of manufacturer reserve programs. *J Health Econ* 29: 438–444.

Herrmann M (2010). Monopoly pricing of an antibiotic subject to bacterial resistance. *J Health Econom* 29: 137–150.

Ide H, Mollahaliloglu S (2009). How firms set prices for medical materials: A multi-country study. *Health Policy* 92: 73–78.

Koskinen H, Martikainen JE, Maljanen T (2009). Antipsychotics and antidepressants: An analysis of cost growth in Finland from 1999 to 2005. *Clin Ther* 31: 1469–1477.

Levaggi R, Orizio G, Domenighini S, *et al.* (2009). Marketing and pricing strategies of online pharmacies. *Health Policy* 92: 187–196.

Lim D, Emery J, Lewis J, *et al.* (2009). A systematic review of the literature comparing the practices of dispensing and non-dispensing doctors. *Health Policy* 92: 1–9.

Mason AR, Drummond MF (2009). Public funding of new cancer drugs: Is NICE getting nastier? *Eur J Cancer* 45: 1188–1192.

Morgan S, McMahon M, Greyson D (2008). Balancing health and industrial policy objectives in the pharmaceutical sector: Lessons from Australia. *Health Policy* 87: 133–145.

Tetteh EK (2008). Providing affordable essential medicines to African households: The missing policies and institutions for price containment. *Soc Sci Med* 66: 569–581.

8

Health policy and regulatory actions – focus on tobacco

Introduction

In the USA over the past 50 years there has been no more contentious debate and reaction than that carried out over tobacco and its regulation. Federal government regulators, elected officials, disease advocacy organizations, manufacturing entities, smoking cessation advocacy groups, and state and local government units have focused their efforts on tobacco regulation. Some were in support, some opposed, and some vigorously opposed (tobacco manufacturers) the effort to increase taxes on tobacco products, restrict where tobacco could be sold, place limits on the minimum age of purchasers, and tightly restrict where tobacco could be used. Regulating nicotine as a drug, limits placed on nicotine and tar content in cigarettes, requirements for manufacturers to place health warnings on packaging, and restrictions on providing free goods have all been tried as a remedy for the scourge of tobacco use in the USA. The percentage of smokers has steadily decreased, but the sheer number of smokers is greater than it has ever been because of the increase in the total population of the country.

These health policy debates concerning tobacco use, sale, and regulation will continue as this book is published, and on into the foreseeable future.

Tobacco regulation as a health policy issue

Impacts upon tobacco have been in place for almost 400 years in the USA (Morison 1965). These influences have been on growers, manufacturers, and users of tobacco. Tobacco was first grown in the Americas by Native Americans and exported to Europe starting in the late 15th century. In the USA, the most prominent use of tobacco until the mid to late 19th century was smoking (Brooks 1952). Since that point in the USA and abroad, tobacco ingestion via cigarette smoking is by far and away the most predominant form of tobacco consumption. Cigarette smoking by individuals in the USA as a percentage has decreased from over 50% during the 1950s to 18.4% in 2010

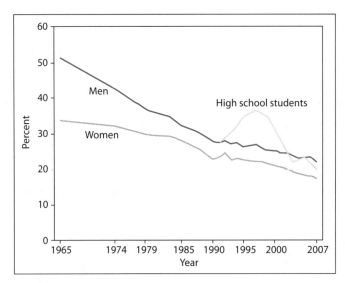

Figure 8.1 Trends among select population groups over a 42-year period. Source: CDC/NCHS, Health, United States, 2009, Figure 6. Data from the National Health Interview Survey and the Youth Risk Behavior Survey.

(State of Tobacco Control 2010). Figure 8.1 chronicles the trends over 42 years and graphically shows that the percentage of US smokers has decreased across the population, but the trends are not uniform across population subgroups, e.g., men, women, and high school groups. Despite this decrease, there are more smokers in number than ever before in the USA, again due to the country's increasing total population. Also, a troubling percentage of youths are smoking in the USA; latest data indicate that over 10% (10.1%) of youths have smoked in the past month. The number of new adolescent smokers beginning to use cigarettes is estimated to be 1000 per day in the USA.

The regulatory aspects that impact tobacco are presented in Table 8.1, and discussed below.

Table 8.1 Regulations impacting tobacco
Regulation of production
Revenue generation
Consumption
State regulations
Health warnings
Bans on advertising

Regulation of production

The colonial era saw tobacco growing regulated in the late 18th century (Morison 1965). Initially, Virginia exported tobacco almost exclusively to England. Commissions placed on growers on the sale of tobacco by the English were cripplingly high. Production controls allowed this practice to be managed to the advantage of the English.

Revenue generation

The states and federal government have taxed tobacco products for an extended period of time. This revenue has been a major budgetary-generating device for over a century. These funds have been used for any number of purposes from general funds to promotion of tobacco cessation efforts. The current average state tax is $1.34 per pack of cigarettes.

Consumption

Age limits on the purchase of tobacco products have sought to curb the epidemic of teenage, and younger, smoking that is seen in the USA and elsewhere. Increases in consumption have been seen both by tobacco manufacturers seeing a growth in tobacco consumed (Gottsegen 1940) and public health advocates, who see increasing morbidity and mortality accompanying increases in tobacco use.

State regulations

Restrictions on where individuals may smoke have come about as a result of so-called Clean Indoor Air Acts which targeted stopping cigarette use indoors and later outdoors at public events or in public places.

Health warnings

Health warnings explicitly cautioning on the use of cigarettes have focused on cancer, heart disease, lung disease, and sexual performance. Abroad, much more graphic and intense warnings against use have been placed on cigarette packaging as opposed to the US-style warnings.

Bans on advertising

Recently in the USA, bans on billboard, television, radio, and certain print advertising have been implemented.

Detrimental aspects of tobacco use

If there was a drug contained within a delivery device provided through pharmacies that had a mortality associated with its use amounting to over 450 000 annual deaths in the USA, and was a leading contributor to untold morbidity, would not our collective voice be heard to eliminate this product from our pharmacy milieus? The product is nicotine-wrapped in the deadly delivery mechanism of cigarettes and other tobacco products.

Of the roughly 60 000 pharmacies in the USA about 70% are chain community pharmacies or food market-based pharmacies. Tobacco is sold in virtually every one of these pharmacies, with a few exceptions. Traditional chains, mass merchandiser and food market-based pharmacies have been suggested to sell more tobacco products than other types of pharmacies (Hickey *et al.* 2006). As a percentage of total sales, tobacco products account for much less than 1% of total sales. A major inducement for some pharmacies to continue to sell cigarettes is the significant promotional funding provided by US tobacco manufacturers. This is over and above their meager tobacco profits from sales.

In a replicated study of tobacco sales in pharmacies in the San Francisco area, Eule *et al.* (2004) found that, in 2003, 61% of surveyed pharmacies sold cigarettes; this figure was down from 89% of pharmacies selling cigarettes in 1976. Over 8 of 10 of the pharmacies continuing to sell cigarettes also displayed cigarette advertising. Over-the-counter nicotine replacement products were sold by 78% of pharmacies. And, in a bizarre placement scheme, in 55% of pharmacies selling cigarettes, these nicotine replacement products were displayed immediately next to the cigarettes (Eule *et al.* 2004).

What do pharmacy colleagues around the globe have to say about tobacco sales in pharmacy? In 2004, in New Orleans, the Fédération Internationale Pharmaceutique (FIP), representing pharmacists worldwide, recommended that pharmaceutical organizations diligently pursue policies stating that tobacco products should not be sold in pharmacies, and that licensing bodies should not license pharmacies that are located in premises in which such products are sold. FIP also recommended that smoking should not be permitted in pharmacies (International Pharmacy Federation 2004). The Pharmaceutical Society of Australia supports the Quality Care Pharmacy Program which includes a mandatory pharmacy accreditation standard under which stocking or selling tobacco products is prohibited (Quality Care Pharmacy Program 2004).

Some pharmacies have exited from selling tobacco

Some chains allow individual store managers to make the decision to sell or not to sell cigarettes. The Target Corporation pulled tobacco from shelves over a decade ago for economic reasons. The low profit margins and potential for high theft and expensive-to-implement ordinances to control sales to minors have made selling cigarettes much less appealing to retailers. Some mass merchandisers have pulled cigarettes from shelves in one country while continuing to promote tobacco sales heavily in developing countries.

Most recently the Wegmans' regional food market chain made the decision to stop selling cigarettes (Veale and Wallace 2008). In a letter to employees, chief executive officer Danny Wegman and daughter Colleen Wegman (company president) noted: "We believe there are few of us who would introduce our children to smoking" (Veale and Wallace 2008). This action is noteworthy in and of itself, but in addition the food market retailer is providing smoking cessation programs for company employees.

Some cities have also expressly prohibited health care providers from selling tobacco. For example, the city of Newton, Massachusetts, in November 2009 passed the following (Newton, Massachusetts Aldermen 2009):

> The Revised Ordinances of the City of Newton, Massachusetts 2007 are hereby amended by inserting the following provision in Section 20-2 after paragraph (g) thereof, and renumbering paragraphs (h) through (i) thereof, respectively, as paragraphs (i) through (j):

> (h) Prohibition of the Sale of Tobacco Products by Health Care Providers:

> No health care provider located in the City of Newton shall sell tobacco products or cause tobacco products to be sold. No retail establishment that operates, maintains or employs a health care provider within it, such as a pharmacy or drug store, shall sell tobacco products or cause tobacco products to be sold.

A global crisis and epidemic

The World Health Organization estimates that, worldwide, tobacco has been estimated to have killed 100 million individuals in the past century; this total could reach 1 billion in the current century (World Health Organization 2008). Alarmingly, roughly 50% of the world's children live in countries that do not ban free distribution of tobacco products (World Health Organization 2008). Many of the cigarettes marketed and sold worldwide are from US-based tobacco manufacturers. Evidence shows that around one-half of those who start smoking in adolescence continue to smoke for 15–20 years (Cai 2006). Between 80 000 and 100 000 children worldwide start smoking every day (Cai 2006; World Health Organization 2008). Of this number, approximately half of them live in Asia (Cai 2006). In the Philippines, 14% of children start smoking before 10 years of age. Also, in China, 20–40% of children start smoking before age 10 years (Cai 2006; World Health Organization 2008). The World Health Organization notes that a person dies every 6 seconds due to cigarette smoking.

From Table 8.2 it can be seen that the largest tobacco manufacturer in the world is a Chinese corporation, one of the major companies (Philip Morris) is American, two are British (BAT and Imperial Tobacco), and one is Japanese (Japan Tobacco International). As is the case in the USA and elsewhere, taxes on Chinese cigarettes are used to pay for other societal services. As the pressure on tobacco companies has ratcheted up significantly in the USA, American-based tobacco manufacturers have marketed their wares successfully globally.

According to Mathers and Loncar (2006), tobacco use is a risk factor for six of the eight leading causes of death in the world (ischemic heart disease; cerebrovascular disease; lower respiratory infections; chronic obstructive pulmonary disease; tuberculosis; and trachea and bronchus lung cancers). No doubt tobacco use is a co-factor in other morbidity-inducing diseases as well.

A total of 30% of the world's smokers live in China – 350 million Chinese smoke, a significant number and much more than the entire US population. There is a perverse incentive for the People's Republic of China to encourage its citizens to smoke: tobacco sales in China are controlled by the government, with an estimated profit of $30 billion yearly. An estimated 2 million Chinese will die from cigarette smoking annually by the year 2020. In China, 60% of males smoke and cigarettes offered to employees by employers or colleagues are difficult to turn away because of societal mores.

Table 8.2 World's five largest tobacco companies

	% World market share (2007)	Profits (US $ millions) (2008)
China National Tobacco Corporation (China)	32	
Philip Morris (USA)	18.7	13 400
British American Tobacco (BAT) (UK)	17.1	5223
Japan Tobacco International	10.8	7692
Imperial Tobacco	5.6	3412

Source: Adapted from *The Tobacco Atlas* (2010) available online at: http://www.tobaccoatlas.org/companies.html?iss=14&country=0.

The 2008 World Health Organization report on the global tobacco epidemic promotes an "mpower" movement. mpower seeks to implement six components:

1   Monitor tobacco use and prevention policies.
2   Protect people from tobacco smoke.
3   Offer to help others to quit tobacco use.
4   Warn about the dangers of tobacco.
5   Enforce bans on tobacco advertising, promotion, and sponsorship.
6   Raise taxes on tobacco.

Need for health professional advocacy of smoking cessation

Dr. LEE Jong-wook, former director of the World Health Organization, noted (World Health Organization 2008):

> Doctors, nurses, midwives, dentists, pharmacists, chiropractors, psychologists and all other professionals dedicated to health can help people change their behaviour. They are on the front line of the tobacco epidemic and collectively speak to millions of people (p. 37).

Since this declaration, there is a feeling that we have not done what we can and should do to stem the deaths resultant from tobacco use.

Miller (2010), writing about a report released on the state of smoking in the world, noted that World Health Organization Chief Margaret Chan suggests "that tobacco-related deaths among women will likely rise from 1.5 million in 2004 to 2.5 million by 2030." Miller also notes that projections point to 75% of these projected deaths occurring in low- and middle-income countries.

Selected milestones in tobacco influences in the past 50 years in the USA

> 1956: Drs. Richard Doll and A. Bradford Hill, publish a landmark paper (Doll and Hill 1956) in the *British Medical Journal* confirming the relation between lung cancer and smoking cigarettes.
> 1964: The first US Surgeon General's report on smoking is published. Called *Smoking and Health – Report of the Advisory Committee to the Surgeon General of the Public Health Service* (http://profiles.nlm.nih. gov/NN/B/B/M/Q/_/nnbbmq.pdf), this report recognized the proven link between smoking and lung cancer. Each successive year, this thoroughly detailed linkage of smoking to health, cancer, and other disease states has been a prominent reference for smoking cessation and tobacco control advocates at the federal, state, association, and corporate level.

1966: Health warnings (Caution – cigarette smoking may be hazardous to your health) make their first appearance on packages of cigarettes in the USA.

1975: The state of Minnesota becomes the first state to limit smoking in indoor spaces to separate areas with the passage and implementation of The Minnesota Clean Indoor Air Act.

1984: Nicotine polacrilex gum (marketed by Lakeside Pharmaceuticals) is approved by the US Food and Drug Administration (FDA) for marketing in the USA. This product had been available in Europe for several years before entry into the US market.

1986: The 19th US Surgeon General's report on *The Health Consequences of Involuntary Smoking* is published (http://profiles.nlm.nih.gov/NN/B/C/P/M/_/nnbcpm.pdf). This report focuses on the health effects of second-hand (sidestream) involuntary ingestion of cigarette smoke. It is the first report to do so in the USA.

1987: The US Congress institutes a ban on smoking on domestic flights of less than 2 hours. The ban is set to become law in 1988.

1987: The R.J. Reynolds Tobacco Company (Winston-Salem, NC) debuts the inaugural "Joe Camel" character in its US advertisements. This cartoon character is claimed to have introduced millions of adolescents to Camel tobacco products. A landmark and disturbing study published in 1991 (Fischer *et al.* 1991) indicated that the Joe Camel was more recognizable than Mickey Mouse in a sample of 3–6-year-old children.

1988: Californians approve Proposition 99, which increased the cigarette tax by 25 cents, and dedicated some of the revenue to create the first comprehensive statewide tobacco control program in California (State of Tobacco Control 2010). It was also the first time a state dedicated proceeds from tobacco taxes to help prevent and stop smoking (State of Tobacco Control 2010). The American Lung Association was instrumental in the passage of this proposition and subsequent support for the California Tobacco Control Program (State of Tobacco Control 2010).

1988: Tobacco Free America (American Lung Association, American Heart Association and American Cancer Society) publishes *State Legislated Actions on Tobacco Issues* (http://slati.lungusa.org/reports/SLATI_2009_Final_Web.pdf). This document tracks tobacco control policies – such as tobacco taxes, smokefree air laws, and tobacco control program funding – for each of the 50 US states (State of Tobacco Control 2010).

1989: A bill co-sponsored by Senator Frank Lautenberg (D-NJ) and Representative Dick Durbin (D-IL) passes both houses of Congress. This bill bans smoking on all domestic airlines. The American Lung Association is one of many public health groups leading efforts to pass this law (State of Tobacco Control 2010).

1990: San Luis Obispo, California, becomes the first city in the world to eliminate smoking in all public buildings, including bars and restaurants (State of Tobacco Control 2010).

1993: The US Environmental Protection Agency publishes *Respiratory Health Effects of Passive Smoking – Lung Cancer and Other Disorders* (State of Tobacco Control 2010). The report concludes that secondhand smoke is responsible for approximately 3000 lung cancer deaths each year in non-smoking adults and impairs the respiratory health of hundreds of thousands of children (State of Tobacco Control 2010).

1994: A group of seven US tobacco company executives testify before Representative Henry Waxman's (D-CA) congressional committee that they can state that they do not believe nicotine is addictive (State of Tobacco Control 2010).

1995: The US FDA asserts jurisdiction over tobacco products by declaring nicotine a drug. President Clinton approves this proposal in 1996, giving the agency authority to regulate cigarettes as a "drug delivery device."

1996: US FDA asserts jurisdiction, but in 2000 the Supreme Court holds that only Congress can give FDA authority over tobacco (see related item below from 2000).

1996: FDA establishes nationwide standards requiring retailers to verify age for over-the-counter sales and provides funds for states to enforce.

1998: Attorneys General from 46 states and the tobacco industry reach the landmark Master Settlement Agreement to reimburse state government for tobacco-related health care costs. The billions of dollars were supposed to be used to prevent smoking and help people quit smoking; unfortunately states have used most of this money for other unrelated purposes (State of Tobacco Control 2010).

1999: The US Centers for Disease Control and Prevention releases the first edition of *Best Practices for Comprehensive Tobacco Control Programs* (State of Tobacco Control 2010). This document details how state tobacco control programs should be structured to best prevent smoking and help smokers quit.

2000: The US Supreme Court rules in a 5–4 decision that the US FDA could not assert authority over tobacco products without being given the power to do so by Congress (State of Tobacco Control 2010).

2004: The United States signs the Framework Convention on Tobacco Control Treaty, the first global tobacco control treaty, and establishes international guidelines for countries to implement and control tobacco use and addiction (State of Tobacco Control 2010). The treaty has not yet been sent to the US Senate for ratification.

2006: The US Surgeon General releases *The Health Consequences of Involuntary Exposure to Tobacco Smoke* (State of Tobacco Control

2010). The report states unequivocally that the "debate is over" – secondhand smoke in any form at any level is harmful to health.
2006: Judge Kessler releases her final ruling in the US Department of Justice's federal suit against the tobacco companies. She finds that the tobacco industry has lied for 50 years and deceived the American public on health issues and marketing to children (State of Tobacco Control 2010).
2009: FDA Regulatory Authority Bill passes House again 298–112 on April 2; Senate by a vote of 97 to 17 on June 11; House passes Senate version June 12; President Barack Obama signs into law June 22, 2009.
2009: US President Obama signs legislation granting the US FDA regulatory authority over tobacco products (State of Tobacco Control 2010). Tobacco products are now no longer exempt from basic oversight (State of Tobacco Control 2010).

Master Tobacco Settlement Agreement

The major tenets of the 1998 Master Tobacco Settlement Agreement, mentioned above, between 46 state Attorneys General and the major US tobacco companies are listed in Table 8.3. The settlement amount was $192.4 billion. The settlement amounts for the additional four non-participating states are as follows: Florida $11.3 billion, Minnesota $6.1 billion, Mississippi $3.6 billion, and Texas $15.3 billion (Lacombe and Winter 2004).

The intent of this settlement was to provide funding for health expenditures downstream for states' expected expenses to treat smoking-related morbidity in state-funded Medicaid programs. In addition, funding was to be placed into programs to assist smokers in quitting. Many states implemented programs to this end, and were successful in their efforts from a smoking cessation standpoint. However, as the economies in states waxed and waned over the years, this money was diverted to other general fund expenditure requirements. This in and of itself did not violate the legal components of the settlement. However, there can be little doubt that these diversions into other spending programs did indeed violate the spirit of the settlement. The intent to spend money on smoking cessation activities would remove the need for Medicaid expenditures in the future to deal with the many expensive and predictable sequelae associated with continued smoking. The states taking a time value approach to money today versus money tomorrow or in the future do not take into consideration that the expenses necessary to pay for additional health costs due to smoking morbidity will exceed these settlement dollars.

The issue of global tobacco morbidity and mortality will be further examined in succeeding chapters on international health issues and impacts.

Table 8.3 Key provisions of the Master Tobacco Settlement Agreement

Prohibition on youth targeting
Ban on use of cartoons
Limitation of tobacco brand-name sponsorships
Elimination of outdoor advertising and transit advertisements
Prohibition on payments related to tobacco products and media
Ban on tobacco brand-name merchandise
Ban on youth access to free samples
Ban on gifts to underage persons based on proof of purchase
Limitation on third-party use of brand names
Ban on non-tobacco brand names
Minimum pack size of 20 cigarettes
Corporate culture commitments related to youth access and consumption
Limitations on lobbying
Restriction on advocacy concerning settlement proceeds
Dissolution of the Tobacco Institute, the Council for Tobacco Research–USA, and the Center for Indoor Air Research
Regulation and oversight of new tobacco-related trade associations
Prohibition on agreements to suppress research
Prohibition on material misrepresentations

Source: http://www.ag.ca.gov/tobacco/pdf/1msa.pdf.

US federal smoking cessation health policy components

Department of Health and Human Services (HHS)

The US HHS has multipronged efforts in play to impact tobacco use in the USA. One such effort is through HHS Secretary Kathleen Sebelius' Strategic Initiatives (Sebelius 2010). An initiative is reprinted below and is in the public domain in the USA:

> Smoking harms nearly every organ of the body, causing many diseases and affecting the health of smokers in general. Quitting smoking has both immediate and long-term benefits for you and your loved ones. Despite progress in reducing tobacco use, more than 20% of Americans still smoke (Thorne *et al.* 2008) and smoking rates that

have been falling for decades have now stalled. The good news is that we know what it will take to get those numbers dropping again – comprehensive, sustained, and accountable tobacco control efforts based on evidence-based interventions.

We have identified the following set of actions to accelerate our efforts to prevent and reduce tobacco use.

- **Strengthen the Implementation of Evidence-based Tobacco Control Interventions and Policies in States and Communities**
  HHS will work to accelerate adoption of comprehensive smoke-free laws in every state and will continue to support efforts to build state and local capacity to implement proven policy interventions. HHS will support comprehensive quit line services; focus greater attention on populations with a disproportionate burden of use and dependence; and increase local, state, and Tribal enforcement of tobacco regulation.
- **Change Social Norms Around Tobacco Use**
  HHS will develop a comprehensive communication agenda to promote a culture change around tobacco use, including national campaigns to prevent and reduce youth tobacco use and increase knowledge about the evidence-base for and availability of treatment options. HHS will unify communication and education campaigns employed across HHS agencies.
- **Accelerate Research to Expand the Science Base and Monitor Progress**
  HHS will develop and implement new research and surveillance activities to address gaps in knowledge about what works in tobacco prevention and control, including in regulatory science, evolving product changes, industry practices, and public perception. We will also develop new prevention and treatment interventions for high-risk populations.
- **Leverage HHS Systems and Resources to Create a Society Free of Tobacco-related Disease and Death**
  HHS will provide comprehensive cessation treatment across all its facilities and require HHS-funded programs to have or provide a plan for implementing tobacco-free campus policies. HHS will ensure that HHS health care providers offer cessation advice and referrals; enhance health care professionals' knowledge and adoption of effective treatments; and provide more powerful incentives to health care providers and others to promote cessation treatment.

Secretary Sebelius' prominent comments regarding the prevalence and importance of intervention efforts aimed at cigarette smoking are important health policy pronouncements and carry the weight of a US federal cabinet officer.

FDA regulation of tobacco

The passage of the Family Smoking Prevention and Tobacco Control and Federal Retirement Reform

Public law 111–31 – June 22, 2009, which was passed and signed into law in 2010, allows the US FDA to regulate several aspects of the manufacturing, marketing, sales, and content of tobacco products in the USA. The bill has the following preface:

> An Act
>
> To protect the public health by providing the Food and Drug Administration with certain authority to regulate tobacco products, to amend title 5, United States Code, to make certain modifications in the Thrift Savings Plan, the Civil Service Retirement System, and the Federal Employees' Retirement System, and for other purposes.

Key substantive elements of the Family Smoking Prevention and Tobacco Control Act include the following components:

1   Requires tobacco companies to provide information to the federal government so as to allow the federal government to better inform consumers regarding the dangers of tobacco consumption
2   Restricts tobacco company marketing that is focused on appeals to children, misleads adults, and in intent deceptively encourages tobacco use:
   a   Ban remaining tobacco brand sponsorships of sports and entertainment events
   b   Ban free giveaways of any non-tobacco items with the purchase of a tobacco product or in exchange for coupons
   c   Ban free samples of cigarettes and the sale of cigarettes in packages that contain fewer than 20 cigarettes
   d   Ban outdoor tobacco advertising near schools and playgrounds after further FDA review
3   Strengthen the restrictions on tobacco sales to youth:
   a   Limit in-store point-of-sale tobacco advertising to black-and-white text only
   b   Limit advertising in publications with significant teen readership (more than 15% or 2 million) to black-and-white text only
   c   Restrict vending machines and self-service displays to adult-only facilities
4   Grants states broader powers of influence on marketing of tobacco products, expands power of states:
   a   Permits states to restrict time, place, and manner of tobacco marketing

b   Imposes specific limits on industry marketing, sales, and promotions, including but not limited to marketing that appeals to young people

5   More accurately informs tobacco consumers

6   Improved cigarette and tobacco warning labels

7   Improved accuracy in testing of tar, nicotine, and other harmful substances

8   Setting of standards to prohibit unsubstantiated health claims. What must be shown is that the product: (1) as it is used by consumers (2) will significantly reduce the risk of tobacco-related disease (3) to individual tobacco users; and (4) benefit the health of the population as a whole, taking into account both users of tobacco products and persons who do not currently use tobacco products.

9   Regulation of the contents of tobacco products in order to protect consumers.

Section 904 requires disclosures to the FDA and the general public. The bill requires tobacco companies to disclose to the FDA anything they add and chemicals found in both the product and the product's smoke, whether added or occurring naturally, by quantity, including nicotine. The bill requires tobacco companies to notify the FDA of changes to a product, and allows for regulation of the content of tobacco products.

The bill does not allow the FDA to ban all cigarettes, all smokeless tobacco products, or all roll-your-own tobacco products, or require the reduction of nicotine yields of a tobacco product to zero.

For cigarettes, the bill requires replacement of the current small, hard-to-read warning labels with larger, more specific warning labels covering 50% of the top half of the front and back of each pack with graphics depicting the health consequences of tobacco use. This style of graphic material is common elsewhere in the world, e.g., the UK, Canada, and Australia. For smokeless tobacco products, the bill requires replacement of the current small, hard-to-read warning labels with larger, more specific warning labels covering 30% of the top half of the front and back of each package.

Summary

The health policy influences on tobacco use in the USA have come from many sources. Although tobacco use is higher due to increases in the US population, the percentage of smokers in the USA has steadily declined over the past 50 years. The morbidity and mortality associated with tobacco use exceed that caused from any other source, and tobacco-related mortality exceeds 500 000 deaths per year in the USA. Second- and third-hand smoke further adds to tobacco's illness reach.

Smokeless tobacco was the predominant form of tobacco use in the 19th century until the cigarette-rolling machine was invented. This device allowed for mass production of cigarettes and ease of use for smokers of tobacco products. In addition, in both World Wars I and II, cigarettes were provided in food ration kits to soldiers.

The issues surrounding tobacco use, control, marketing, manufacturing, and sales have been contentious for centuries. Vehemence is still in play when these issues are discussed; they will no doubt continue to be dealt with from many angles from many sides.

Discussion questions

1 What health policy factors have impacted tobacco use in the USA to the greatest extent?

2 Assume you are a marketing manager for a pharmaceutical company that has developed a new non-addictive nicotine polymer congener (Niconomore) to be used as prescription-only smoking cessation therapy. Where do you feel that you and your company would benefit from the most impact, from a health policy standpoint, on smoking cessation and tobacco control efforts?

3 Is it ethical for a drug company to benefit monetarily from helping patients stop smoking using drug therapy?

4 What role do professional associations play in stemming tobacco use in the USA?

5 When viewing federal and state smoking cessation legislative efforts, which level of government has had the most influence?

6 The state tax on a pack of cigarettes now averages $1.34 across the USA. Is it ethical to tax cigarette consumption for individuals when this money is not used for smoking cessation impacts?

7 What else might be done by the US FDA to regulate nicotine use?

8 Why have the US Master Settlement Agreement funds been directed to general tax revenue applications?

9 How credible are the tobacco company efforts to promote smoking cessation and reduce youth tobacco use?

10 From a health policy perspective, how have coalitions of many smoking cessation advocacy groups impacted federal and state policy activities in the USA?

11 Which of the following had the most impact upon tobacco use in the USA:

a The Master Settlement Agreement between tobacco companies and the states?

b The Family Smoking Prevention and Tobacco Control and Federal Retirement Reform Act?

Health policy and regulatory actions – focus on tobacco | **181**

References

Brooks JE (1952). *The Mighty Leaf: Tobacco Through the Centuries*. Boston: Little, Brown.

Cai C (2006). Globalization and its impact on youth health in Asia. Presentation, 30 March 2006. Regional Expert Group Meeting Development challenges for young people in Asia 28–30 March 2006, Bangkok, Thailand.

Doll R, Hill AB (1956). Lung cancer and other causes of death in relation to smoking. *Br Med J* 2: 1071–1081.

Eule B, Sullivan MK, Schroeder SA, *et al.* (2004). Merchandising of cigarettes in San Francisco pharmacies: 27 years later. *Tobacco Control* 13: 429–432.

Family Smoking Prevention and Tobacco Control and Federal Retirement Reform (2009). Public Law 111–31 – June 22, 2009; 123 Stat. 1776.

Fischer PM, Schwartz MP, Richards JW Jr, *et al.* (1991). Brand logo recognition by children aged 3 to 6 years. Mickey Mouse and Old Joe the Camel. *JAMA* 266: 3145–3148.

Gottsegen JJ (1940). *Tobacco – A Study of its Consumption in the United States*. New York: Pittman, pp. 8–10, 28, 87, 147, 153, 155.

Hickey LM, Farris KB, Peterson NA, *et al.* (2006). Predicting tobacco sales in community pharmacies using population demographics and pharmacy type. *J Am Pharm Assoc* 46: 385–390.

International Pharmaceutical Federation (2004). FIP calls for ban on tobacco sales and smoking in pharmacies: press release. Available online at: http://www.fip.org/projectsfip//pharmacists-againsttobacco/.

Lacombe DJ, Winter H (2004). In or out? Explaining state shares of the Tobacco Master Settlement Agreement. *Int J Econ Business* 11: 279–285.

Mathers CD, Loncar D (2006). Projections of global mortality and burden of disease from 2002 to 2030. *PLoS Medicine* 3: e442.

Miller T (2010). World no tobacco day focuses on rising number of female smokers. PBS Newshour, 31 May 2010. Available online at: http://www.pbs.org/newshour/updates/health/jan-june10/smoking_05-31.html (accessed 31 May 2010).

Morison SE (1965). *The Oxford History of the American People*. New York: Oxford University Press, pp. 93–94.

Newton, Massachusetts Aldermen (2009). Available online at: http://www.ci.newton.ma.us/Aldermen/Programs%20and%20Services/2009/11-04-09ProgandServReport.pdf (accessed 5 May 2010).

Quality Care Pharmacy Program (2004). *Pharmacy Stock* [STO-5]. Canberra: The Pharmacy Guild of Australia.

Sebelius K (2010). Secretary's strategic initiatives: prevent and reduce tobacco use. Available online at: http://www.hhs.gov/secretary/about/prevent.html (accessed 6 May 2010).

State of Tobacco Control (2010). American Lung Association, Washington, DC. Available online at: http://www.stateoftobaccocontrol.org/2009/our-fight/tobacco-timeline.html (accessed 5 May 2010).

Thorne SL, Malarcher A, Maurice E, *et al.* (2008). Cigarette smoking among adults – United States, 2007. *MMWR* 57: 1221–1226.

Veale S, Wallace D (2008). Wegmans snuffs tobacco sales. Ithica Journal, Gannett News Service January 5, 2008. Available online at: www.theithicajournal.com (accessed 14 February 2008).

World Health Organization (2008). *WHO Report on the Global Tobacco Epidemic, 2008: The MPOWER Package*. Geneva: World Health Organization.

Further reading

Bell K, Salmon A, Bowers M, *et al.* (2010). Smoking, stigma and tobacco 'denormalization': Further reflections on the use of stigma as a public health tool. *Soc Sci Med* 70: 795–799.

Bolliger CT (2009). Smoking cessation should have more emphasis within tobacco control? The case for. *Health Policy* 91 (suppl. 1): S31–S36.

Burgess DJ, Fu SS, van Ryn M (2009). Potential unintended consequences of tobacco-control policies on mothers who smoke: A review of the literature. *Am J Prevent Med* 37 (suppl. 1): S151–S158.

Chen C, Isabelle LM, Pickworth WB, *et al.* (2010). Levels of mint and wintergreen flavorants: Smokeless tobacco products vs. confectionery products. *Food Chem Toxicol* 48: 755–763.

Clancy L (2009). Progress in tobacco control. *Health Policy* 91 (suppl. 1): S3–S14.

Colilla SA (2010). An epidemiologic review of smokeless tobacco health effects and harm reduction potential. *Regul Toxicol Pharmacol* 56: 197–211.

Córdoba R, Nerín I (2009). Strategies for reducing risks in smoking: Opportunity or threat?. *Arch Bronconeumol (English Edn)* 45: 611–616.

Cruz TB (2009). Monitoring the tobacco use epidemic IV. The vector: Tobacco industry data sources and recommendations for research and evaluation. *Prevent Med* 48 (suppl. 1): S24–S34.

Dewhirst T (2010). Gender, extreme sports, and smoking: A case study of export 'A' cigarette brand marketing. In: Fuller LK (ed.) *Sexual Sports Rhetoric: Global and Universal Contexts.* New York, NY: Peter Lang, pp. 263–275.

Dinno A, Glantz S (2009). Tobacco control policies are egalitarian: A vulnerabilities perspective on clean indoor air laws, cigarette prices, and tobacco use disparities. *Soc Sci Med* 68: 1439–1447.

Farrelly MC (2009). Monitoring the tobacco use epidemic V: The environment: Factors that influence tobacco use. *Prevent Med* 48(suppl. 1): S35–S43.

Gallet CA, Catlin JR (2009). The determinants of tobacco control in Europe: A research note. *Soc Sci J* 46: 143–149.

Gartner C, Hall W (2010). Harm reduction policies for tobacco users. *Int J Drug Policy* 21: 129–130.

Germain D, Wakefield MA, Durkin SJ (2010). Adolescents' perceptions of cigarette brand image: Does plain packaging make a difference?. *J Adolesc Health* 46: 385–392.

Giovino GA, Biener L, Hartman AM, *et al.* (2009). Monitoring the tobacco use epidemic I. Overview: Optimizing measurement to facilitate change. *Prevent Med* 48 (suppl. 1): S4–S10.

Gray N, Hecht SS (2010). Smokeless tobacco – proposals for regulation. *Lancet* 375: 1589–1591.

Greaves LJ, Hemsing NJ (2009). Sex, gender, and secondhand smoke policies: Implications for disadvantaged women. *Am J Prevent Med* 37 (suppl. 1): S131–S137.

Hammond D, Dockrell M, Arnott D, *et al.* (2009). Cigarette pack design and perceptions of risk among UK adults and youth. *Eur J Public Health* 19: 631–637.

Healton CG, Vallone D, Cartwright J (2009). Unintended consequences of tobacco policies: Implications for public health practice. *Am J Prevent Med* 37 (suppl. 1): S181–S182.

Henningfield JE, Shiffman S, Ferguson SG, *et al.* (2009). Tobacco dependence and withdrawal: Science base, challenges and opportunities for pharmacotherapy. *Pharmacol Ther* 123: 1–16.

Hopkins DP, Razi S, Leeks RD, *et al.* (2010). Smokefree policies to reduce tobacco use: A systematic review. *Am J Prevent Med* 38 (suppl. 1): S275–S289.

Hyland A, Cummings KM (2010). Using tobacco control policies to increase consumer demand for smoking cessation. *Am J Prevent Med* 38 (suppl. 1): S347–S350.

Kan M-Y, Lau M (2010). Minor access control of Hong Kong under the framework convention on tobacco control. *Health Policy* 95: 204–210.

Kysar DA, Salzman J (2008). Symposium: Harnessing the power of information for the next generation of environmental law. Foreword: Making sense of information for environmental protection. *Texas Law Review* 86: 1347.

Ling PM, Neilands TB, Glantz SA (2009). Young adult smoking behavior: A national survey. *Am J Prevent Med* 36: 389–394.

McGoldrick DE, Boonn AV (2010). Public policy to maximize tobacco cessation. *Am J Prevent Med* 38 (suppl. 1): S327–S332.

Osypuk TL, Acevedo-Garcia D (2010). Support for smoke-free policies: a nationwide analysis of immigrants, US-born, and other demographic groups, 1995–2002. *Am J Public Health* 100: 171–181.

Panzano VC, Wayne GF, Pickworth WB, *et al.* (2010). Human electroencephalography and the tobacco industry: a review of internal documents. *Tobacco Control* 19: 153–159.

Pennel JL (2008). Big food's trip down tobacco road: What tobacco's past can indicate about food's future. *Buffalo Public Interest Law J* 27: 101.

Prochaska JJ (2010). Failure to treat tobacco use in mental health and addiction treatment settings: A form of harm reduction?. *Drug Alcohol Depend* 110: 177–182.

Rasmussen N, Seevers M (2010). The stimulants and the political economy of addiction in American biomedicine. *BioSocieties* 5: 105–123.

Rychlak R (2009). Cards and dice in smoky rooms: Tobacco bans and modern casinos. *Drake Law Rev* 57: 467.

Stellman SD, Djordjevic MV (2009). Monitoring the tobacco use epidemic II: The agent: Current and emerging tobacco products. *Prevent Med* 48 (suppl. 1): S11–S15.

Stokes AQ, Rubin D (2010). Activism and the limits of symmetry: the public relations battle between Colorado GASP and Philip Morris. *J Public Relat Res* 22: 26–48.

Verdonk-Kleinjan WMI, Knibbe RA, Tan FE, *et al.* (2009). Does the workplace-smoking ban eliminate differences in risk for environmental tobacco smoke exposure at work? *Health Policy* 92: 197–202.

9

Global public health and ethical issues

Introduction

In May 2007, ignoring health officials' advice, a man infected with an extremely drug-resistant form of tuberculosis flew from Atlanta to Paris. After traveling in Europe, he took a flight from Prague to Montreal and then returned to the USA by land – all in a span of about 3 weeks. Authorities in North America and Europe scurried to track down about 80 passengers who sat near him in the two transatlantic flights to ensure no one was infected.

Driven by changes in the human environment, behaviors, and lifestyle in the last half-century, there has been a dramatic rise in the rates of obesity and type 2 diabetes in both developed and developing nations worldwide. The combination of obesity and diabetes is one of the major threats to human life today (Zimmet *et al.* 2005).

Once considered a mild illness only seen in the tropics, dengue fever is resurgent in more than 100 low-latitude countries, putting about 2.5 billion people at risk; the speed of spread and the escalating seriousness of its complications have made it a serious public health concern (Phillips 2008; De Blij 2009), particularly in urban areas (De Blij 2009).

All three descriptions above are examples of global public health issues. The global nature of the problem is apparent in each, for different reasons. The targets and levels (local, national, international, and global) of intervention needed and the incentives to address the problems are also different from each other. Perspectives of global health also vary by disciplinary backgrounds and the interests of the actors involved. There are also inconsistencies in use of the terms "global health" and "global public health." Recently, there have been concerted efforts to clearly define and advocate consistent use of the terms, which are described later in this chapter. It is important, however, first to explore the various frameworks for global public health. The term "global health" has different meanings for different users. Stuckler and McKee (2008) described five leading metaphors for global health (reprinted from Stuckler D,

McKee M (2008). Five metaphors about global-health policy. *Lancet* 372: 95–97, with permission from Elsevier):

1   Global health as foreign policy, where the goal is to create alliances, exert influence, spur economic growth, enhance reputation, etc. These foreign policy goals determine the global health priorities of a country. Therefore, engagement in global health activities is used as a means to create trade alliances, enhance international reputation, promote economic growth and democracy in other countries, and open new markets for trade. Infectious diseases typically get priority under this approach.

2   Global health as security focuses where the primary interest of health policy is to protect one's own population. The focus is on issues such as bioterrorism, infectious diseases, and drug resistance. The policies are guided by a country's interest to protect its own population. Consequently, usually the diseases of poor countries that get attention are the ones with the potential to threaten populations of affluent countries. Recent examples of such diseases include severe acute respiratory syndrome (SARS), H5N1 influenza (avian flu), drug-resistant tuberculosis, and H1N1 influenza (swine flu).

3   Global health as charity, where promotion of health is considered a major factor in the fight against poverty. Non-governmental organizations dependent on philanthropic donations take the lead in these efforts. Thus, issues target health as a means to fight poverty. Issues considered deserving by the donors, such as maternal and child health, malnutrition, malaria, and HIV/AIDS [human immunodeficiency virus/acquired immunodeficiency syndrome], get priority. Large philanthropic and non-governmental organizations are typically involved.

4   Global health as investment treats health as a means to maximize economic development and consequently targets diseases that afflict young and working-age people. Diseases that can affect economic productivity, such as tuberculosis, malaria, and HIV/AIDS, get priority. International organizations such as the World Health Organization (WHO) and some large private sector companies are usually involved.

5   Global health as public health takes the most expansive perspective with the goal of reducing the global burden of disease. Attention is focused on risk factors and diseases that contribute most to the global burden. The WHO and disease-specific non-governmental organizations are involved in such efforts. Although not dominant in the recent progress of global public health, this approach "has the potential to produce most equitable and sustainable health improvement" (Beaglehole and Bonita 2008, p. 1988).

In practice, the policies and motivations are not always as discrete as described above and in many instances different actors pursue different goals and contradictory policies on the same issue (Stuckler and McKee 2008). Given the varied uses and perspectives of global health, it has been a difficult concept to define. The term is also often used interchangeably with public health and international health. Two definitions of global health have been proposed to address these issues and to distinguish it from the established disciplines of public health and international health. The Consortium of Universities for Global Health (CUGH) offers the following definition: "global health is an area for study, research, and practice that places a priority on improving health and achieving equity in health for all people worldwide" (Koplan *et al.* 2009, p. 1995). Beaglehole and Bonita (2010) modified the definition to: "collaborative transnational research and action for promoting health for all." Both definitions focus on health equity and emphasize the transnational nature of global health issues and the importance of collaboration. Beaglehole and Bonita (2010) also justify the use of the term "global health" rather than "global public health" to underscore that the efforts are broader than country-focused public health actions. This use is consistent with the CUGH definition and is increasingly being used in the literature. These definitions are also tacit recognition of the increasingly powerful roles global forces are playing in shaping the world.

Global forces and health

Globalization is a ubiquitous topic in the public discourse today. It is increasingly being used to describe the economic, political, social, and cultural atmosphere of the current times in the same vein that "roaring twenties," "cold war," or "digital age" has been used to describe eras in recent history. For some it holds the promise of growth and prosperity and for others it represents a major threat. The supporters of globalization see it as the key to eliminating world poverty whereas its opponents see it as contributing to increasing international inequality (Jenkins 2004). Yet, there is widespread disagreement on what globalization means. Indeed, the meaning varies according to perspective and context. Regardless of whether the connotation is economic, political, or cultural, a major driver of the changes brought about by globalization is the rapid growth in flow of information across national boundaries aided by advances in communication and information technology. In his much-acclaimed book *The World is Flat,* Thomas Friedman (2005) illustrates how such technology has reduced the distances between people and created new economic opportunities, enhanced productivity, better standard of living, and in many respects leveled the playing field for people in different parts of the world. In what Friedman describes as "flattening of the world," there is increased flow of goods, services, capital, ideas, technology, and people across national boundaries. Such global marketplaces "lead increasingly to economic decisions being influenced by global conditions" (Jenkins 2004, p. 1).

What are the implications of the flattening of the world for health care systems and population health globally? Does global health take a new meaning in the era of globalization? It is arguable whether the world is becoming flat when it comes to population health and health care systems. However, there are new challenges in terms of lifestyle, health behaviors, disease transmission, health care delivery, access to care, health workforce, climate change, security, governance, and myriad other issues. Many of these challenges are global in scope. There are also pervasive disparities in health, well-being, and longevity among the world's populations, both between and within countries. In some instances globalization has exacerbated these inequalities (Commission on Social Determinants of Health 2008). The already proven drugs and vaccines and the advances in medical knowledge are yet to benefit people in all parts of the world and there are many economic, structural, and political barriers to the world becoming "flat" in that respect. Because of the interconnected and interdependent nature of the world today, nations can ill afford to ignore these disparities and have to depend on each other for resources, expertise, and experience to deal with health problems. Health of populations is also not immune to events taking place outside their national boundaries. The growing recognition of the need for collective action for health is reflected in the inclusion of multiple goals, targets, and indicators directly relating to health in the United Nations Millennium Development Goals (MDGs). Moreover, some argue that health should be considered a global public good and there is a need for a global value system to deal with global health issues (Fidler 2001).

The influences of global forces on health are complex and multisectoral. Consequently, the relationships between global forces, determinants of health, and health are also complex and varied. Understanding such relationships is a difficult undertaking because of the complexity and the multidisciplinary approach, and amount of data, time, and resources needed to explore the linkages fully. In many instances, data are not available or are incorrect or incomplete, and the infrastructure to collect data may be deficient (Sibai 2004). Exploration of these linkages has begun only recently (Lee 2000). Various conceptual frameworks have been proposed to analyze the health impacts of globalization (Woodward *et al.* 2001; Huynen *et al.* 2005; Labonté and Schrecker 2007). All the frameworks suggest direct and indirect pathways of influence through various tiers of determinants of health.

Determinants of health

At the basic level, as described in *Healthy People 2010,* individual and community health is determined by an array of critical influences (US Department of Health and Human Services 2000). At the core of these are individual biology and behavior, which interact with each other and with the individual's physical and social environments to influence health. Health policies and interventions targeting specific health behaviors or elements of the physical or social environment can have a profound effect on health. Access to quality health care, both in the form of services received from health care providers and services and information received from other venues in the community, can significantly enhance quality of life and reduce health disparities.

Biology includes one's genetic makeup, hereditary risk factors, and alterations in physical and mental status due to illness and disability during the course of life. Genetic makeup is the rather immutable aspect of one's biology, but behavior can have protective, enhancing, or damaging effects on biology. One can engage in preventive behavior and make lifestyle choices such as diet and exercise that protect against hereditary risk factors and/or enhance health. On the other hand, one can engage in behaviors such as smoking, unhealthy diet, and drug use, or make lifestyle choices that are harmful to health.

Behavior includes health behavior and lifestyle choices that can have either positive or negative effects on health. Changes in biology can also have an effect on one's behavior. For example, one may start exercising after being diagnosed with high blood pressure, or a person suffering from depression may abuse alcohol.

Physical environment refers to the characteristics and conditions of an individual's physical surroundings that can positively or negatively affect health. This includes air and water quality, pollution, disease vectors, and the built environment.

Social environment includes, among other things, family and community structure and relationships, social institutions, availability of services, and safety and security.

Social determinants of health

As the determinants of health described above indicate, the conditions of the places where people live and work have a significant influence on their opportunities to lead a healthy life. These conditions are shaped by political, social, and economic forces on which individuals, communities, or even countries may not have direct control. Globally, the distribution of health status generally resembles the distribution of power and wealth – the poorest and weakest populations are also the sickest (De Blij 2009). Knowledge of the roles of political, social, and economic forces in determining health is important in fully understanding variations in health. In 2005, the WHO convened the Commission on Social Determinants of Health to assemble evidence on social determinants of health (SDH) and to identify ways to promote health equity globally and within countries. The Commission considered issues beyond the immediate causes of disease, focusing on "fundamental global and national structures of social hierarchy and the socially determined conditions these create" (Commission on Social Determinants of Health 2008, p. 42). The following statement in the Commission's report underscores the importance of SDH:

> lack of health care is not the cause of the huge global burden of illness: water-borne diseases are not caused by lack of antibiotics but by dirty water, and by the political, social, and economic forces that fail to make clean water available to all; heart disease is caused not by a lack of coronary care units but by the lives people lead, which are shaped by the environments in which they live; obesity is not caused by moral failure on the part of individuals but by the excess availability of high-fat and high-sugar foods. The main action on social determinants of health must therefore come from outside the health sector (p. 45).

The conceptual framework (Solar and Irwin 2007) used by the Commission identified two broad areas of SDH that can be targets for interventions to address health inequity: the circumstances of daily life and the structural drivers. These areas captured the influences included in the *Healthy People 2010* framework described above; however, issues further distal to the individual were also considered and social stratification and factors within a socioeconomic and political context were more explicitly identified.

The circumstances of daily life refer to the conditions in which people are born, grow, live, work, and age. These conditions play a significant role in determining one's opportunities to lead a healthy life and consequently health status. Variations in conditions are largely determined by variations in two sets of factors:

1   Circumstances that make one more or less vulnerable to poor health – material circumstances, social cohesion, psychosocial support, behavioral options, and biological factors. These circumstances are in turn influenced by factors associated with social stratification, such as early childhood experiences, physical and social environment, and nature of employment and working conditions. Therefore, inequalities in health are rooted in social policies and programs, distribution of resources, and economic and political arrangements. The influences of these determinants on one's life start long before birth and continue for the entire lifespan.

2   Characteristics of the health care system, including preventive, curative, and palliative interventions directed at individuals and populations. The distribution and availability of health care services, distribution of health

care personnel, whether or not health care coverage is equitable and universal, whether or not access to health care is equitable and universal, the degree of emphasis on health promotion and prevention, and the capability to adapt to changing needs due to demographic changes are among the characteristics of the health care system that determine one's ability to lead a healthy life.

The structural drivers encompass social, economic, and political systems and functions locally, nationally, and globally. These structures and processes, manifested in the distribution of power, money, and resources, are at the root of inequities in circumstances of daily life. Most social policies potentially have health implications, even when the aim of a particular policy is something other than health, such as finance, education, employment, housing, or transportation. Although structural drivers operate mainly within the confines of a country under the authority of various levels of government, the influence of global forces on these drivers is increasing. The broad areas of structural drivers are:

1   The nature and degree of stratification in the society by education, occupation, income, gender, and ethnicity/race. A person's social position determines his or her ability to take the actions and procure the goods and services necessary to lead a healthful life as well as vulnerability and exposure to health-compromising conditions. Throughout the world, there is a notable gradient in health by socioeconomic status. Low socioeconomic position in many cases means lack of education, amenities, safety, and security, poorer working conditions, material deprivation, and vulnerability to natural disasters. Therefore, addressing such inequalities is necessary in order to address health disparities successfully.

2   Socioeconomic and political context

> refers to the spectrum of factors in society that cannot be directly measured at the individual level . . . encompasses a broad set of structural, cultural and functional aspects of a social system whose impact on individuals tends to elude quantification but which exert a powerful formative influence on patterns of social stratification and thus on people's health opportunities (Solar and Irwin 2007, p. 21).

Those aspects include:

a   Cultural and societal norms and values. The value placed on health by a society is reflected in the priority given to health in the societal agenda, whether financing and organization of health care are viewed as collective responsibility, and the degree of acceptability of societal involvement in the distribution of health resources. The values vary from society to society and are important in shaping health policies and the organization of the health care delivery system of a country. Similarly, norms, such as gender biases and role expectations, lead to differential treatment and availability of power and resources.

b   Economic and social policy. A country's economic policies, such as fiscal, trade, market regulation, and labor policies and social policies such as social welfare, housing, infrastructure, and workforce distribution policies, have significant health ramifications. Health determinants are also affected by the relative strength of the public sector, tax capacity, intersectoral coherence in policy and action, and whether distribution of resources is equitable. Global trade agreements, global aid (for example, proportion of aid tied to the donor country's trade and security interests), and issues such as whether development assistance for health is targeted at treatment or prevention and whether development assistance is available to address a health issue comprehensively, also influence a country's public policies.

c   Governance processes at the global, national, and local level. Fairness, accountability and transparency, attention to public needs and equity, and civil society and community participation are among the characteristics of governance process that can affect health and health equity in a country. On the same token, equitable and participatory global policy-making is necessary for global health equity.

Globalization and determinants of health

With rapid globalization, forces that transcend national boundaries are increasingly shaping the economic, social, environmental, and cultural factors that influence health. The current phase of globalization has been largely driven by rapid growth of the global market, which, for the most part, has not been accompanied by corresponding developments in global governance and economic and social institutions. Consequently, the recent effect has been increasing inequity in health between countries as well as within countries. Yet, globalization has great potential to bring about health equity through effective governance (Commission on Social Determinants of Health 2008). As stated earlier, influences of global forces on health operate through complex interactions between multiple sectors. A widely accepted comprehensive explanatory framework for the mechanisms and pathways of such influences is yet to emerge. However, there is little consensus on the mechanisms and pathways of these influences.

Analytical frameworks also vary in the features of globalization included as influencers. Knowledge of the relative strengths of the linkages under different social and economic contexts is also limited at this point.

Woodward *et al.* (2001) proposed a framework for analyzing the impact of economic aspects of globalization on health. The framework considers the impact of globalization on proximal determinants of population health – population-level health influences (environmental, social, cultural, infectious), individual-level health risks, and the health care system. The model suggests five key linkages between globalization and these determinants:

1 direct effects on health systems and policies, such as effects of increasing international trade in health (which includes cross-border delivery of services and movement of health workforce, consumers, and capital (Chanda 2001)) or impacts of internationally determined quality and safety standards for health care services
2 direct effects on health systems and policies through international markets, such as changes in pharmaceutical prices due to international trade or intellectual property right agreements
3 direct effects on population-level health influences, such as cross-border transmission of infectious diseases or marketing of tobacco
4 indirect effects on health systems operating through national economy, such as changes in resources available for health care or costs of health care inputs due to trade liberalization, trade agreements, global fiscal crisis, or volatility in currency exchange rates
5 indirect effects on individual health risks operating through national economy, such as changes in household income resulting in changes in nutrition or living conditions.

The model proposed by Huynen *et al.* (2005) considers the impacts of six main features of the globalization process operating at the contextual level on distal and proximal determinants of population health:

1 Global governance structure: International organizations such as the WHO and the World Bank, as well as public–private partnerships, are increasingly gaining importance, particularly in low-income countries, in formulating health policies and health-related policies, which in turn determine the delivery and distribution of health services.
2 Global markets: Increased global trade and economic globalization can facilitate economic development. Yet, exclusion from the global market can be detrimental to nations and persons. These can affect health through changes in the health services and the social and physical environmental factors.

3   Global communication and diffusion of information make sharing of knowledge and experiences on common problems possible, and this can result in changes in health services, lifestyle, and the social and physical environment.
4   Global mobility: Increased movements of people, both in the forms of travel and migration, have implications for economic, political, social, and physical environments as well as the health systems.
5   Cross-cultural interaction can affect cultural norms, lifestyles, health behaviors, and social environment.
6   Global environmental changes can have a profound impact on the ecosystem resulting in alterations in the supply of food, clean air, and clean water, the patterns of spread of diseases, and the supply of biological resources.

Both models demonstrate the profound changes globalization can bring about in society. However, empirical evidence of many of the suggested linkages is needed to understand fully the impact of globalization on health.

Global health status and challenges

With an unprecedented level of interest and involvement of major international agencies in global health in recent years, important achievements have been made on many issues in many parts of the world; yet much remains to be achieved. There is wide variation in the major health issues affecting different countries and regions of the world, as there is variation in responses to these issues. However, there is also greater recognition of health as a development issue, and global responses to health issues are increasingly being coordinated. One of the driving forces behind such activities has been the United Nations MDG. The most recent report on achievements on the health-related MDGs shows mixed results (World Health Organization 2010a). Highlights include:

• The risk of malnutrition, particularly among children, increased during 2009 due to rising food prices coupled with falling incomes. After the decline in percentage of children globally under 5 years old who are underweight, from 25% in 1990 to 18% in 2005, progress has slowed down and in some countries the prevalence of undernutrition has increased.
• Child mortality has continued to decline globally and 2008 data show a 27% reduction in mortality in children under 5 years old from 90 per 1000 live births in 1990 to 65 per 1000 live births. However, the reductions were greatest in wealthier households and in urban areas, underscoring significant disparities in child mortality.

- Between 1990 and 2005, no WHO region achieved a decline in maternal mortality at a rate sufficient to meet the MDG goals and in some regions the situation stagnated or worsened. Among all health indicators, maternal mortality shows the greatest disparity between the richer and the poorer, both between and within countries.

- Several countries are on course to meet the MDG targets for reduction of malaria burden. However, availability of insecticide-treated mosquito nets and access to treatment are inadequate almost everywhere.

- Incidence rates of tuberculosis continued to decline, as did the prevalence of all tuberculosis cases. The case detection rate of new smear-positive tuberculosis also improved globally. However, multidrug-resistant tuberculosis and HIV-associated tuberculosis continued to be serious challenges, with a large proportion of all multidrug-resistant tuberculosis cases globally concentrated in only a few countries.

- There has been a reduction in new HIV infections and expansion of preventive interventions and availability of treatment and care globally. However, there were regional disparities in availability of treatment.

- Use of "improved" drinking water sources increased from 77% of the world's population in 1990 to 87% in 2008. However, there were regional variations, with the WHO Africa region lagging behind others.

Beaglehole and Bonita (2008) portrayed the state of global public health by identifying five key areas for the global health agenda and assessing the response of global public health to each area. The areas were: (1) maternal, newborn, and child health; (2) infectious diseases; (3) chronic non-communicable diseases; (4) global environmental changes; and (5) SDH. Global public health responses were assessed along four dimensions: (1) leadership; (2) infrastructure; (3) evidence for action based on availability of data and cost-effective intervention; and (4) the health systems' response. In their opinion, global leadership – in terms of both advocacy and inclusion in the agenda – fully met the criteria of success in the child health component of the maternal, newborn, and child health area and the infectious disease area. There was evidence of advocacy in other areas, but none was firmly in the global public health agenda. In the infrastructure dimension, financial resources met the criteria in maternal, newborn, and child health and infectious disease areas; human resources were deficient in all five areas. Availability for evidence for action fully or partially met criteria for success in most areas, although the areas of global environmental changes and SDH were lacking in feasible cost-effective interventions. The health systems' response – in terms of both strengthening of the system to give attention to the area and integration into the national health plan – partially met the criteria of success in maternal, newborn, and child health and the infectious disease areas and did not meet criteria in any other area. The assessment once again demonstrated that, despite success in some areas, there is substantial room for improvement in the global public health response to global health issues.

In addition to the specific diseases and issues identified above, there are several major challenges related to health that are global in scope, have potentially global implications, or affect a significant portion of the world's population.

Disparities

The foremost challenging issue in global health today is perhaps none other than health disparities between and within countries along various dimensions. Some of those dimensions were outlined in the discussion of achievements in health-related MDGs above. The global disparity in health is reflected in the fact that 90% of global medical expenditure is spent on diseases comprising 10% of the global burden of diseases (World Health Organization 1999). A widely used indicator of health disparities is life expectancy. Despite dramatic increases in life expectancy at birth worldwide for more than a century, significant disparities exist throughout the world. Life expectancy at birth is 80 years in countries with a high human development index, whereas it is 51 years in countries with a low human development index (United Nations Development Programme 2009). Until recently, HIV/AIDS pushed life expectancy down – to 30 years in some countries in Africa. There are also significant regional and social group differences in life expectancy within both developed and developing countries. For example, while average life expectancy continued to improve in the USA, it stagnated or declined among the worst-off segments of the population in the 1980s and 1990s (Ezzati *et al.* 2008); in Brazil, variation in life expectancy among states has been found to be associated with variations in the degree of income inequality, illiteracy rate, and gross domestic product per capita (Messias 2003). Similar disparities can be found in access to care, chronic disease outcomes, obesity rates, immunization rates, vulnerability to natural disasters, and myriad other issues. At the core of many of these disparities is unequal distribution of income and resources – good social policies and smaller income differences between the rich and the poor, rather than great national wealth, seem to be more important for achieving excellent health (Wilkinson 1996; Commission on Social Determinants of Health 2008).

International aid and local health systems

The increase in interest and attention to global health issues in recent decades has been accompanied by substantial increase in funding for developing nations from both government and private sources in developed nations as well as international agencies. Yet, there is concern that global health efforts are uncoordinated and largely focused on certain high-profile diseases rather than public health, and that development assistance allocations do not match burden of disease and may not reflect priorities in the recipient countries (MacKellar 2005; Garrett 2007). These concerns also reflect the dichotomy between medical relief and health development approaches (also known as the vertical and horizontal approaches respectively) to international health assistance. While the medical relief approach is not driven by considerations of sustainability, it is a major consideration in the health development approach aiming for improved health systems. For many poor countries, provision of adequate levels of health care is not possible without more national and international financial commitments to the health sector. Such commitments are also needed for the long term to improve public health substantially. However, sustainability considerations (and perhaps shorter time horizons) lead development agencies to advocate the cheapest interventions and in turn contribute to maintaining the status quo of inadequate public health funding (Ooms 2006). The medical relief approach aims for disease-specific results, and high level of donor attention to certain high-profile diseases such as HIV/AIDS has possibly diverted attention and displaced aid from other health issues (Shiffman 2007). The major criticism of this approach is that much of the disease-specific aid is delivered outside the recipient countries' planning and budgeting systems, resulting in distortion of the countries' efforts to deal with their problems and leaving little international funding for strengthening developing countries' health care systems (England 2007b). The countries' health systems also suffer because workforce and talent are moved from other health programs to the better-funded disease-specific programs (England 2007a; Garrett 2007). On the other hand, many argue that the direct and indirect effects of disease-focused programs, particularly on economic development and infrastructure, end up helping the counties' health care systems. There is evidence for the argument on each side and the effects are somewhat mixed: in many instances, focus on high-profile diseases has raised awareness for the need of a robust public health system, benefited the basic health infrastructures, and enhanced the overall service delivery capacity of the country's health system; in other situations, it indeed has resulted in workforce and priority shifts as described above (Yu *et al.* 2008). The vertical and horizontal approaches are not necessarily incompatible. There are increasing calls for the recognition that priority disease approaches also need to focus on the vitality of the underlying health system in order to be effective, and to adopt the "diagonal approach" where explicit intervention priorities are used to drive needed improvements into the health care system (Ooms *et al.* 2008; Sepúlveda *et al.* 2006).

Workforce

Health outcomes are closely associated with the quality, size, and distribution of the health workforce. Unfortunately, over a billion people worldwide have limited or no access to the services or advice of health workers (Crisp *et al.* 2008). The *World Health Report 2006* estimated a shortage of 4.3 million health care workers worldwide, with the most acute shortages being in poor countries. There is a critical shortage – workforce density below the threshold necessary for high coverage of essential interventions – in 57 countries and considerable mismatch between workforce density and disease burden globally. For example, 37% of the world's health care workers reside in the region of the Americas, which has only 10% of the global disease burden, whereas Africa, with 24% of the global disease burden, has only 3% of the global health workforce. There is also geographical maldistribution with a disproportionately higher concentration of health care workers in urban and wealthier areas in many countries. Many factors, including the global rise of chronic diseases, aging of the population, poor local conditions, and migration, are responsible for the health worker crisis. Although migration of health workers takes place within countries, regionally, and across continents, many developing nations, particularly in Africa, are hard hit by "brain drain" to the developed nations. For example, 33% of physicians working in the UK were trained abroad and 23% of the physicians trained in sub-Saharan African countries work abroad. Notwithstanding the enormous variations among countries, health profession education institutions are not producing enough graduates to meet the worldwide need for health workers (World Health Organization 2006). Almost all countries have shortages and skill imbalances in their health workforce – many due to lack of capacity and resources to train health workers, but many also due to poor planning and inadequate investment in health workforce education (Chen *et al.* 2004; Kuehn 2007). The WHO established the critical shortage threshold at 2.28 health care professionals (physicians, nurses, and midwives) per 1000 population, which may not be attainable by many developing countries without devoting a significantly greater share of their gross national product to health, in some cases as high as 50% (Bossert and Ono 2010). Political commitment of the country's leadership combined with significant national and international long-term funding for education and training and subsequent employment opportunities are necessary for a country to address health workforce shortages (Crisp *et al.* 2008). However, one country's own action may not be sufficient to do this; international cooperation

(McGee *et al.* 2005), including treaties and actions to address the dynamics of global labor markets affecting health workers, is needed (World Health Organization 2006).

Urbanization

Currently more than half of the world's population lives in urban areas and the proportion is expected to grow to 70% by the year 2050 (World Health Organization 2010b). Rapid urbanization is posing unique health challenges and reshaping the population health picture in many parts of the world. "Health challenges particularly evident in cities relate to water, environment, violence and injury, noncommunicable diseases (cardiovascular diseases, cancers, diabetes and chronic respiratory diseases), unhealthy diets and physical inactivity, harmful use of alcohol as well as the risks associated with disease outbreaks" (World Health Organization 2010b, p. 245). More than a billion people – one in every three urban dwellers – live in the trying conditions of slums (United Nations Human Settlements Programme 2006). Urban air pollution is responsible for an estimated 800 000 deaths annually, and in poorer countries urban residents face the double burden of infectious diseases and the chronic diseases associated with urban living – the so-called diseases of modernity (Worldwatch Institute 2006). Poor urban living conditions are associated with the resurgence of diseases such as dengue (Phillips 2008). Built and social environment also affect physical activity and health behaviors; decreased energy expenditure along with increasing availability and consumption of energy-dense foods, a common feature of urban living, has contributed to the rising rates of obesity, particularly among the socially disadvantaged in many cities of the world (Popkin 2006). Violence and crime are also major urban health challenges in both developing and developed nations. Unabated urbanization in the current pattern will give rise to social, health, and environmental challenges of unprecedented scale. A new approach to urbanization is needed with prevention and amelioration of health impacts of physical, social, and natural environments at the forefront of planning and design of cities.

Overweight and obesity

An estimated 1 billion adults worldwide are overweight, with at least 300 million among them obese. As a major risk factor for chronic diseases such as type 2 diabetes, cardiovascular disease, and certain forms of cancer, the increasing global prevalence of overweight and obesity has created a significant public health threat (World Health Organization n.d.). The rise in the prevalence of obesity in many western countries has been evident since the early 1980s and it is fast becoming a public health challenge for developing nations as well (Friel *et al.* 2007; James 2008). Rapidly increasing rates of obesity and the metabolic syndrome – a cluster of conditions that increase the risk of several chronic diseases – are evident in both adults and children in the developing countries, many of which are still also dealing with undernutrition (Kelishadi 2007; Misra and Khurana 2008). The recent trend toward increased obesity and non-communicable diseases is the reflection of "nutrition transition" characterized by a shift towards an increasingly energy-dense and sweeter diet, the replacement of high-fiber foods by processed versions, and reduced energy expenditure at work, during travel, at leisure, and at home (Popkin 2006). A multisectoral and integrated approach with the involvement of non-health sectors such as trade, education, agriculture, and urban planning at local, national, and international levels is needed to address this issue since most of the interconnected determinants of overweight and obesity lie outside the scope and capabilities of the health sector (Friel *et al.* 2007).

Emerging infectious diseases

The Institute of Medicine defines emerging infectious diseases as "diseases of infectious origin whose incidence in humans has increased within the past two decades or threatens to increase in the near future" (Institute of Medicine 1992). In the recent past, increase in the incidence of several new infectious diseases and re-emergence of some diseases previously thought to be eradicated or controlled have become global health threats. A closely related concern is the development and spread of microorganisms resistant to antimicrobial agents. Drug-resistant infections have increased in both frequency and scope in recent decades, resulting in increased morbidity, mortality, and health care costs in many parts of the world. Increased global travel and trade, migration, internal displacement of populations, urban crowding, poverty, and poor sanitation are among the factors that facilitate transmission of microorganisms or provide conditions conducive to spread of infection: the ability of the organisms to adapt to new environments and replicate, incorrect use and misuse of antibiotics, and incomplete drug regimens are key contributors to drug resistance (Kombe and Darrow 2001). The growing trend of medical tourism has also increased the risk of global transmission of infections (Kumarasamy *et al.* 2010). Recent experiences with emerging infectious diseases such as H5N1 influenza, H1N1 influenza, SARS, and West Nile virus are vivid reminders of the world's collective vulnerability to pandemic diseases and the global nature of these threats. The speed and frequency of global travel today mean that disease-causing agents can spread globally faster than ever before. The majority of emerging infectious diseases are caused by organisms of non-human animal origin and the interface between humans and animals plays an important role in the emergence process (Jones *et al.* 2008;

Pike *et al.* 2010). Experts consider the ability of current global disease surveillance systems to be inadequate to identify emergent diseases early and highlight the fact that, although disease surveillance systems are robust in industrialized nations, such systems are weak in developing nations from where most of the recent diseases have emerged (Institute of Medicine and National Research Council 2009). The majority of nations also lack the capacity to handle a pandemic (Garrett 2005). With the current global disease control efforts focused mostly on responding to the global spread of pandemics, it is imperative that attention is refocused on developing systems to prevent pandemics before they become established (Pike *et al.* 2010). Socioeconomic, environmental, and ecological factors correlated with origins of emerging infectious diseases can provide important indications about regions predisposed to disease emergence, and surveillance and research efforts should be focused on those "hotspots" (Jones *et al.* 2008). As with many other global health issues, multisectoral cooperation at local, national, and international levels in research, surveillance, prevention, and intervention is needed to address this threat.

United Nations Educational, Scientific and Cultural Organization (UNESCO)

UNESCO is a component of the United Nations that has developed significant policy statements on bioethics and human rights. Bioethics and human rights statements can be found at: http://www.unesco.org/new/en/social-and-human-sciences/themes/bioethics/bioethics-and-human-rights/; http://www.unesco.org/new/en/social-and-human-sciences/themes/bioethics/; and http://www.unesco.org/new/en/social-and-human-sciences/themes/global-ethics-observatory/.

Ethical imperative

As one would expect, the complex, multifactorial, and multisectoral nature of global health issues, the multitude of stakeholders involved, the multifarious competing and overlapping interests, and the myriad approaches to these issues give rise to many ethical and moral dilemmas. The ethical challenges are also often complex and encompass competing values. In other instances, there may be broad agreement on the importance of an issue, yet divergent perspectives on how to address that. Perhaps the most prominent moral challenge in global health today is health disparity. The discussions on determinants of health in this chapter highlight the enormous political, social, and structural changes and the degree of cooperation at local, national, and global levels necessary to achieve equity. Yet, there is no consensus on the basis of equity – is it equity of health outcomes or equity of capability for good health?

What is the appropriate measure for either of these? Should there be a minimum threshold for determining inequality? What is considered just and fair also varies by moral perspectives, societal values, and political ideologies. Often, parties or issues involved in a problem have competing moral claims. Is it acceptable to pursue other valuable social needs such as construction of dams or irrigation projects when there might be negative public health consequences? Is it acceptable to restrict health professionals' migration citing regional or national interest? Is it morally justified for developed countries to recruit health care workers internationally and consequently strain the health care systems of poor countries? Is medical tourism acceptable when development of such a sector might compromise the capacity of the health care system available to the population of the host country? Many similar questions can be asked about competing interests in global health. Power imbalances between and within countries and influences of powerful interests also raise ethical concerns from the global health perspective. The medical research agenda is increasingly influenced by the interests of powerful nations and market forces and has a profound impact on health services worldwide. Most medical research is focused on diseases and conditions afflicting only a small minority of the world's population. Many new discoveries have the potential to increase disparity by benefiting only the privileged minority (Benatar 2000). There also seems to be a tendency to prefer the acquisition of new knowledge over appropriate use of existing knowledge (Trouiller *et al.* 2002). In global health research funding too, the interests of donor nations and organizations rather than the impact of the new knowledge seem to dictate allocations. Globalization of trade has put the corporate interests of transnational companies at odds with population health interests of many countries, as seen in the global spread of tobacco and "junk food" markets or debates surrounding intellectual property rights over pharmaceutical products in recent times. As the influence of global forces on health continues to grow and there is recognition that development aid is necessary but not sufficient to improve global health, the need for ethical values to guide actions for addressing global health issues is paramount.

Indeed, ethical claims is a powerful tool mobilizing support for global health actions and holding the parties involved accountable for achieving common goals (Ruger 2006). Alkire and Chen (2004) described four major moral positions commonly used in global health initiatives (reprinted from Alkire S, Chen L (2004). Global health and moral values. *Lancet* 364: 1069–1074, with permission from Elsevier):

- Humanitarianism: It is the most common ethical basis of global health action in which "people respond to human suffering and realize human fulfillment by acting in a virtuous manner based on compassion" (p. 1070). This approach does not address underlying structural issues responsible for the problems and may be more appropriate for catastrophic situations.

- Utilitarianism: In this approach, valuation of health is on the basis of the utility it creates for an individual. Therefore, it is a good framework for underscoring the effects of improving the health of the deprived on other utility-generating states and the aggregate utility of the society. The limitation of this approach, however, is in the difficulties in measuring and aggregating utilities and the lack of direct sensitivity to distributional concerns.

- Equity: In this approach, the ethical assessment is done on the basis of distributional characteristics of the variable of interest. In the recent health equity discourse, one prominent question is whether equity in the means or in the ends is desirable. Nobel laureate Amartya Sen (2002) has argued that health capabilities and achievements, not health care activities, should form the basis of health equity evaluations and thus be informed by equitable social processes that expand conditions under which individuals have the freedom to choose healthier life strategies.

- Rights: This approach is rooted in the concept of fundamental human rights – entitlement to certain inalienable rights merely because of one's existence as a human being. The modern conception of human rights is captured in the Universal Declaration of Human Rights adopted by the United Nations (UN) General Assembly in 1948 and several subsequent UN declarations. Conferral of rights also invokes duties and obligations on the part of others. A right to a minimum level of health necessary for maintaining human dignity is assumed in this perspective.

According to Alkire and Chen (2004), no single school of moral values dominates global health actions, and oftentimes several schools are relevant to a particular initiative. They argue that, while consensus on the central moral value behind a particular initiative may not be attainable or practicable and everyone should not have to agree on one ethical justification for global health, ethical analyses should be conducted to "clarify what, which, and how global health initiatives can best proceed" (p. 1074). Others have however called for the development of global health ethics:

> a set of values that combines genuine respect for dignity of all people with a desire to promote the idea of human development beyond that conceived within the narrow individualistic "economic" model of human flourishing . . . extend beyond the rhetoric of human rights to include greater attention to duties, social justice, and interdependence (Benatar *et al.* 2003, p. 108).

Nevertheless, strong global governance rooted in clear ethical values is needed to face the global health challenges.

Discussion questions

1   What limitations should be placed on travel for individuals with drug-resistant strains of tuberculosis? If you suggest limitations, how can this be ethically justified?
2   What health policies should be instituted at macro and micro levels to deal with the convergence of diabetes and obesity that is of epidemic proportions globally?
3   Of the five descriptors of global health presented early in this chapter, which is the most significant in your view? Why?
4   What are your views on the current time in history assessed as a time of "globalization"?
5   Thomas Friedman's *The World is Flat* suggests that the current state of mobility allows for an "equaling of the playing field" for individuals in differing parts of the world. Do you feel that health and health resources are equally available globally? If so, why?
6   How can the physical environment positively and negatively impact health policies?
7   How will the BP Gulf of Mexico oil disaster impact global health and global health policy?
8   What health policy impacts can positively influence global efforts, enhancing health promotion?
9   How can international trade agreements dealing with pharmaceutical products influence health policies from one part of the world to other parts?
10   What influence can global mobility have upon health care systems in developing countries?

References

Alkire S, Chen L (2004). Global health and moral values. *Lancet* 364: 1069–1074.
Beaglehole R, Bonita R (2008). Global public health: a scorecard. *Lancet* 372: 1988–1996.
Beaglehole R, Bonita R (2010). What is global health? *Global Health Action* 3: 5142.
Benatar SR (2000). Human rights in the biotechnology era: a story of two lives and two worlds. In: Bhatia GS, O'Neil JS, Gall GL, *et al.* (eds) *Peace, Justice and Freedom: Human Rights Challenges in the New Millennium*. Edmonton: University of Alberta Press, pp. 245–257.
Benatar SR, Daar AS, Singer PA (2003). Global health ethics: The rationale for mutual caring. *Int Affairs* 79: 107–138.
Bossert TJ, Ono T (2010). Finding affordable health workforce targets in low-income nations. *Health Affairs* 29: 1376–1382.
Chanda R (2001). Trade in health services. *Bull W H O* 80: 158–163.
Chen L, Evans T, Anand S, *et al.* (2004). Human resources for health: overcoming the crisis. *Lancet* 364: 1984–1990.
Commission on Social Determinants of Health (2008). *Closing the Gap in a Generation: Health Equity Through Action on the Social Determinants of Health*. Geneva: World Health Organization.

Crisp N, Gawanas B, Sharp I, *et al.* (2008). Training the health workforce: scaling up, saving lives. *Lancet* 371: 689–691.

De Blij HJ (2009). *The Power of Place: Geography, Destiny, and Globalization's Rough Landscape.* New York: Oxford University Press.

England R (2007a). Are we spending too much on HIV? *Br Med J* 334: 344.

England R (2007b). The dangers of disease specific aid programmes. *Br Med J* 335: 565.

Ezzati M, Friedman AB, Kulkarni SC, *et al.* (2008). The reversal of fortunes: Trends in county mortality and cross-county mortality disparities in the United States. *PLOS Med* 5: 4.

Fidler DP (2001). The globalization of public health: the first 100 years of international health diplomacy. *Bull W H O* 79: 842–849.

Friedman TL (2005). *The World is Flat.* New York: Picador.

Friel S, Chopra M, Satcher D (2007). Unequal weight: quality oriented policy responses to the global obesity epidemic. *Br Med J* 335: 1241–1243.

Garrett L (2005). The next pandemic? *Foreign Affairs* 84: 3–23.

Garrett L (2007). The challenge of global health. *Foreign Affairs* 86: 14–38.

Huynen MM, Martens P, Hilderink HB (2005). The health impacts of globalisation: a conceptual framework. *Global Health* 1: 14.

Institute of Medicine (1992). *Emerging Infections: Microbial Threats to Health in the United States.* Washington, DC: National Academy Press.

Institute of Medicine and National Research Council (2009). *Sustaining Global Surveillance and Response to Emerging Zoonotic Diseases.* Washington, DC: National Academies Press.

James WP (2008). The epidemiology of obesity: the size of the problem. *J Intern Med* 263: 336–352.

Jenkins R (2004). Globalization, production, employment and poverty: debates and evidence. *J Int Dev* 16: 1–12.

Jones KE, Patel NG, Levy MA, *et al.* (2008). Global trends in emerging infectious diseases. *Nature* 451: 990–993.

Kelishadi R (2007). Childhood overweight, obesity, and the metabolic syndrome in developing countries. *Epidemiol Rev* 29: 62–76.

Kombe GC, Darrow DM (2001). Revisiting emerging infectious diseases: The unfinished agenda. *J Commun Health* 26: 113–122.

Koplan JK, Bond TC, Merson MH, *et al.* (2009). Towards a common definition of global health. *Lancet* 373: 1993–1995.

Kuehn BM (2007). Global shortage of health workers, brain drain stress developing countries. *JAMA* 298: 1853–1855.

Kumarasamy KK, Toleman MA, Walsh TR, *et al.* (2010). Emergence of a new antibiotic resistance mechanism in India, Pakistan, and the UK: a molecular, biological, and epidemiological study. *Lancet Infect Dis* 10: 597–602.

Labonté R, Schrecker T (2007). Globalization and social determinants of health: introduction and methodological background (part 1 of 3). *Global Health* 3: 5.

Lee K (2000). The impact of globalization on public health: implications for the UK faculty of Public Health Medicine. *J Public Health Med* 22: 253–262.

MacKellar L (2005). Priorities in global assistance for health, AIDS, and population. *Population Dev Rev* 31: 293–312.

McKee M, Gilmore AB, Schwalbe N (2005). International cooperation and health. Part I: issues and concepts. *J Epidemiol Commun Health* 59: 628–631.

Messias E (2003). Income inequalty, illiteracy rate, and life expectancy in Brazil. *Am J Public Health* 93: 1294–1296.

Misra A, Khurana L (2008). Obesity and the metabolic syndrome in developing countries. *J Clin Endocrinol Metab* 93: s9–s30.

Ooms G (2006). Health development versus medical relief: The illusion versus the irrelevance of sustainibility. *PLoS Med* 3: e345.

Ooms G, Van Damme W, Baker BK, *et al.* (2008). The 'diagonal' approach to Global Fund financing: a cure for the broader malaise of health systems? *Global Health* 4: 6.

Phillips ML (2008). Dengue reborn: widespread resurgence of a resilient vector. *Environ Health Perspect* 116: A382–A388.

Pike BL, Saylors KE, Fair JN, *et al.* (2010). The origin and prevention of pandemics. *Clin Infect Dis* 50: 1636–1640.

Popkin BM (2006). Global nutrition dynamics: the world is shifting rapidly toward a diet linked with noncommunicable diseases. *Am J Clin Nutr* 84: 289–298.

Ruger JP (2006). Ethics and governance of global health inequalities. *J Epidemiol Commun Health* 60: 998–1003.

Sen AK (2002). Why health equity? *Health Econ* 11: 659–666.

Sepúlveda J, Bustreo F, Tapia R, *et al.* (2006). Improvement of child survival in Mexico: the diagonal approach. *Lancet* 368: 2017–2027.

Shiffman J (2007). Has donor prioritization of HIV/AIDS displaced aid for other health issues? *Health Policy Planning* 23: 95–100.

Sibai AM (2004). Mortality certification and cause-of-death reporting in developing countries. *Bull W H O* 82: 83.

Solar O, Irwin A (2007). *A Conceptual Framework for Action on the Social Determinant of Health.* Geneva: World Health Organization.

Stuckler D, McKee M (2008). Five metaphors about global-health policy. *Lancet* 372: 95–97.

Trouiller P, Olliaro P, Torreele E, *et al.* (2002). Drug development for neglected diseases: a deficient market and a public-health policy failure. *Lancet* 359: 2188–2194.

United Nations Development Programme (2009). *Human Development Report 2009.* New York: Palgrave Macmillan.

United Nations Human Settlements Programme (2006). *The State of the World's Cities Report 2006/2007.* London: Earthscan.

US Department of Health and Human Services (2000). *Healthy People 2010.* Washington, DC: US Government Printing Office.

Wilkinson RG (1996). *Unhealthy Societies: The Affllictions of Inequality.* New York: Routledge.

Woodward D, Drager N, Beaglehole R, *et al.* (2001). Globalization and health: a framework for analysis and action. *Bull W H O* 79: 875–881.

World Health Organization (n.d.). *Obesity and Overweight.* Available online at: http://www. who.int/dietphysicalactivity/media/en/gsfs_obesity.pdf (accessed 15 August 2010).

World Health Organization (1999). *Investing in Health Research and Development: Report of the ad hoc Committee on Health Research Relating to Future Intervention Options.* Geneva: WHO.

World Health Organization (2006). *The World Health Report 2006: Working Together for Health.* Geneva: World Health Organization.

World Health Organization (2010a). *World Health Statistics 2010.* Geneva: WHO.

World Health Organization (2010b). Urbanization and health. *Bull W H O* 88: 245–246.

Worldwatch Institute (2006). *State of the World 2007: Our Urban Future.* New York: WW Norton.

Yu D, Souteyrand Y, Banda MA, *et al.* (2008). Investment in HIV/AIDS programs: Does it help strengthen health systems in developing countries? *Global Health* 4: 8.

Zimmet P, Magliano D, Matsuzawa Y, *et al.* (2005). The metabolic syndrome: A global public health problem and a new definition. *J Atherosclerosis Thrombosis* 12: 295–300.

Further reading

Bornemisza O, Ranson MK, Poletti TM, *et al.* (2010). Promoting health equity in conflict-affected fragile states. *Soc Sci Med* 70: 80–88.

Brunk KH (2010). Exploring origins of ethical company/brand perceptions – A consumer perspective of corporate ethics. *J Bus Res* 63: 255–262.

du Toit LC, Pillay V, Choonara YE (2010). Nano-microbicides: Challenges in drug delivery, patient ethics and intellectual property in the war against HIV/AIDS. *Adv Drug Del Rev* 62: 532–546.

Gilley KM, Robertson CJ, Mazur TC (2010). The bottom-line benefits of ethics code commitment. *Bus Horizons* 53: 31–37.

Gostin L (2010). The unconscionable health gap: A global plan for justice. *Lancet* 375: 1504–1505.

Hanlon P, Carlisle S, Reilly D, *et al.* (2010). Enabling well-being in a time of radical change: Integrative public health for the 21st century. *Public Health* 124: 305–312.

Macaluso M, Wright-Schnapp TJ, Chandra A, *et al.* (2010). A public health focus on infertility prevention, detection, and management. *Fertil Steril* 93: 16.e1–16.e10.

Martin Hilber A, Hull TH, Preston-Whyte E, *et al.* (2010). A cross cultural study of vaginal practices and sexuality: Implications for sexual health. *Soc Sci Med* 70: 392–400.

Milstien JB, Kaddar M (2010). The role of emerging manufacturers in access to innovative vaccines of public health importance. *Vaccine* 28: 2115–2121.

Numminen OH, Leino-Kilpi H, von der Arend A, *et al.* (2010). Nurse educators' teaching of codes of ethics. *Nurse Educ Today* 30: 124–131.

Pike IL, Straight B, Oesterle M, *et al.* (2010). Documenting the health consequences of endemic warfare in three pastoralist communities of northern Kenya: A conceptual framework. *Soc Sci Med* 70: 45–52.

Razzouk D, Sharan P, Gallo C, *et al.* (2010). Scarcity and inequity of mental health research resources in low-and-middle income countries: A global survey. *Health Policy* 94: 211–220.

Warren A, Bell M, Budd L (2010). Airports, localities and disease: Representations of global travel during the H1N1 pandemic. *Health Place* 16: 727–735.

Wieser B (2010). Public accountability of newborn screening: Collective knowing and deciding. *Soc Sci Med* 70: 926–933.

Yip WC, Hsiao W, Meng Q, *et al.* (2010). Realignment of incentives for health-care providers in china. *Lancet* 375: 1120–1130.

10

Key policy issues

Introduction

Health policy decisions based upon regulatory guideline interpretation have had a profound influence on the US health care system and subcomponents. This is not a uniquely American phenomenon: differing and sometimes similar regulations passed through health policy influences have altered health care delivery elsewhere in the world as well. This chapter will focus on selected items that have been influenced by health policy-directed legislation or regulations. Each of these has influenced or will influence the manner in which patients use the health care system.

These decisions related to health care delivery and processes and regulations of such are often impacted by numerous groups exerting influence. These groups may or may not be successful, but groups rarely give up and they continue to press an agenda. Table 10.1 gives a timeline of specific US Food and Drug Administration (FDA) (Food and Drug Administration 2010) milestones over more than a century of influence and/or regulatory impacts that were often the result of decades'-long attempts to address a specific health or safety concern from a regulatory standpoint (About FDA 2010).

US Food and Drug Administration

Many of the successes listed in Table 10.1 were the result of health policy efforts aimed at processes or manufactured goods that caused tragic harm. One of the fundamental guiding principles of government is to protect populations from harm. The formation of the FDA was no doubt controversial at the time, and controversy has been an ever present fact for the FDA for over a century. Adulterated and/or misbranded products being marketed on a widespread basis led to the initial passage of the 1906 legislation. Concerns about safety and efficacy led to further passage of legislation after deaths due to inactive substrates that caused lethal consequences, e.g., the elixir of sulfanilamide tragedy. And in the 1960s and 1970s concerns about the lack of information patients were receiving from health professionals or other sources led to the regulatory health policy decision to promote patient package inserts (PPIs) as a remedy for misinformation or lack of information about prescription drugs (Vander Stichele 2004).

Patient package inserts in the USA and elsewhere

Shortly after passage of the 1938 Federal Food, Drug and Cosmetic Act in the USA (Table 10.1), the FDA issued regulations that created "prescription drugs," a class of drugs that could only be prescribed and obtained via a prescription (Temin 1980). Then in 1951, the Kefauver–Harris Drug Amendments were passed to ensure drug efficacy and greater drug safety. For the first time, drug manufacturers were required to prove to the FDA the effectiveness of their products before marketing them. In addition the 1951 amendments further delineated the difference between prescription (or legend) drugs and over-the-counter (OTC) drugs. The legend refers to the requirement that, on the manufacturers' label, the phrase "Rx only" must appear.

The differentiation of prescription drugs (prescribed by physicians and only available via prescription) from OTC drugs allowed manufacturers to focus their marketing efforts on physicians, knowing that physicians would be the gatekeepers for the use of drugs by patients. So, based on this health policy decision to differentiate prescription from OTC products, the whole marketing of pharmaceuticals and focus on the channels of distribution of prescriptions drugs evolved as the clear delineation of OTC and legend (prescription) drugs was codified (Temin 1980).

From the early stages of prescription drug differentiation, the package insert that accompanied the drug was nothing more than the legal document affirming the material approved by the FDA for inclusion in such. This material was not written, nor intended for patient use. Patient information regarding the proper use of medications has always been less than optimum. Physicians, pharmacists, and other health professionals all have been incomplete in properly counseling patients on proper drug use (Javitt *et al.* 2008; Keshishian *et al.* 2008; Storm *et al.* 2008; Donohue *et al.* 2009). The results of this lack of proper counseling on drug use have led to problems of noncompliance, adverse drug reactions and effects, and drug misadventures (Katz 2010). Also, the tragic sequealae of the thalidomide crisis in continental Europe and the UK fostered a need for patient information on a much broader scale to describe drug risks. As seen in Table 10.1, Dr. Frances Kelsey, an FDA medical officer, was largely responsible for keeping the drug thalidomide off the US market.

The lack of adequate information that patients receive about the drugs they take has prompted the federal government to become involved in mandating the provision of information to patients. The Omnibus Budget

Table 10.1 Significant dates in US food and drug law history

Date	Event
1820	Eleven physicians meet in Washington, DC, to establish the US Pharmacopeia, the first compendium of standard drugs for the USA
1848	Drug Importation Act passed by Congress requires US Customs Service inspection to stop entry of adulterated drugs from overseas
1862	President Abraham Lincoln appoints a chemist, Charles M. Wetherill, to serve in the new Department of Agriculture. This was the beginning of the Bureau of Chemistry, the predecessor of the Food and Drug Administration (FDA)
1880	Peter Collier, chief chemist, US Department of Agriculture, recommends passage of a national food and drug law, following his own food adulteration investigations. The bill was defeated, but during the next 25 years more than 100 food and drug bills were introduced in Congress
1883	Dr. Harvey W. Wiley becomes chief chemist, expanding the Bureau of Chemistry's food adulteration studies. Campaigning for a federal law, Dr. Wiley is called the "crusading chemist" and "father of the pure Food and Drugs Act." He retired from government service in 1912 and died in 1930
1902	The Biologics Control Act is passed to ensure purity and safety of serums, vaccines, and similar products used to prevent or treat diseases in humans
1906	The original Food and Drugs Act is passed by Congress on June 30 and signed by President Theodore Roosevelt. It prohibits interstate commerce in misbranded and adulterated foods, drinks, and drugs. The Meat Inspection Act is passed the same day. Shocking disclosures of insanitary conditions in meat-packing plants, the use of poisonous preservatives and dyes in foods, and cure-all claims for worthless and dangerous patent medicines were the major problems leading to the enactment of these laws
1911	In US v. Johnson, the Supreme Court rules that the 1906 Food and Drugs Act does not prohibit false therapeutic claims but only false and misleading statements about the ingredients or identity of a drug
1912	Congress enacts the Sherley Amendment to overcome the ruling in US v. Johnson. It prohibits labeling medicines with false therapeutic claims intended to defraud the purchaser, a standard difficult to prove Mrs Winslow's soothing syrup for teething and colicky babies, unlabeled yet laced with morphine, kills many infants
1914	The Harrison Narcotic Act requires prescriptions for products exceeding the allowable limit of narcotics and mandates increased record-keeping for physicians and pharmacists who dispense narcotics
1933	The FDA recommends a complete revision of the obsolete 1906 Food and Drugs Act. The first bill is introduced into the Senate, launching a 5-year legislative battle
1937	Elixir of sulfanilamide, containing the poisonous solvent diethylene glycol, kills 107 persons, many of whom are children, dramatizing the need to establish drug safety before marketing and to enact the pending food and drug law

(continued overleaf)

Date	Event
Table 10.1 *(continued)*	
1938	The Federal Food, Drug, and Cosmetic Act of 1938 is passed by Congress, containing new provisions: • requiring new drugs to be shown safe before marketing – starting a new system of drug regulation • eliminating the Sherley Amendment requirement to prove intent to defraud in drug-misbranding cases • providing that safe tolerances be set for unavoidable poisonous substances • authorizing factory inspections • adding the remedy of court injunctions to the previous penalties of seizures and prosecutions Under the Wheeler–Lea Act, the Federal Trade Commission is charged with overseeing advertising associated with products otherwise regulated by the FDA, with the exception of prescription drugs
1945	Penicillin amendment requires FDA testing and certification of safety and effectiveness of all penicillin products. Later amendments extended this requirement to all antibiotics. In 1983 such control was found to be no longer needed and was abolished
1950	In Alberty Food Products Co. v. US, a court of appeals rules that the directions for use on a drug label must include the purpose for which the drug is offered. Therefore, a worthless remedy cannot escape the law by not stating the condition it is supposed to treat
1951	Durham–Humphrey Amendment defines the kinds of drugs that cannot be safely used without medical supervision and restricts their sale to prescription by a licensed practitioner
1962	Thalidomide, a new sleeping pill, is found to have caused birth defects in thousands of babies born in western Europe. News reports on the role of Dr. Frances Kelsey, FDA medical officer, in keeping the drug off the US market, arouse public support for stronger drug regulation
1962	Kefauver–Harris Drug Amendments passed to ensure drug efficacy and greater drug safety. For the first time, drug manufacturers are required to prove to the FDA the effectiveness of their products before marketing them
1965	Drug Abuse Control Amendments are enacted to deal with problems caused by abuse of depressants, stimulants, and hallucinogens
1966	FDA contracts with the National Academy of Sciences/National Research Council to evaluate the effectiveness of 4000 drugs approved on the basis of safety alone between 1938 and 1962
1968	FDA Bureau of Drug Abuse Control and Treasury Department Bureau of Narcotics are transferred to the Department of Justice to form the Bureau of Narcotics and Dangerous Drugs, consolidating efforts to police traffic in abused drugs The FDA forms the Drug Efficacy Study Implementation to implement recommendations of the National Academy of Sciences investigation of effectiveness of drugs first marketed between 1938 and 1962
1970	The FDA requires the first patient package insert: oral contraceptives must contain information for the patient about specific risks and benefits
1972	Over-the-Counter Drug Review begun to enhance the safety, effectiveness, and appropriate labeling of drugs sold without prescription

(continued overleaf)

Date	Event
1982	Tamper-resistant Packing Regulations issued by FDA to prevent poisonings such as deaths from cyanide placed in Tylenol capsules. The Federal Anti-Tampering Act, passed in 1983, makes it a crime to tamper with packaged consumer products
1983	Orphan Drug Act passed, enabling the FDA to promote research and marketing of drugs needed for treating rare diseases
1984	Drug Price Competition and Patent Term Restoration Act expedites the availability of less costly generic drugs by permitting the FDA to approve applications to market generic versions of brand-name drugs without repeating the research done to prove them safe and effective. At the same time, the brand-name companies can apply for up to 5 years' additional patent protection for the new medicines they developed to make up for time lost while their products were going through the FDA approval process
1988	The Prescription Drug Marketing Act bans the diversion of prescription drugs from legitimate commercial channels. Congress finds that the resale of such drugs leads to the distribution of mislabeled, adulterated, subpotent, and counterfeit drugs to the public. The new law requires drug wholesalers to be licensed by the states; restricts reimportation from other countries; and bans the sale, trade, or purchase of drug samples, and traffic or counterfeiting of redeemable drug coupons
1992	Generic Drug Enforcement Act imposes debarment and other penalties for illegal acts involving abbreviated drug applications Prescription Drug User Fee Act requires drug and biologics manufacturers to pay fees for product applications and supplements, and other services. The Act also requires the FDA to use these funds to hire more reviewers to assess applications
1993	A consolidation of several adverse reaction reporting systems is launched as MedWatch, designed for voluntary reporting of problems associated with medical products to be filed with the FDA by health professionals
1994	FDA announces it could consider regulating nicotine in cigarettes as a drug, in response to a Citizen's Petition by the Coalition on Smoking OR Health Uruguay Round Agreements Act extends the patent terms of US drugs from 17 to 20 years
1995	FDA declares cigarettes to be "drug delivery devices." Restrictions are proposed on marketing and sales to reduce smoking by young people. A series of proposed reforms to reduce the regulatory burden on pharmaceutical manufacturers is announced, including an expansion of allowable promotional material on approved uses of drugs that firms can distribute to health professionals, streamlining certain elements in the documentation of investigational drug studies, and a reduction in both environmental impact filings and preapproval requirements in tablet manufacture
1997	Food and Drug Administration Modernization Act reauthorizes the Prescription Drug User Fee Act of 1992 and mandates the most wide-ranging reforms in agency practices since 1938. Provisions include measures to accelerate review of devices, regulate advertising of unapproved uses of approved drugs and devices, and regulate health claims for foods
1999	ClinicalTrials.gov is founded to provide the public with updated information on enrollment in federally and privately supported clinical research, thereby expanding patient access to studies of promising therapies A final rule mandates that all over-the-counter drug labels must contain data in a standardized format. These drug facts are designed to provide the patient with easy-to-find information, analogous to the nutrition facts label for foods

(continued overleaf)

Table 10.1 (continued)	
Date	Event
2000	The US Supreme Court, upholding an earlier decision in Food and Drug Administration v. Brown & Williamson Tobacco Corp. et al. ruled 5–4 that FDA does not have authority to regulate tobacco as a drug. Within weeks of this ruling, FDA revokes its final rule, issued in 1996, that restricted the sale and distribution of cigarettes and smokeless tobacco products to children and adolescents, and that determined that cigarettes and smokeless tobacco products are combination products consisting of a drug (nicotine) and device components intended to deliver nicotine to the body
2003	The Medicare Prescription Drug Improvement and Modernization Act requires, among other elements, that a study be made of how current and emerging technologies can be utilized to make essential information about prescription drugs available to the blind and visually impaired
2004	Deeming such products to present an unreasonable risk of harm, FDA bans dietary supplements containing ephedrine alkaloids based on an increasing number of adverse events linked to these products and the known pharmacology of these alkaloids

Adapted from: http://www.fda.gov/AboutFDA/WhatWeDo/History/Milestones/ucm128305.htm, updated April, 2009. This material is in the public domain and can be freely printed.

Reconciliation Act of 1990 (OBRA '90) guidelines stipulate that certain information should be offered to patients among other tenets. Some pharmacies go above and beyond the minimum requirements specified in these guidelines. Others simply follow the basic letter of the law.

These governmental efforts are not lacking in cause; patients simply do not understand enough about the drugs they take. Efforts to institute mandated PPIs in the 1970s and 1980s were aimed at the lack of patient drug knowledge and receipt of such from health professionals. However, written information alone is not the answer. There needs to be individualized assessment and interventions aimed at particular and specific patient needs. The usual side-effect information that is provided in these leaflets, although it may be useful, is often limited. The worth of these leaflets has been subject to much discussion and analysis. The information is inadequate if the leaflet is all the counseling received about prescriptions. If it complements what has been told verbally by a pharmacist or physician, the written information can be useful supplemental material.

The most useful type of information that patients receive is a combination of verbal and written information (Fincham 1998). Here face-to-face counseling can be augmented by written materials to reinforce the information transmitted verbally.

The important party in this counseling scenario is always the patient. Patients must be ready to hear and read what is meant for them; if they are too busy to wait at the pharmacy to be counseled, a time should be set up with the pharmacist that is more convenient for them. This can be either in person or via the telephone. If medications are dispensed by a mail-order pharmacy, the pharmacy must provide a 1-800 tollfree phone number for patients to call in order to have questions answered. This is a right, and patients should expect no less than all the information necessary, whether in person or via the phone.

One method of attempting to address patient misinformation or the lack of information provided to patients was through providing written information. As indicated in Table 10.1, the first required PPIs were for oral contraceptives in 1970. The 50th anniversary of the approval of the oral contraceptive or "birth control pill" for marketing in the USA (June 23, 1960) has now passed. When the FDA granted approval of the first oral contraceptive to G.D. Searle (Enovid 10 mg), probably over 500 000 women had been prescribed this drug for menstrual irregularities – it was obviously being used off-label as a birth control pill. Searle was granted approval for Enovid 5 mg. When the drug was marketed in the early 1960s, it was widely used, as it has been in succeeding decades. In 1970, a PPI was required for inclusion along with birth control packages for the first time. This regulation was in response to concern about a link between birth control pills and breast cancer. The PPI was to provide consumers with information to allow them to be informed about taking oral contraceptives. Oral contraceptives must contain information for the patient about specific risks and benefits. A PPI had been required for isoproterenol in the late 1960s to explain how to administer the drug. In the late 1970s, the FDA required a PPI for supplemental estrogen products as well.

The then FDA Commissioner, Dr. Jere Goyan, was enmeshed in the controversy surrounding mandatory inclusion of PPIs with all prescriptions dispensed (Goyan 1981). In 1979, and before Goyan became FDA Commissioner, the FDA had decided to mandate PPIs for all prescriptions. This created a backlash from health professionals regarding the suitability of for all patients and for all prescriptions. There was a "feeling" that this mandating of PPIs would somehow damage the patient–provider relationship. Goyan was the face of the FDA and of the PPI controversy. According to Goyan (1981), some felt that the FDA was moving too slowly, some felt the pace of the evaluative process was just right, and others expressed dismay at the requirement for mandatory inclusion of PPIs with prescriptions. The FDA PPI program was halted by President Ronald Reagan from an executive order that required reconsideration of any regulations that might cost at least $100 million, increase product costs, or adversely affect competition.

The controversy surrounding PPIs continued, but as of this date, in the USA and elsewhere, virtually every prescription dispensed is provided along with a leaflet that describes the drug and cautions about side-effects and how to take the product. Further controversy surrounds the print font size of these materials and the perhaps confusing information that they contain. These PPIs are voluntary, but nevertheless widely used. Their inclusion is a result of OBRA '90 patient counseling requirements, discussed in Chapter 1. A curious fact about PPIs and their use is that for the most part the major adoption of PPIs has occurred in continental Europe and the UK, where PPIs have been widely required and used for decades. The research on the rationale for use of PPIs as a means of patient education has largely been based in the USA, where PPIs have been most controversial. Many products in the USA at present are also accompanied by an information section to be provided to patients for patient use, which is voluntary on the part of manufacturers. Liederman (2009) notes that there are perhaps over 200 PPIs in use as of 2002, but distribution of PPIs is only required for two categories of drug products: oral contraceptives and estrogen replacement therapies.

Another FDA program is the risk management plan (RiskMAP). RiskMAPs for selected drugs have been implemented for drugs such as iso-tretinoin, a drug used for severe acne, but one which has severe teratogenic effects when taken by women of child-bearing age. The RiskMAP for isotret-inoin seeks to avoid fetal exposure to the drug through the prevention of pregnancy.

Liederman (2009) presents PPIs as but one health policy, risk management segment of the FDA pertaining to drug products. Other policies pertaining to the closed pharmacy dispensing of clozapine (an atypical antipsychotic agent) restricted who could dispense the drug and requires mandatory blood work for dispensing (a clozapine registry and a "blood for drug" requirement for patient use).

FDA efforts regarding drug importation

According to the FDA (Food and Drug Administration 2010), the Food, Drug and Cosmetic Act states that prescription drugs made in the USA and exported to a foreign country can only be reimported by the drug's original manufacturer. Even when original manufacturers reimport drugs, the drugs must be real, properly handled, and relabeled for sale in the USA if necessary.

Although importing unapproved prescription drugs is illegal, the FDA's guidance on importing prescription drugs for personal use recognizes that there may be circumstances in which the FDA can exercise discretion not to take action against illegal importation (Food and Drug Administration 2010).

The current policy is not a law or a regulation, but serves as guidance for FDA personnel (Food and Drug Administration 2010). The importation of certain unapproved prescription medications for personal use may be allowed in some circumstances if all of these factors apply:

- if the intended use is for a serious condition for which effective treatment may not be available domestically
- if the product is not considered to represent an unreasonable risk
- if the individual seeking to import the drug affirms in writing that it is for the use of the patient and provides the name and address of the US-licensed doctor responsible for his or her treatment with the drug or provides evidence that the drug is for continuation of a treatment begun in a foreign country
- if the product is for personal use and is a 3-month supply or less and not for resale, since larger amounts would lend themselves to commercialization
- if there is no known commercialization or promotion to US residents by those involved in the distribution of the product (Food and Drug Administration 2010).

The health policy implications of use of imported drugs from Canada entered the political realm in the US presidential election of 2008. As long as the same drugs are being sold by the same USA-based pharmaceutical companies in different countries for a price that is less than paid in the USA, reimportation of prescription drugs from Canada and elsewhere will be a political issue.

Plan B emergency contraception

According to the FDA (2006), emergency contraception is a method of preventing pregnancy to be used after a contraceptive fails or after unprotected sex. It is not for routine use. Drugs used for this purpose are called emergency contraceptive pills, postcoital pills, or morning-after pills. Emergency contraceptives contain the hormones estrogen and progestin (levonorgestrel), either separately or in combination. The FDA has approved two products for prescription use for emergency contraception – Preven (approved in 1998) and Plan B (approved in 1999).

According to the FDA (2006):

> Plan B is emergency contraception, a backup method to birth control. It is in the form of two levonorgestrel pills (0.75 mg in each pill) that are taken by mouth after unprotected sex. Levonorgestrel is a synthetic hormone that has been used in birth control pills for over 35 years. Plan B can reduce a woman's risk of pregnancy when taken as directed if she has had unprotected sex. Plan B contains only progestin, levonorgestrel, a synthetic hormone used in birth control pills for over 35 years. It is currently available only by prescription. Plan B works like other birth control pills to prevent pregnancy. Plan B acts primarily by stopping the release of an egg from the ovary (ovulation).

It may prevent the union of sperm and egg (fertilization). If fertilization does occur, Plan B may prevent a fertilized egg from attaching to the womb (implantation). If a fertilized egg is implanted prior to taking Plan B, Plan B will not work.

The FDA received an application to switch Plan B from prescription to non-prescription status in 2002. FDA staff reviewed the scientific data contained in the application which included, among other data, an actual-use study and a label comprehension study. On December 16, 2003, the FDA held a public advisory committee meeting with a panel of medical and scientific experts from outside the federal government. The members of the Nonprescription Drugs Advisory Committee (NDAC) and the Advisory Committee for Reproductive Health met jointly to consider the safety and effectiveness data of non-prescription use of Plan B. The author of this book (JEF) served on the FDA NDAC during this time.

Although the joint committee recommended via a strongly positive vote to the FDA that this product be sold without a prescription, some members of the committee, including the Chair, raised questions concerning whether the actual-use data could be generalized to the overall population of non-prescription users, chiefly because of inadequate sampling of younger age groups.

Following the advisory committee meeting, the FDA requested additional information from the sponsor pertaining to adolescent use (Food and Drug Administration 2006). The sponsor submitted this additional information to the FDA in support of its pending application to change Plan B from a prescription to an OTC product.

Again, according to the FDA (2006):

Now FDA has completed its review of the supplemental application and concluded that the application could not be approved at this time because (1) adequate data were not provided to support a conclusion that young adolescent women can safely use Plan B for emergency contraception without the professional supervision of a licensed practitioner and (2) a proposal from the sponsor to change the requested indication to allow for marketing of Plan B as a prescription-only product for women under 16 years of age and a nonprescription product for women 16 years and older was incomplete and inadequate for a full review. Therefore, FDA concluded that the application was not approvable.

There was a significant level of disagreement within the FDA concerning this issue. Kaufman (2005), in an article in the *Washington Post*, detailed the resignation of a former FDA employee, Susan F. Wood, assistant FDA commissioner for women's health and director of the Office of Women's Health. Dr. Wood in an e-mail to her staff and colleagues at the FDA noted:

I can no longer serve as staff when scientific and clinical evidence, fully evaluated and recommended for approval by the professional staff here, has been overruled (Kaufman 2005).

Although the true facts may never come to light, it was generally assumed that political pressure was exerted via the Executive Branch of the US government to restrict this drug from general availability by pro-life elements. Although this drug is not an abortifacient, it has been portrayed as such. This drug had been approved as a prescription-only product since the late 1990s.

Eventually the FDA (2006) did approve a revised application for OTC availability of Plan B. The US FDA approved Plan B One-Step, a single-dose emergency contraceptive containing levonorgestrel 1.5 mg in a single tablet. The FDA also announced a change in the labeling of Plan B, currently marketed as an emergency contraceptive consisting of two levonorgestrel 0.75 mg tablets taken 12 hours apart. Plan B had been available to women 18 years of age and older without a prescription and to women younger than 18 years of age only by prescription since August 2006.

With the FDA's action, both Plan B One-Step and Plan B will be available without a prescription to women 17 years of age and older. Both will be available for women younger than 17 years of age only by prescription.

OTC children's medication recall 2010, McNeil

In May 2010, McNeil, a division of Johnson & Johnson, initiated a recall of 43 children's and infant liquid formulations of branded OTC products such as Tylenol, Motrin, Zyrtec, and Benadryl. This recall was instituted despite the fact that no injuries or deaths had been connected to the 43 products recalled. The recall came as a result of an FDA inspection of the McNeil plan in Fort Washington, PA, on April 19, 2010. The recall notice stated that affected lots may:

- contain more than the stated concentration amount of active ingredient
- contain inactive ingredients that do not meet quality standards
- contain particulate matter.

This action could not have been possible without Food, Drug and Cosmetic Laws that stipulated that manufacturing plants could be inspected by FDA personnel. Many such inspections have occurred in the decades since these laws have been enacted, challenged, and supported in the legal system. Health policy impacts such as these would not have been possible without the legacy of these laws, passed in the previous century. Also, the FDA recommendation during the 2010 recall to avail use of generic formulations of these products could not have been possible without approval of prescription to OTC switches of many of these products, and subsequent approval of generic manufacturers marketing generic formulations of each of these products. These products are not only sold in the USA, but also in Canada, the Dominican Republic, Dubai, Fiji, Guam, Guatemala, Jamaica, Kuwait, Panama, and Puerto Rico (McNeil Product Recall Information 2010). In instances such as this, if voluntary recalls are not implemented, the FDA does not have the regulatory power to require such recalls.

Further complicating this messy recall is the allegation that a contractor was hired as early as 2008 to buy up lots of ibuprofen liquid, and not tell retailers why, to check for suspected problems, thus circumventing a public relations disaster if this were to appear in the press.

Counterfeit drugs

Fake drugs, or counterfeit drugs, are continuing to emerge as a major public health crisis issue. In January 2010, the World Health Organization (WHO) published an updated newsletter on counterfeit drugs. Within the newsletter the following was presented:

> Counterfeit medicines are medicines that are deliberately and fraudulently mislabelled with respect to identity and/or source.

- Use of counterfeit medicines can result in treatment failure or even death.
- Public confidence in health-delivery systems may be eroded following use and/or detection of counterfeit medicines.
- Both branded and generic products are subject to counterfeiting.
- All kinds of medicines have been counterfeited, from medicines for the treatment of life-threatening conditions to inexpensive generic versions of painkillers and antihistamines.
- Counterfeit medicines may include products with the correct ingredients or with the wrong ingredients, without active ingredients, with insufficient or too much active ingredient, or with fake packaging.

Counterfeit medicines are found everywhere in the world. They range from random mixtures of harmful toxic substances to inactive, ineffective preparations. Some contain a declared, active ingredient and look so similar to the genuine product that they deceive health professionals as well as patients. But in every case, the source of a counterfeit medicine is unknown and its content unreliable. Counterfeit medicines are always illegal. They can result in treatment failure or even death. Eliminating them is a considerable public health challenge (World Health Organization 2010).

Counterfeit medications are not a new phenomenon, but the extent of the problem extends worldwide and potentially affects every citizen globally. Estimates of counterfeit medications as 10% of the drug supply worldwide are simply that – estimates. The scope is much more severe in developing countries, but the true extent is unknown. Incidence may be underestimated by a factor of 50% in actuality.

Precipitating factors may include, but are not limited to, the following:

- The high cost of pharmaceuticals, which leads to attempts at profiteering by unscrupulous and unethical elements in societies.
- There is a large market for counterfeit drugs due to lack of access to legitimate pharmaceuticals by many.
- There may be corruption at high levels of government agencies charged with overseeing the drug use process within and between countries.
- There may be organized crime involvement.
- Restrictive patent laws may favor branded pharmaceutical products.
- Unscrupulous generic manufacturers may seek profits at any cost and not assure consistency and quality standards for substrate products.
- Secondary wholesalers may be gaming the system for profits.
- Unscrupulous health professionals may be exhibiting the worst form of ethical behavior, looking for profits above anything else.

As noted, problems have occurred everywhere. Published reports note the specific toll on India (Chatterjee 2010). Neighboring Pakistan has suffered and the problem has been exacerbated by sectarian violence (Varley 2010). These and other instances (Newton and Green 2010) point to populations with problems compounded by lack of access to health care services. Particularly troubling is the abhorrent targeting of drugs used to treat diseases with specific foci in children (Crawley and Chu 2010). One would not expect counterfeiters to have ethical principles, but this is unconscionable.

The WHO through the International Medical Product Anti-Counterfeit Taskforce has worked to stimulate action against counterfeit medications. Gopakumar and Shashikant (2010), in *Unpacking the Issue of Counterfeit Medicines*, suggest that:

> WHO's approach has resulted in concerns that legitimate generic medicines may get caught up in the web of definitions and enforcement of "counterfeit products," with adverse consequences for access to medicine as well as legitimate trade.

One of the issues Gopakumar and Shashikant (2010) address is the problem of using the term "counterfeit" (in connection with intellectual property rights violations) to refer to products with compromised quality, safety, and efficacy issues against a background of anticounterfeiting initiatives in the context of intellectual property. The concern is that the use of generic drugs may be compromised, or has been compromised, in the context of anticounterfeiting measures.

A contributing factor to the growth in counterfeit medication availability and access has been the internet as a source of sale of counterfeit drugs. In February 2010, the search engine Google changed its policy on advertising internet pharmacies. It refined its advertising model through its search program AdWords to accept only advertisements from online pharmacies in the USA that are accredited by the National Association Boards of Pharmacy's Verified Internet Pharmacy Practice Sites program.

Pseudoephedrine

A discussion of the health policy implications of pseudoephedrine must start with a discussion of methamphetamine. Methamphetamine is a compound that has been around for close to 80 years. It is an amphetamine derivative that was first synthesized by the Germans and used in World War II by the Nazis as a drug to keep pilots awake and alert. The Americans and others have used the drug for this purpose as well. Legitimate uses for methamphetamine include the treatment of narcolepsy, attention deficit disorder, and obesity.

According to the National Institute of Drug Abuse (NIDA) (2006):

> Methamphetamine is a highly addictive central nervous system stimulant that can be injected, snorted, smoked, or ingested orally. Methamphetamine users feel a short yet intense "rush" when the drug is initially administered. The immediate effects of methamphetamine include increased activity and decreased appetite.

> Most amphetamines distributed to the black market are produced in clandestine laboratories. Methamphetamine laboratories are, by far, the most frequently encountered clandestine laboratories in the United States. The ease of clandestine synthesis, combined with tremendous profits, has resulted in significant availability of illicit methamphetamine. Large amounts of methamphetamine are also illicitly smuggled into the United States from Mexico.

According to the 2008 National Survey on Drug Use and Health (Substance Abuse and Mental Health Services Administration 2009), approximately 12.6 million Americans aged 12 or older reported using methamphetamine at least once during their lifetime, representing 5% of the population aged 12 or older. Approximately 850 000 (0.3%) reported past-year methamphetamine use and 314 000 (0.1%) reported past-month methamphetamine use (National Institute on Drug Abuse 2008). Common street names for methamphetamine are listed in Table 10.2.

Methamphetamine is a very addictive drug, and treatment for methamphetamine addiction is difficult to carry through and reach a symptomfree state. Methamphetamine abuse leads to addiction, anxiety, insomnia, mood

Table 10.2 Methamphetamine street names	
Biker's coffee	Methlies quick
Chalk	Poor man's cocaine
Chicken feed	Shabu
Crank	Speed
Crystal meth	Stove top
Glass	Trash
Go-fast	Yellow bam
Ice	

Source: Methamphetamine facts and figures (2010) US Office of National Drug Control Policy, 2010. White House, Washington DC. Available online at: http://www.whitehousedrugpolicy.gov/publications/asp/topics.asp?txtTopicID=8&txtSubTopicID=22 (accessed 21 December 2010).

disturbances, and violent behavior (National Institute on Drug Abuse 2008). Additionally, psychotic symptoms such as paranoia, hallucinations, and delusions (such as the sensation of bugs crawling under the user's skin) can occur and do so frequently. The psychotic symptoms can last for months or years after methamphetamine use has ceased (National Institute on Drug Abuse 2008).

Ephedrine, phenylpropanolamine (now both difficult to obtain as OTC products in the USA), and pseudoephedrine are precursors in the chemical formation of methamphetamine. A methamphetamine "cooker" using the Nazi method (common in the Midwest) brings about this chemical reaction by combining the ephedrine or pseudoephedrine with two other ingredients: anhydrous ammonia (a liquified fertilizer) and lithium (a metal extracted from lithium batteries). A methamphetamine "cooker" using the red-P method produces methamphetamine by combining ephedrine or pseudoephedrine with red phosphorus, iodine crystals, and water. Often a toxic solvent such as acetone or kerosene is used to melt the pseudoephedrine tablets (sugar-coated formulation) into pseudoephedrine. Obviously this melted substrate also contains impurities from the solvent and also the inert ingredients in the pseudoephedrine tablets. Cooking a batch of meth can be very dangerous due to the fact that the chemicals used are volatile and the byproducts are toxic. Methamphetamine laboratories present a danger to the methamphetamine "cooker," the community surrounding the lab, and the law enforcement personnel who discover the laboratory (Office of Community Oriented Policing Services 2002).

The majority of the methamphetamine supply in the USA has been home-made; an increased amount of methamphetamine is also smuggled into the

USA from Mexico by drug cartels. The tremendous increase in gang warfare activity and other armed conflicts along the USA–Mexico border is a result of drug activity and smuggling efforts. As limits on the sale of pseudoephedrine and law enforcement crackdowns have hampered methamphetamine "cooking" operations in the USA, a rise in imported methamphetamine from Mexico and South and Central America has offset this decrease in US production. There has been a 400% decrease in the number of methamphetamine laboratory seizures in the USA from 2002 through 2007 (from over 9000 to 1800) (National Institute on Drug Abuse 2008).

Methamphetamine is a Schedule II narcotic under the Controlled Substances Act, Title II of the Comprehensive Drug Abuse Prevention and Control Act of 1970 (Drug Enforcement Administration 1996). The chemicals that are used to produce methamphetamine are also controlled under the Comprehensive Methamphetamine Control Act of 1996. This legislation broadened the controls on listed chemicals used in the production of methamphetamine, increased penalties for the trafficking and manufacturing of methamphetamine and listed chemicals, and expanded the controls of products containing the licit chemicals ephedrine, pseudoephedrine, and phenylpropanolamine (Drug Enforcement Administration 1996).

As previously noted, three precursor chemicals have been tightly restricted in order to gain a foothold in stemming the illegal manufacture of methamphetamine: ephedrine, phenylpropanolamine, and pseudoephedrine. Ephedrine and phenylpropanolamine are both sympathomimetic amines, used as nasal decongestants. Phenylpropanolamine was also included in some OTC weight loss formulations up until the 1990s. Pseudoephedrine, also a sympathomimetic amine, has been the most widely available and effective nasal decongestant for 50 years. Pseudoephedrine is a drug that has been used for many years to treat nasal and sinus congestion. It has now been restricted to behind-the-counter sale in pharmacies, in a "third class" of drugs, meaning that you have to ask for it specifically from the pharmacy. You will not find it available in non-pharmacy outlets. As described here, pseudoephedrine has received a "bad rap" due to its use as a precursor chemical for the illegal manufacturing or cooking of methamphetamine.

Pseudoephedrine is safe when used as directed. Patients with unstable high blood pressure, hyperthyroidism, diabetes, closed-angle glaucoma, urinary retention, uncontrolled cardiac heart failure, cardiomyopathy, cardiac arrhythmias (tachycardia), or other cardiac disease should not use the drug without physician approval. Patients taking a class of drugs called monoamine oxidase inhibitors for depression should not take pseudoephedrine at all. For the above groupings of patients, the use of a saline nasal spray (Ocean, or a generic equivalent) will sometimes provide relief.

Pseudoephedrine is known to cause excitability in some patients, especially infants and young children. If nervousness, insomnia, or dizziness occurs, discontinue pseudoephedrine and consult a physician. The drug should not be given to infants and young children less than 4 years of age.

Pseudoephedrine is classified as a pregnancy category C drug. No adequate or well-controlled pregnancy studies have been done in humans. Use of pseudoephedrine during pregnancy should be avoided unless the potential benefits outweigh the unknown potential risks to the fetus: this is a decision for the patient and her physician. Pseudoephedrine is excreted into breast milk. The American Academy of Pediatrics has considered the use of pseudoephedrine to be compatible with lactation. Lactating women may want to avoid breast-feeding during times of peak concentrations (i.e., within 1–2 hours of a dose) when possible.

Some pseudoephedrine products contain aspartame and thus contain phenylalanine. Use with caution in those patients with phenylketonuria. For example, Sudafed children's chewable tablets contain phenylalanine 0.78 mg per tablet. There are also many OTC cold and sinus formulas that contain pseudoephedrine and other ingredients: ask your pharmacist what is contained in the products if you are unsure.

From a health policy standpoint, as the products containing pseudoephedrine were moved to a third class of drugs, the formulations of some cold products were reformulated to include a drug called phenylephrine. Phenylephrine in the author's opinion does not work nearly as well as pseudoephedrine when taken orally. When drugs are reformulated in the USA, often the same trade name may be part of the name of the drug, even though the ingredients may have been totally changed.

Abuse of prescription drugs

The US NIDA monitors drug abuse with prescription medications along with illicit drugs of abuse. This abuse of legitimately prescribed medications has emerged as a significant problem in the USA (National Institute on Drug Abuse 2008). The NIDA estimates the numbers of abusers of prescription drugs and the drugs abused:

- In 2006, approximately 7.0 million persons were current users of psychotherapeutic drugs taken non-medically (2.8% of the US population). This class of drugs is broadly described as those targeting the central nervous system, including drugs used to treat psychiatric disorders (Substance Abuse and Mental Health Services Administration 2009).
  - pain relievers: 5.2 million
  - tranquilizers: 1.8 million
  - stimulants: 1.2 million
  - sedatives: 0.4 million

- Abuse of prescription drugs is particularly problematic among adolescents.
  - NIDA's 2007 Monitoring the Future Survey (drugabuse.gov/drugpages/MTF.html) found continued high rates of non-medical use of the prescription pain relievers Vicodin and OxyContin in each grade. In 2007, many 12th grade students reported non-medical use of Vicodin and OxyContin during the past year– 9.6% and 5.2%, respectively.
  - Levels reported remain high. For the past year, non-medical use of amphetamines, 7.5% of 12th graders reported abuse; for Ritalin, 3.8% reported abuse; and for methamphetamine, 1.7% reported abuse.
- It is generally believed that the broad availability of prescription drugs (e.g., via home medicine cabinets, the internet, and willingly prescribing physicians) and misperceptions about their safety make prescription medications particularly prone to abuse.
- Among those who abuse prescription drugs, high rates of other risky behaviors, including abuse of other drugs and alcohol, have also been reported (National Institute on Drug Abuse 2008).

Varying risks associated with prescription drug abuse

The National Institute on Drug Abuse (2008) lists varying risks associated with prescription drug abuse.

Opioids

- High risk for addiction and overdose. This is a major concern, particularly for recently synthesized slow-release formulations, which abusers override by crushing the pills and injecting or snorting the contents, heightening their risk for respiratory depression and death.
- Dangerous combination effects. Combining opioids with other drugs, including alcohol, can intensify effects such as respiratory depression and distress.
- Heightened human immunodeficiency virus (HIV) risk. Injecting opioids increases the risk of HIV and other infectious diseases through the use of unsterile or shared needles and syringes (National Institute on Drug Abuse 2008).

Stimulants

- They have a reputation as performance enhancers. Incorrectly perceived as safe for enhancing academic achievement and weight loss, these drugs are highly addictive and potentially harmful.

- There is a range of risky health consequences, including risk of dangerously high body temperature, seizures, and cardiovascular complications (National Institute on Drug Abuse 2008).

Recent reports have highlighted the use of stimulants such as methylphenidate and Adderall by college-aged students for performance enhancement purposes. This was mentioned above in general, but it is important to focus on this subset of users (Staufer and Greydanus 2005; McCabe and Teter 2007; Ford and Arrastia 2008).

Health policy decisions intended to stem drug abuse of legitimate prescription drugs

Health policy decisions over 70 years have guided how prescriptions are written by physicians, processed by pharmacists, and how patients are able to access prescription medications in the USA. The controls on scheduling of prescriptions into five classes, four of which are eligible for prescribing, dispensing, and access by patients in the USA, have been in place since the 1970s. Originally guided at the federal level by the Bureau of Narcotics and Dangerous Drugs, the agency overseeing this at the federal level is now the Drug Enforcement Agency (DEA). DEA has been stressed the past decade to deal with illicit drug use and availability in the USA. State boards of pharmacy also guide requirements within states pertaining to use of narcotic and non-narcotic scheduled drugs. The federal guidelines regarding the scheduling of these drugs take precedence over state laws pertaining to Schedules I–IV. States may also place certain drugs within Schedule categories as well, e.g., anabolic steroids. Schedule I drugs are used for restricted purposes only; drugs such as peyote, marijuana, and mescaline are in Schedule I.

The limits on refilling prescriptions within Schedules II–V are controlled throughout the USA. Schedule II prescriptions may not be refilled, and there are limits on how the prescriptions are transferred from physicians to pharmacies for filling and dispensing. All of these processes have been guided by health policy decisions. These policies have evolved over time and will continue to evolve in the milieu in which these medications are consumed, and abused perhaps.

Developing countries and health policy needs

The purpose of this section is not to highlight the deficiencies of developing countries from a health policy standpoint, but rather to highlight the issues surrounding developing countries as they may lack health policy constructs that guide health care systems, health professionals, and financing for health care services. The purpose is to focus on how health policy decision-making is so crucial in controlling health care and morbidity and mortality. So, the intent is not to criticize; it is to explore and rejoice in the process of change and the influence of health policy on structures and outcomes of health care.

Vietnam

Vietnam has been in numerous wars over an extended period of time. The Vietnamese were at war with the Chinese for centuries before the war with the French, which ended in 1954 at Dien Bien Phu. The war between Vietnam and the USA lasted through 1975, and after this period, the Vietnamese were at war with the Cambodians and then again with the Chinese. From the end of the Vietnam War in 1975 through 1996, the USA had an embargo in place against Vietnam, which included restrictions on the importation of medicines and pharmaceutical precursors or substrates. Thus the Vietnamese health care system was in a state of flux until the late 1990s.

Vietnam is a developing nation with a rapidly expanding economy and an energetic and engaged workforce. Vietnam is one of the fastest-growing economies in the world, and certainly in Southeast Asia. The Vietnamese spend 5–6% of their gross domestic product on health care (WHO website for Vietnam 2010). This amount is significantly lower than many Asian countries, but higher than others around the world. Laos spends 3.1% and Cambodia spends 11.8%. A total of 25% of this expenditure is in the public sector (WHO website for Vietnam 2010).

The Vietnamese health care system has made recent improvements, and many challenges remain pertaining to health care, health care systems, and health professional involvement. Several improvements in Vietnamese health care practices have produced tangible rewards. Vietnam ranks 116 of 191 WHO organizations in adjusted life expectancy (Adams 2005) (much better than many wealthier countries). There have been significant decreases in infant and under-5 mortality rates. Also, progress has been seen in providing vaccinations for many preventable diseases (measles, diphtheria, and tetanus). Polio was completely eradicated in 1996 (Adams 2005).

Tran (2004) notes the improvements in Vietnamese health care practices. These enhancements have included an emphasis on active prevention at "grassroots" level (communes and health care structures), expansion of privatized medical care, and insurance coverage (1992) (Tran 2004).

The study by Tran (2004) reveals a high level of self-medication, greater access to private than public services, and less use of public services or any health care services by the poor in comparison to those who are better off. Self-funded purchases of drugs for self-medication and use of private curative services were even common in those with health insurance. Finally, the percentage of ill people with no access to any health care providers during their illness episode was high, regardless of their wealth or health insurance status.

The main features of the current rural health care system in Vietnam identified from the community-based evidence found in Tran's (2004) research were: (1) primary health care services are available and there is equality in physical access; (2) financial resources for the Commune Health Center system are diversified, with the Vietnamese government resources the key contributors; (3) there are private health care providers for outpatient services, and public providers for inpatient services; (4) quality of treatment services is below the national standard; (5) public services are available but underutilized; (6) the rural health care system is not a pro-poor system; (7) direct payment is the main component of total health care expenditure; and (8) the economic relationship of the rural health care system is a user–provider model rather than a health care triangular model (e.g., one that would incorporate a health insurance component).

For the initiative, Strategy for People's Health Care and Protection, 2001–2010, specific goals included:

- Improve equality in access to and use of health care services.
- Improve quality of health care services at all levels.
- These goals were very similar to those in the *Healthy People 2010* and *Healthy People 2020* initiatives in the USA.

Specific barriers to effective delivery of health care include:

- an absence of actively enforced drug policy
- incomplete integration of technology
- incomplete coverage of health services under socialized medicine
- absence of formal professional standards for some health care professionals.

A considerable problem for developing countries is the prevalence of smoking by the population; Vietnam is not different in this regard. Four of the top 10 areas with dramatic tobacco consumption increases include: Malaysia, Indonesia, Pakistan, and Vietnam (Mackay and Eriksen 2004). The smoking prevalence in Vietnam is 70% for males and 5% for females. This smoking activity has led to an estimated 40 000 deaths per year. It is projected that 10% of the Vietnamese population will die prematurely due to smoking. The average (annual) salary is $300, and of this, $40 will be spent on cigarettes (Mackay and Eriksen 2004).

Nguyen (1999) has described the pharmacy practice arena in Vietnam. In 1986, and in response to population demands, the Vietnamese government eased restrictions on business operations to allow for private ownership of businesses, including pharmacies in Vietnam. This process of change is called "Doi Moi." Pharmacy in Vietnam is unique in a number of ways. There is a much greater emphasis on the use of herbal agents compared to the western world. Retail pharmacies are not covered under the national program of socialized medicine (Nguyen 1999). Pharmacies are owned by pharmacists, but most pharmacies are not operated under their direct supervision, and as such, drugs are sold without prescriptions, and there is not a requirement for prescriptions to be presented for dispensing to occur. There are no formal record-keeping system or patient profiles in place. Improper drug storage appears to be a large problem. An estimated 90% of drugs dispensed are released without a prescription (Nguyen 1999). An estimated 50% of antibiotics dispensed are dispensed with 2.5 days' supply or less. This has led to antibiotic resistance and exacerbation of symptoms (Larsson *et al.* 2000). There is also not a well-defined system of drug distribution throughout the country; the channels of distribution are imperfectly formed and wholesale to pharmacy distribution of medications and supplies is crude at best.

In Vietnam, the role of a pharmacist is certainly not recognized. The WHO states that "the pharmacist is expected to be a communicator, a quality drug supplier, a trainer and supervisor, a collaborator, and a health promoter." Many professionals and patients are unaware of pharmacists' capabilities (Olsson *et al.* 2002).

Cambodia

In April 2010, news was disseminated that Cambodia had taken action to fight substandard and counterfeit medicines by forcing the closure of upwards of 65% of illegal pharmacy outlets over a 5-month period (United States Pharmacopeia 2010). The evidence gathered to proceed with these forced closures was generated from medicines quality-monitoring activities conducted in Cambodia by the Promoting the Quality of Medicines Program, a US Agency for International Development-funded program implemented by the US Pharmacopeial Convention, with additional support from the Global Fund to Fight AIDS, Tuberculosis, and Malaria and the WHO (United States Pharmacopeia 2010). This recent activity by the Cambodian government has resulted in a reduction of illegal outlets from 1081 in November 2009 to 379 in March 2010, or a 64.9% reduction, according to an April report by the Cambodian Ministry of Health. As part of this effort, the government banned sales of products from five manufacturers in the country (United States Pharmacopeia 2010).

Summary

Health policy decisions are rarely static. Within established health care systems, changes are instituted frequently and are affected by many constituent groups seeking parochial enhancements of delivery systems, financing of health care, or the structure of health care systems. In developing countries, often with rudimentary-functioning health care systems, health policy enactments must often start from scratch. International agencies have proven helpful to developing countries as they seek to enhance the delivery of care to patients almost from ground zero. So, the degree of sophistication of a health care system or the length of time that one has been in place does not obfuscate the need for health policy to play a prominent role in how health care is accessed, delivered, and paid for within countries.

Discussion questions

1   Why did it take so many health crises before the US FDA was formed in the early part of the 20th century?
2   Choose one of the many milestones in the history of the US FDA, and describe why this event had health policy ramifications.
3   Why was the approval of oral contraceptives so controversial in the USA?
4   Similarly, why was the switching of Plan B from prescription to OTC status in the USA so controversial?
5   What would you do as a product manager for a treatment of attention deficit disorder to best position your product within the channels of distribution? How would you as a product manager and a company address the issues surrounding potential abuse of the drug from your company?
6   What health policy enactments can possibly stem the illicit abuse of legitimately prescribed and dispensed medications in the USA?
7   How would you structure the channels of distribution for pharmaceuticals in a developing country?
8   Recently, Cambodia was successful over a 6-month period in closing illegal pharmacy operations. Do you feel this success will continue? How can similar illegal pharmacies be halted before they are in business?
9   What role should international pharmaceutical manufacturers play in health policy formation and deliberations in developing countries?
10 Comment on the ethics of pricing of pharmaceuticals in developing countries.

References

About FDA (2010). Available online at: http://www.fda.gov/AboutFDA/WhatWeDo/History/Milestones/ucm128305.htm (accessed 14 May 2010).

Adams S (2005). *Vietnam's Healthcare System: A Macroeconomic Perspective*. Hanoi, Vietnam: International Monetary Fund.

Chatterjee P (2010). India combats confusion over counterfeit drugs. *Lancet* 375: 542.

Crawley J, Chu C (2010). Malaria in children. *Lancet* 375: 1468–1481.

Donohue JM, Huskamp HA, Wilson IB, *et al.* (2009). Whom do older adults trust most to provide information about prescription drugs? *Am J Geriatr Pharmacother* 7: 105–116.

Drug Enforcement Administration (1996). Office of Diversion Control. Provisions of the Comprehensive Methamphetamine Control Act of 1996. Washington, DC: US Government Printing Office.

Fincham JE (1998). The drug use process. In: Fincham JE, Wertheimer AI (eds) *Pharmacy and the US Health Care System,* 2nd edn. Binghamton, NY: Haworth Press, pp. 395–438.

Food and Drug Administration (2006). Plan B: questions and answers. Available online at: http://www.fda.gov/Drugs/DrugSafety/PostmarketDrugSafetyInformationforPatientsandProviders/ucm109783.htm.

Food and Drug Administration (2010). Resources for you. Available online at: http://www.fda.gov/Drugs/ResourcesForYou/Consumers/ucm143561.htm (accessed 15 May 2010).

Ford JA, Arrastia MC (2008). Pill-poppers and dopers: A comparison of non-medical prescription drug use and illicit/street drug use among college students. *Addict Behav* 33: 934–941.

Gopakumar KM, Shashikant S (2010). *Unpacking the Issue of Counterfeit Medicines.* Penang, Malaysia: Third World Network.

Goyan J (1981). Fourteen fallacies about patient package inserts. *West J Med* 134: 463–468.

Javitt JC, Rebitzer JB, Reisman L (2008). Information technology and medical missteps: Evidence from a randomized trial. *J Health Econ* 27: 585–602.

Katz MD (2010). Evaluation of adverse drug reactions. In: Stuart BM, Harry LG (eds) *Decision Making in Medicine,* 3rd edn. Philadelphia: Mosby, pp. 698–699.

Kaufman M (2005). FDA official quits over delay on Plan B. Women's health chief says commissioner's decision on contraceptive was political. *Washington Post,* September 1, 2005. Available online at: http://www.washingtonpost.com/wp-dyn/content/article/2005/08/31/AR2005083101271.html (accessed 15 May 2010).

Keshishian F, Colodny N, *et al.* (2008). Physician–patient and pharmacist–patient communication: Geriatrics' perceptions and opinions. *Patient Educ Counsel* 71: 265–284.

Larsson M, Kronvall G, Chuc NT, *et al.* (2000). Antibiotic medication and bacterial resistance to antibiotics: a survey of children in a Vietnamese community. *Trop Med Int Health* 5: 711–721.

Liederman DB (2009). Risk management of drug products and the US Food and Drug Administration: Evolution and context. *Drug Alcohol Depend* 105 (suppl. 1): S9–S13.

Mackay J, Eriksen M (2004). *The Tobacco Atlas.* Geneva: World Health Organization.

McCabe SE, Teter CJ (2007). Drug use related problems among nonmedical users of prescription stimulants: A web-based survey of college students from a Midwestern university. *Drug Alcohol Depend* 91: 69–76.

McNeil Product Recall Information (2010). Available online at: www.mcneilproductrecall.com/ (accessed 21 December 2010).

National Institute on Drug Abuse (2006). *Research Report: Methamphetamine Abuse and Addiction.* Washington, DC: National Institutes of Health.

National Institute on Drug Abuse (2008). *Prescription Drug Abuse,* March 2008. Washington, DC: National Institutes of Health.

Newton PN, Green MD (2010). Impact of poor-quality medicines in the 'developing' world. *Trends Pharmacol Sci* 31: 99–101.

Nguyen T (1999). "Doi moi" and private pharmacies: a case study on dispensing and financial issues in Hanoi, Vietnam. *Eur J Clin Pharmacol* 55: 325–332.

Office of Community Oriented Policing Services (2002). Problem-oriented guides for police series no. 16. Available online at: http://www.cops.usdoj.gov/pdf/e02021446.pdf (accessed 15 May 2010).

Olsson E, Tuyet LT, Nguyen HA, *et al.* (2002). Health professionals' and consumers' views on the role of the pharmacy personnel and the pharmacy service in Hanoi, Vietnam – a qualitative study. *J Clin Pharm Ther* 27: 273–280.

Staufer WB, Greydanus DE (2005). Attention-deficit/hyperactivity disorder psychopharmacology for college students. *Pediatr Clin North Am* 52: 71–84.

Storm A, Andersen SE, Benfeld E, *et al.* (2008). One in 3 prescriptions are never redeemed: Primary nonadherence in an outpatient clinic. *J Am Acad Dermatol* 59: 27–33.

Substance Abuse and Mental Health Services Administration (2009). *Results from the 2008 National Survey on Drug Use and Health: National Findings.* Washington, DC: US Department of Health and Human Services, Substance Abuse and Mental Health Services Administration, Office of Applied Studies.

Temin P (1980). Regulation and the choice of prescription drugs. *Am Econ Rev* 70: 301–305.

Tran T (2004). *Community-Based Evidence About the Health Care System in Rural Vietnam.* PhD Dissertation. Newcastle, Australia: School of Medicine Practice and Population Health, The University of Newcastle.

United States Pharmacopeia (2010). Promoting the quality of medicines in developing countries, Available online at: http://www.usp.org/worldwide/ (accessed 17 May 2010).

Vander Stichele RH (2004). *Impact of Written Drug Information in Patient Package Inserts: Acceptance and Impact on Benefit/Risk Perception.* Doctor of Medical Sciences thesis. Ghent University, Faculty of Medicine and Health Sciences, Heymans Institute of Pharmacology. Ghent, Belgium: Academia Press Scientific Publishers.

Varley E (2010). Targeted doctors, missing patients: Obstetric health services and sectarian conflict in Northern Pakistan. *Soc Sci Med* 70: 61–70.

WHO website for Vietnam (2010) Available online at: http://www3.who.int/whosis/country (accessed 17 May 2010).

World Health Organization (2010). Medications: Counterfeit medications. Available online at: http://www.who.int/mediacentre/factsheets/fs275/en/ (accessed 15 May 2010).

WHO website for Vietnam (2010) Available online at: http://www3.who.int/whosis/country (accessed 17 May 2010).

Further reading

Ali MM, Cleland J (2010). Oral contraceptive discontinuation and its aftermath in 19 developing countries. *Contraception* 81: 22–29.

Baker BK, Ombaka E (2009). The danger of in-kind drug donations to the Global Fund. *Lancet* 373: 1218–1221.

Behague D, Tawiah C, Rosato M, *et al.* (2009). Evidence-based policy-making: The implications of globally-applicable research for context-specific problem-solving in developing countries. *Soc Sci Med* 69: 1539–1546.

Bertoldi AD, de Barros AJD, Wagner A, *et al.* (2009). Medicine access and utilization in a population covered by primary health care in Brazil. *Health Policy* 89: 295–302.

Buxton JA, Haden M, Mathias R (2008). The control and regulation of currently illegal drugs. In: Kris H (ed.) *International Encyclopedia of Public Health.* Oxford: Academic Press, pp. 7–16.

Criel B, Waelkens MP, Soors W, *et al.* (2008). Community health insurance in developing countries. In: Kris H (ed.) *International Encyclopedia of Public Health.* Oxford: Academic Press, pp. 782–791.

DiazGranados CA, Cardo DM, McGowan JE Jr (2008). Antimicrobial resistance: international control strategies, with a focus on limited-resource settings. *Int J Antimicrob Agents* 32: 1–9.

Ensor T (2008). Universal coverage in developing countries, transition to. In: Kris H (ed.) *International Encyclopedia of Public Health.* Oxford: Academic Press, pp. 441–452.

Fry CL, Cvetkovski S (2008). The regulation of drugs and drug use: public health and law enforcement. In: Kris H (ed.) *International Encyclopedia of Public Health.* Oxford: Academic Press, pp. 501–505.

Fuller CM, Ford C, Rudolph A (2009). Injection drug use and HIV: past and future considerations for HIV prevention and interventions. In: Kenneth HM, Hank FP (eds) *HIV Prevention.* San Diego: Academic Press, pp. 305–339.

Krüsi A, Wood E, Montaner J, *et al.* (2010). Social and structural determinants of HAART access and adherence among injection drug users. *Int J Drug Policy* 21: 4–9.

Lockhart M, Babar ZU, Garg S (2010). Evaluation of policies to support drug development in New Zealand. *Health Policy* 96: 108–117.

Lucas H (2008). Information and communications technology for future health systems in developing countries. *Soc Sci Med* 66: 2122–2132.

Maïga D, Akanmori BD, Chocarro L (2009). Regulatory oversight of clinical trials in Africa: Progress over the past 5 years. *Vaccine* 27: 7249–7252.

Newton PN, Green MD, Fernández FM (2010). Impact of poor-quality medicines in the 'developing' world. *Trends Pharmacol Sci* 31: 99–101.

Nyika A (2009). Ethical and practical challenges surrounding genetic and genomic research in developing countries. *Acta Trop* 112 (suppl. 1): S21–S31.

Ritter A (2010). Illicit drugs policy through the lens of regulation. *Int J Drug Policy* 21: 265–270.

Sacks LV, Behrman RE (2008). Developing new drugs for the treatment of drug-resistant tuberculosis: a regulatory perspective. *Tuberculosis* 88 (suppl. 1): S93–S100.

Tetteh EK (2008). Providing affordable essential medicines to African households: The missing policies and institutions for price containment. *Soc Sci Med* 66: 569–581.

Tetteh E (2009). Creating reliable pharmaceutical distribution networks and supply chains in African countries: Implications for access to medicines. *Res Soc Admin Pharm* 5: 286–297.

Tetteh EK (2009). Policies and institutional arrangements for rationalizing drug selection and consumption patterns in African healthcare systems. *Res Soc Admin Pharm* 5: 274–285.

van Roey J, von Schoen-Angerer T, Ford N, *et al.* (2008). How developing world concerns need to be part of drug development plans: a case study of four emerging antiretrovirals. *Drug Discov Today* 13: 601–605.

Vayena E, Peterson HB, Adamson AD, *et al.* (2009). Assisted reproductive technologies in developing countries: are we caring yet? *Fertil Steril* 92: 413–416.

Wellman-Labadie O, Zhou Y (2010). The US Orphan Drug Act: Rare disease research stimulator or commercial opportunity? *Health Policy* 95: 216–228.

11

Health impacts and health policy influencers

Introduction

The topics of this chapter are disparate and may be considered to have no influence upon each other. While this may be the case, what in fact creates an overlap among the topics is the importance of health policy, ethics, and health-planning considerations and needs occurring and recurring as a result of each of these issues.

Influence of war and violence on health policy

There are major distinctions that must be made at the outset regarding global health, health policy, and war and/or violence (Table 11.1). The differences are starkly apparent. Perhaps we do not think of war in this regard, but examine for a minute how the devastating effects of war play havoc on health policy deliberations, health care systems, and the health of populations affected by war.

Devastating effects of war and the resultant devastation affecting health care systems

War extracts a tremendous toll on health, health care, and public health. Levy and Sidel (2007) write:

> War accounts for more death and disability than many major diseases combined. It destroys families, communities, and sometimes whole cultures (p. 3).

Kruk *et al.* (2010) note that violent conflicts claim lives, disrupt livelihoods, and halt the delivery of essential services, such as health care and education. Furthermore, health systems are often devastated in conflicts as health professionals flee, infrastructure is destroyed, and the supply of drugs and supplies is halted.

Table 11.1 Differences between global health and war/violence

Global health seeks to:

- save lives
- reduce suffering
- build infrastructure
- invest in health for economic improvement
- improve education and understanding
- enhance collaboration for common goals
- use technology to create security for a better future

War/violence has as goals:

- to kill people, both combatants and civilians, while gaining land
- to maim people both physically and mentally
- to destroy infrastructure that was so hard to get in the first place
- to create poverty
- to exacerbate hate and intolerance
- to make it difficult to see our common humanity
- to destroy the future

As noted, wars and political violence present a negative impact upon health care systems. Kurtz (2008) points out that, as wars cease, there are numerous opportunities from a health policy standpoint to develop new systems, provide innovation in design and structures of health care delivery processes, and incorporate new technologies. These opportunities are also in competition with other infrastructural needs (housing, roads, electricity, and other social services). Kurtz (2008) also notes the positive influence of international efforts, including non-governmental organizations (NGOs) in rebuilding and restructuring efforts.

Impact of war on health policy

Paton and Heggenhougen (2008), when discussing health policy in the context of public policy, highlight factors that dramatically affect health policy formation, such as periods of violence and/or war. Green et al. (2008a) point to war and violence as challenges that greatly influence health planning currently.

Despite an armistice signing in 1953 between North and South Korea, the Republic of Korea (South Korea) has had to exist in a state of war readiness for over 50 years. Health reform in Korea, specifically the Medical-Aid policy, has not achieved the hoped-for goal of increasing access to health care services for the poor in the Republic of Korea (Shin 2006). One of the reasons Shin (2006) suggests for the lack of progress may be government crises that result from activities necessary for war readiness in the Republic of Korea.

Public health preventive activities can also suffer after war and violent periods (Markovic *et al.* 2005). In Serbia, inadequate public health education, lack of patient-friendly health services, sociocultural health beliefs, gender roles, and personal difficulties were the most salient barriers to screening (Markovic *et al.* 2005).

Effects of war on subpopulations

Women

The Kaiser Family Foundation (2004) has posted materials indicating the toll war takes on females, who suffer from a lack of protection from violence, and who experience increased rates of human immunodeficiency virus (HIV)/ acquired immunodeficiency syndrome (AIDS) after sexual assaults, which are common. Iqbal (2010) has noted that all violent conflicts damage many components of population health. Specific damage to infrastructure segments such as health facilities, disruption of food supplies, and forcing internal or external refugee movements spread the collateral damage of war to an extensive degree.

Children

Heller (2006) points out that armed conflicts affect civilians in a prominent fashion, and women and children disproportionately. Heller calls for pediatricians to advocate for children globally at the United Nations and similar levels.

Mental health issues

Miller and Rasmussen (2010), when examining war exposure and mental health outcomes, propose a model in which daily stressors partially mediate the relationship of war exposure to mental health. They further suggest a sequenced approach to intervention in which daily stressors are first addressed, and specialized interventions are then provided for individuals whose distress does not abate with "the repair of the social ecology."

Soldiers

Mays and Heggenhougen (2008) studied health issues affecting soldiers returning from armed conflicts, specifically disease symptoms reported by

Gulf War veterans returning home after active duty. For example, Mays and Heggenhougen note that, following the 1991 Gulf War, there was much controversy surrounding service-related health effects. Drawing on evidence from the Vietnam experience, they suggested that self-reported ill health following that conflict may be related to how service during the conflict is framed as a societal issue. Mays and Heggenhougen concluded that, even in the absence of societal framing of the war issue, a Gulf War-related ill health effect was found.

Communicable diseases in soldiers have accounted for more deaths than battlefield casualties (Sutherland 1919). In World War I pneumonia and influenza epidemics took the lives of 40 000 US soldiers (Sutherland 1919) and over 56 000 American deaths were due to disease, whereas approximately 49 000 were killed in battle (Rickard 2007).

Country-specific, population-specific effects and impacts

Palestine

In a study of 10th- and 11th-grade Palestinian youths in occupied territories, Giacaman and fellow researchers (2007a) found there was a significant association between a high number of subjective health complaints and demographic variables, particularly for females compared with males, and refugee camp dwellers compared with village dwellers. Also, the exposure to humiliation was significantly associated with an increased number of subjective health complaints. The authors conclude that humiliation induced by conflict and war-like conditions constitutes an independent traumatic event that is associated with negative health outcomes in its own right, regardless of exposure to other violent/traumatic events (Giacaman et al. 2007a).

Giacaman and colleagues (2007b) studied Palestinians and found that political freedom, self-determination, participation in democratic processes, and feeling involved in political decision-making are important contributors to individual quality-of-life determinations. This study, conducted in war-torn areas (the Occupied Palestinian Territory), is particularly relevant to societies and cultures in conflict-affected zones and locales where violence and insecurity constitute an important part of life.

Cambodia

A case in point is Cambodia (Hinton Walker et al. 2009), which, after decades of civil war and war with Vietnam, has advanced progressive health policy actions, including health contracting, health financing, and health planning. Results from these activities have included improvements in child mortality rates, although high maternal mortality rates persist. However, health policy decision-making has trailed social changes and societal shifts. As noted in Chapter 10, Cambodia has recently moved to close illegal pharmacies. Health policy has many tentacles. Policies start broad-based and then become more and more specific, dealing with system structure issues, roles and responsibilities, and policies affecting specific professions. This is where gaps may occur, as in Cambodia, when systems are restructured from scratch.

Postconflict and postwar health policy

Zwi *et al.* (2005) discuss the planning and research processes necessary when considering postconflict health needs and planning requirements.

Sandberg and Bjune (2007) also address shortcomings in preventive health activities, specifically vaccinations. They propose the formation of new institutions, the contribution of institutional design to effective implementation, and the interplay between vaccine initiatives and other global institutions.

Unexpected opportunities

As paradoxical as it might seem at first blush, opportunities are presented in a postwar, postconflict environment. These times at the end of conflicts present public health enhancement options that might not have been evident or possible previously.

Paton and Heggenhougen (2008) note health policy changes in emerging countries, changing health care systems and allowing public health professionals new avenues for promotion of messages and ultimate delivery of services.

The influence of pestilence

Introduction: the influence of pestilence on health policy

Martens (2002) presents the concept of transitions as a useful way to address future changes in the health status of the world due to the processes of globalization. Martens presents developments in the health status of populations according to three potential future ages: the age of emerging infectious diseases, the age of medical technology, and the age of sustained health.

Historical perspective

Santow (2001) describes three transitions – the mortality transition, the epidemiological transition, and the health transition – that provide a framework for understanding past, present, and future health care morbidity and mortality trends.

Bashford (2008) has linked public health issues, including pestilence, to colonialism. Public health and colonialism have strongly linked histories. Bashford presents five key areas for discussion:

1   infectious diseases and their management
2   tropical medicine
3   health and missions
4   maternal and infant health
5   health education and promotion.

Selgelid (2009), considering ethical issues and the importance of infectious diseases, has reviewed four major ethical issues:

1   the obligation of individuals to avoid infecting others
2   health care workers' "duty to treat"
3   allocation of scarce resources
4   coercive social distancing measures.

Nutrition

Iyengar and Nair (2000) point out that nearly 800 million of the world's population remain chronically malnourished. Nearly 200 million children are moderately to severely underweight, while 70 million are severely malnourished. The researchers point out that environmental lead, arsenic, mercury, and other heavy metals that enter the food chain can seriously deplete body stores of iron, vitamin C, and other essential nutrients, leading to decreased immune defenses, intrauterine growth retardation, impaired psychosocial faculties, and other disabilities associated with malnutrition (Iyengar and Nair 2000). Increased susceptibilities to communicable diseases, and those provoked by water or insect-borne vectors, are additional risks encountered by malnourished individuals. Careful planning and international cooperation are called for to ameliorate these concerns (Iyengar and Nair 2000).

China and India

China and India are similarly huge nations currently experiencing rapid economic growth, urbanization, and widening inequalities between rich and poor (Dummer and Cook 2008). For both countries, infectious diseases of the past sit alongside emerging infectious diseases and chronic illnesses associated with aging societies, although the burden of infectious diseases is much higher in India. Both countries are seeing a decline in government payment for health care costs (Dummer and Cook 2008).

Cook and Dummer (2004) review the changing health situation in China, which has shown remarkable improvement since the founding of the People's

Republic of China in 1949. China has followed a classical epidemiological model moving from high rates of infectious disease and early mortality (diseases of poverty) in a mainly peasant society to extended morbidity and mortality associated with an aging population in an urban environment. HIV/AIDS has emerged as a rising, major infectious disease, and environmental conditions have spawned additional disease (Cook and Dummer 2004).

Facts regarding malaria

US Centers for Disease Control and Prevention (Malaria Facts 2010) provide an insightful description of the impact of malaria in the USA and globally.

Malaria in the USA

On average, 1500 cases of malaria are reported every year in the USA, even though malaria has been eradicated in this country since the early 1950s (Malaria Facts 2010).

First- and second-generation immigrants from malaria-endemic countries returning to their "home" country to visit friends and relatives tend not to use appropriate malaria prevention measures and thus are more likely to become infected with malaria (Malaria Facts 2010).

Between 1957 and 2009, in the USA, 63 outbreaks of locally transmitted mosquito-borne malaria occurred; in such outbreaks, local mosquitoes become infected by biting persons carrying malaria parasites (acquired in endemic areas) and then transmit malaria to local residents (Malaria Facts 2010).

Of the species of *Anopheles* mosquitoes found in the USA, the three species that were responsible for malaria transmission prior to elimination (*Anopheles quadrimaculatus* in the east, *An. freeborni* in the west, and *An. albimanus* in the Caribbean) are still widely prevalent; thus there is a constant risk that malaria could be reintroduced in the USA.

During 1963–2009, 96 cases of transfusion-transmitted malaria were reported in the USA; approximately two-thirds of these cases could have been prevented if the implicated donors had been deferred from donating according to established guidelines (Malaria Facts 2010).

Malaria globally

A total of 3.3 billion people (half the world's population) live in areas at risk of malaria transmission in 109 countries and territories (Malaria Facts 2010). A mere 35 countries (30 in sub-Saharan Africa and 5 in Asia) account for 98% of global malaria deaths. The World Health Organization (WHO) estimates that in 2008 malaria caused 190–311 million clinical episodes, and 708 000–1 003 000 deaths (Malaria Facts 2010). A total of 89% of the malaria deaths worldwide occur in Africa.

Malaria is the fifth greatest cause of death from infectious diseases worldwide (after respiratory infections, HIV/AIDS, diarrheal diseases, and tuberculosis (TB)) (Malaria Facts 2010). Malaria is the second leading cause of death from infectious diseases in Africa, after HIV/AIDS.

Novel malaria treatments

Yang *et al.* (2010) note that natural products are the most important sources of medicines, and that they have the potential to treat immunological diseases. Also, they speak to the issue of using traditional Chinese medicine to treat other diseases, including cancer and malaria.

Killeen *et al.* (2002) describe malaria control strategies that emphasize domestic protection against adult mosquitoes with insecticides, and improved access to medical services. Malaria prevention by killing adult mosquitoes is generally favored because moderately reducing their longevity can radically suppress community-level transmission (Killeen *et al.* 2002).

Malaria control

Moszynski (2010) points out that efforts to control malaria in Uganda have been undermined by a lack of first-line treatments in public health centers. Investigators from a newly established health-monitoring unit have made dozens of arrests in a crackdown on illicit sales of government-owned drugs, including drugs for malaria.

Health policy and the malaria treatment supply chain

In May 2010, WHO (2010a) published a manual describing the comprehensive elements necessary for proper procurement of artemisinin-based medicines used to treat malaria. This document is complete in providing guidance for all aspects pertaining to the procurement, assurance of quality of ingredients, and quality control aspects of this class of antimalarials. Its aim is to improve understanding of the following aspects of procurement:

- medicines that are recommended in evidence-based treatment guidelines
- common problems with the quality of artemisinin-based antimalarial products
- elements of pharmaceutical product quality
- model product specifications
- documentation supplied to support pharmaceutical product quality
- role, principles, and methods of quality control testing.

The creation of this document is an example of how health policy is translated from a macro to a micro level for use by those who deal with all aspects of a drug used to treat a disease such as malaria. The manual describes the target audience for the publication as follows:

> The target audience for this manual includes programme managers, procurement officers, health officers and supply chain managers in the public and private sectors who are responsible for procuring and distributing artemisinin-based antimalarial medicines (including artemisinin-based combination therapies and artemisinin-based suppositories and injectables) (p. XV).

Tuberculosis

TB is one of the world's deadliest diseases. The US Centers for Disease Control and Prevention (2010) provides the following information regarding TB:

- One-third of the world's population is infected with TB.
- Each year, nearly 9 million people around the world become sick with TB.
- Each year, there are almost 2 million TB-related deaths worldwide.
- TB is the leading killer of people who are HIV-infected.

The US Centers for Disease Control and Prevention (2010) gives the following information regarding TB and pregnancy. Untreated TB represents a greater hazard to a pregnant woman and her fetus than does its treatment. Treatment of pregnant women should be initiated whenever the probability of TB is moderate to high. Infants born to women with untreated TB may be of lower birth weight than those born to women without TB and, rarely, the infant may be born with TB. Although the drugs used in the initial treatment regimen cross the placenta, they do not appear to have harmful effects on the fetus.

Gandy and Zumla (2002) claim that the resurgence of TB is one of the most serious global public health challenges of the 21st century. They conclude that TB research requires a combination of advances in biomedical knowledge with a broader understanding of the evolving relationship between disease and modern societies.

Kaufmann et al. (2010) note the following regarding the development of vaccines for TB:

> After decades of inactivity, research and development for tuberculosis vaccines is slowly increasing, although there is still a substantial shortfall in funding. New partnerships and incentives need to be created (p. 1).

There are approximately a dozen pre-exposure vaccines in various stages of testing (Kaufmann *et al.* 2010), and further postexposure vaccines are being evaluated as well.

Influenza

Mamelund (2008) provides a historical perspective on influenza, and tracks the history of influenza spans for more than 2500 years from Egypt and Ancient Greece to the present. Mamelund notes that there is little evidence of influenza epidemics in the historical literature before the period from 1173 to 1387, and the first generally agreed pandemic occurred in 1580. Hanson *et al.* (2005) describe similar historical perspectives on mucosal infections.

In the summer of 2009, the US Centers for Disease Control and Prevention provided guidance on groups suggested to be vaccinated with the H1N1 vaccination (National Center for Immunization and Respiratory Diseases, CDC 2009).

Initial target groups

When vaccine is first available, the Advisory Committee on Immunization Practices (ACIP) recommends that programs and providers administer vaccine to persons in the following five target groups (not in priority order):

1 pregnant women
2 persons who live with or provide care for infants aged <6 months (e.g., parents, siblings, and daycare providers)
3 health care and emergency medical services personnel
4 persons aged 6 months to 24 years
5 persons aged 25–64 years who have medical conditions that put them at higher risk for influenza-related complications.

These five target groups comprise an estimated 159 million persons in the USA. This estimate does not accurately account for persons who might be included in more than one category (e.g., a health care worker with a high-risk condition). Vaccination programs and providers should begin vaccination of persons in all these groups as soon as vaccine is available.

Subset of target groups during limited vaccine availability

Current projections of initial vaccine supply indicate that it will not be necessary to establish a subset of the five initial target groups in most areas. However, demand for vaccination and initial supply may vary considerably across geographic areas. If the supply of the initially available vaccine is not adequate to meet demand for vaccination among these five target groups, ACIP recommends that the following subset of the initial target groups receives priority for vaccination until vaccine availability increases (order of target groups does not indicate priority):

- pregnant women
- persons who live with or provide care for infants aged <6 months (e.g., parents, siblings, and daycare providers)
- health care and emergency medical services personnel who have direct contact with patients or infectious material
- children aged 6 months to 4 years
- children and adolescents aged 5–18 years who have medical conditions that put them at higher risk for influenza-related complications.

This subset of the five target groups comprises approximately 42 million persons in the USA. Vaccination programs and providers should give priority to this subset only if vaccine availability is too limited to initiate vaccination for everyone in the five initial target groups (National Center for Immunization and Respiratory Diseases, CDC 2009).

Australia and laws regarding public health and pandemics

Pandemic influenza will cause significant social and economic disruption, according to Bennett (2009), who notes that public health laws are also informed by understandings of rights and responsibilities for individuals and communities, and the balancing of public health and public freedoms. Consideration of these issues is an essential part of planning for pandemic influenza.

Global response to H1N1 epidemic

Jordans (2010), in an Associated Press report, described how the WHO had convened a panel to examine its actions regarding the H1N1 influenza outbreak:

> Governments around the world spent millions of dollars (euros) buying antiviral drugs and flu vaccines in anticipation of a serious outbreak that never happened.

Questions regarding access provided by the WHO to decision-makers within governments globally have arisen in the context of an epidemic that was less intense than initially suggested or projected. Governments spent enormous sums of money on vaccinations provided through a limited number of manufacturing entities that reaped significant profits from the sale and distribution of the H1N1 vaccination worldwide.

Jordans concluded:

Among the companies that benefited was Switzerland's Roche Group, which saw sales of its Tamiflu antiviral medication jump by 2 billion Swiss francs ($1.74 billion) last year. British firm GlaxoSmithKline PLC sold both vaccines and its antiviral Relenza, while France's Sanofi-Aventis SA and US-based Baxter International made vaccines. Some companies donated medicine to poor countries.

WHO has confirmed 18 036 deaths from the H1N1 strain over the past year – far fewer than would have died from seasonal flu during the same period.

WHO leaders have indicated that "we were lucky" when observing the extent of the reach of the H1N1 epidemic; others questioned whether expansive projections were premature and resulted in profit windfalls for manufacturers of vaccines as well as treatments approved for active treatment of outbreaks.

Climate, disasters, and the environment

Introduction

Disasters are an unfortunate aspect of human existence. They have been ubiquitous throughout every period of human history. Disasters have had significant effects on the environment, on health functioning, and on individual health and well-being.

Leaning and Kris (2008) note:

Disasters have been part of human experience since the beginning of time. For centuries, people at risk of drought and famine or flood and heavy winds have made individual or small group preparations to try to ward off the worst effects. Agencies and systems dedicated to disaster response have relatively recent origins, however, and can be traced, for most countries, to developments during the nineteenth century and early twentieth century. These years saw governments deploy military units to help people affected by major natural disasters, urban authorities draw on fire departments to assist with emergencies other than fires, and civic organizations founded with the express purpose of taking care of the injured in war (the International Committee of the Red Cross) or the distressed at home (the national Red Cross and Red Crescent Societies). Private or religious groups attended to people affected by emergencies or disaster, within their domestic jurisdictions or internationally (p. 205).

Global warming has been projected to extract the most significant effects of any other impact upon health and health systems. Eastin *et al.* (2010) compare the current debate regarding global warming with the limits of growth discussions of the 1970s. A case is made for focusing on the social, economic, and political dimensions of climate change, as opposed to its excessive emphasis on emission reduction targets.

Hanlon and McCartney (2008) suggest that there is likely to be a significant shortfall in energy supply, resulting in high energy prices and a reversal of many of the aspects of globalization that are currently taken for granted. They suggest that if this happens the restructuring of economies, not unlike the situation in the former Soviet Union, could have a deleterious effect upon health care systems and health in general.

Hübler et al. (2008) estimate an average increase in the number of heat-induced casualties by a factor of more than 3 for the period 2071–2100. Heat-related hospitalization costs increase sixfold, not including the cost of ambulant treatment. Heat also reduces work performance, resulting in an estimated output loss of between 0.1% and 0.5% of gross domestic product (Hübler et al. 2008). Kinney et al. (2008) suggest that projecting the future public health burden of temperature-related health effects can provide valuable information to aid public health and environmental authorities in planning and communicating the risks of climate change to the public.

O'Neill et al. (2009) note that, because of global climate change, the world will, on average, experience a higher number of heat waves, and the intensity and length of these heat waves are projected to increase. O'Neill and colleagues (2009) suggest integrating heat health information into a comprehensive adaptation planning process that can alert local decision-makers to extreme heat risks and provide information necessary to choose strategies that yield the largest health improvements and cost savings.

Shea et al. (2008) point out that climate change is potentially the largest global threat to human health ever encountered. Because of global climate change, the next generations will face more injury, disease, and death related to natural disasters and heat waves, higher rates of climate-related infections, and widespread malnutrition, as well as more allergic and air pollution-related morbidity and mortality. Specific diseases suggested to be most at risk for negative effects are the anticipated increases in prevalence and severity of asthma and related allergic disease mediated through worsening ambient air pollution and altered local and regional pollen production (Shea et al. 2008). The anticipated increases in allergic diseases due to climate change will affect clinical practices as well as health planning.

Urban planning and its role in health policy deliberations

Friel et al. (2008) argue that a shift is needed in priorities in economic development towards healthy forms of urbanization, more efficient and renewable energy sources, and a sustainable and fairer food system.

Stephens *et al.* (2008) suggest that, due to the fact that 50% of the world's population is now urbanized, health-planning efforts need to address urban health issues that include: infectious diseases (caused in part by poor water and sanitation practices), industrial and air pollution and their effects upon health, epidemics of violence, and drug abuse. Stephens *et al.* call for dealing with both industrialization and sustainability in health policy and planning activities. Green and colleagues (2008b) note that for optimal outcomes health policy must be intricately linked to health-planning activities.

Land use planning

Barton (2009) discusses the re-realization that has occurred in the recent past, examining the role planning plays in health outcomes. Barton notes that, in the 19th century, planning was instituted to impact inhumane living conditions, and that this point of view has seen a re-emergence recently. Further it is noted that an urban environment can either exacerbate or mitigate personal health and well-being outcomes (Barton 2009). Blanco *et al.* (2009) also explore the needs for research examining the effects of planning on health outcomes and incorporating the large influence of climate change on environments.

UK efforts

Burns and Bond (2008) describe the UK Strategic Environmental Assessment (SEA) Directive, which established a statutory requirement for the consideration of significant effects on human health in European Union member states. The SEA Directive, along with reforms to the planning system, does provide a framework for improving the consideration of health, but the capacity of the planning system to consider health must be improved, as should be dialogue with health practitioners, and the evidence base for health outcomes.

Richardson *et al.* (2009) examined the UK primary care trusts (PCTs) to determine their incorporation of climate change and resultant health vulnerabilities in their health policy activities. They concluded that evidence of good examples in sustainable development was predominantly limited to policy statements and strategic aims; evidence of action was limited. They suggest that, as champions of the public health agenda, PCT action on sustainability should be integral to all aspects of organizational governance.

Other governments

McCartney *et al.* (2008) suggest that western governments currently prioritize economic growth and the pursuit of profit above alternative goals of sustainability, health, and equality. These authors suggest that public health can make its best contribution by adopting a new mindset, discourse, methodology, and set of tasks.

Food security and climate change

Badjeck *et al.* (2009) pointed out that there is increasing concern over the consequences of global warming for the food security and livelihoods of the world's 36 million fisherfolk and the nearly 1.5 billion consumers who rely on fish for more than 20% of their dietary animal protein.

Vector-borne diseases affected by climate change

Gage *et al.* (2008) suggest that climate change could significantly affect vector-borne disease in humans. Temperature, precipitation, humidity, and other climatic factors are known to affect the reproduction, development, behavior, and population dynamics of the arthropod vectors of these diseases. They also note that adapting to the effects of climate change will require the development of adequate response plans, enhancement of surveillance systems, and the development of effective and locally appropriate strategies to control and prevent the spread of infectious diseases.

The most vulnerable groups affected by climate change

St. Louis and Hess (2008) note that the impact of climate change will disproportionately affect the poor and disadvantaged. They suggest the following: (1) increased awareness among current global health practitioners of climate change and its potential impacts for the most disadvantaged; (2) strengthening of the evidence base; (3) incorporation now of climate change mitigation and adaptation concerns into design of ongoing global health programs; and (4) alignment of current global health program targets and methods with larger frameworks for climate change and sustainable development. St. Louis and Hess (2008) suggest planning should proceed to mitigate climate change in wealthier countries to lessen the impact upon developing countries.

Elsewhere, others agree that greenhouse gas emissions and effects upon health will affect the health of vulnerable populations disproportionately. Younger *et al.* (2008) suggest that working across sectors to incorporate a health promotion approach in the design and development of built environment components may mitigate climate change, promote adaptation, and improve public health.

Health professionals and climate change

Gill and Stott (2009) urge health professionals to play a more proactive role in addressing climate change challenges.

Health workforce issues

There are many health professions and health workers who provide needed care worldwide. Shortages of all of these workers can play havoc with health policy implementations that are placed into planning activities to serve current and future unmet needs. Three professions (medicine, nursing, pharmacy) are addressed in this chapter, but this in no way implies that these are the only professions with shortage components at present and projected into the future.

WHO (2006) suggests that 57 countries, 36 of which are in sub-Saharan Africa, have severe shortages of health workers. More than 4 million additional doctors, nurses, midwives, managers, and public health workers are urgently needed to fill this gap. An adequate health workforce is defined by WHO (2006) as at least 2.3 well-trained health care providers available per 1000 people and balanced in such a way as to reach 80% of the population or more with skilled birth attendance and childhood immunization.

Physicians

The US Health Resources and Services Administration (2006) has published the following information pertaining to physicians:

> The United States continues to debate the adequacy of the current and future supply of physicians. While the general consensus is that overall physician supply per capita will remain relatively stable over the next 15 years, there is less agreement on future demand for physician services. This paper presents projections of physician supply and requirements for 18 physician specialties using the Physician Supply Model (PSM) and the Physician Requirements Model (PRM) developed by the Health Resources and Services Administration (HRSA). In this paper, we describe the data, assumptions and methods used to project the future supply of and requirements for physician services; we present projections from these models under alternative scenarios; and we discuss the implications of these projections for the future adequacy of physician supply.

Accurate projections of physician supply and requirements help preserve a physician supply that is balanced with demand and help the USA achieve its goal of ensuring access to high-quality, cost-effective health care. The length of time needed to train physicians, as well as the time needed to change the US training infrastructure, suggests that we must know at least a decade in advance of major shifts in physician supply or requirements. The US Government Accountability Office noted in its February 2006 report *Health Professions Education Programs – Action Still Needed to Measure Impact* that regular reassessment of future health workforce supply and demand is key to setting policies as US health care needs change (US Government Accountability Office 2006).

Past projections of impending physician shortages and surpluses have influenced policies and programs that, in turn, helped determine the number and specialty composition of physicians being trained. During the 1950s and 1960s, projections of a growing physician shortage helped motivate an expansion of US medical schools, an increase in government funding for medical education, and the creation of policies and programs that encouraged immigration of foreign-trained physicians. Efforts to increase the physician supply proved so successful that, by the late 1970s, many predicted a growing oversupply of physicians (GMENAC 1981).

Rising health care costs paved the way for managed care and its promises to improve the efficiency of the health care system. Enrollment in health maintenance organizations (HMOs) during the 1980s and 1990s prompted re-examination of physician supply adequacy. The greater reliance of HMOs on the use of generalists and the prediction of decreased use of specialist services under managed care led to projections that the USA would have a large surplus of specialists (Council on Graduate Medical Education 1992, 1994; Weiner 1994; Institute of Medicine 1996). However, the perceived limitations of the more restrictive forms of managed care prompted a public backlash against many of the forces predicted to decrease health care use. Also, some researchers have argued that physician projections that relied heavily on HMO staffing patterns underestimated physician requirements by failing to control adequately for out-of-plan care (Hart *et al.* 1997) and systematic differences in the health status of the population enrolled in HMOs and the population receiving care under a traditional fee-for-service arrangement.

Cooper *et al.* (2002) contributed to another round of discussions regarding the adequacy of the future supply of physicians, projecting a significant shortage of physicians – particularly specialists – over the foreseeable future. Other researchers have expressed concerns with the assumptions and conclusions used by Cooper *et al.* (Barer 2002; Grumbach 2002; Reinhardt 2002; Weiner 2002), but a growing consensus is that over the next 15 years, requirements for physician services will grow faster than supply, especially for specialist services and specialties that predominantly serve the elderly. The Council on Graduate Medical Education joined the debate using preliminary projections from Bureau of Health Professions PSM and PRM, adjusted for its own assumptions regarding the effects of key determinants of supply and requirements, projecting a modest shortfall of physicians by 2020. These projections helped influence the Association of American Medical Colleges' decision to encourage growth in US medical school training capacity by approximately 15% (or 3000 physicians per year). The primary contributions of our study are: (1) projections of overall physician supply and requirements to inform the debate on US medical school capacity, and (2) specialty-specific projections of physician supply and requirements under alternative scenarios.

Nursing

Facts pertinent to registered nurses in the USA

From the US Health Resources and Services Administration (2006):

- The USA has more licensed registered nurses (RNs) than ever (an estimated 3 063 163 – a 5.3% increase since the last survey in 2004).
- For every 100 000 people, there are 854 RNs, up from 825 in 2004, but with variations from state to state. Utah has the fewest: 598 RNs for each 100 000 people. The District of Columbia has the most: 1868 per 100 000.
- Most RNs are actively practicing nursing (84.8% – highest in the history of the survey) and most are working full-time (63.2% versus 58.4% in 2004 – the first increase since 1996).
- White, non-Hispanics (65.6% of the US population) comprise 83.2% of licensed RNs, a decrease since 2004, when 87.5% of RNs were white. Asian, Native Hawaiian and Pacific Islanders (non-Hispanic) are the next largest group at 5.8% (4.5% of US population). African-Americans (non-Hispanic) are 5.4% of RNs (12.2% of US population) and Hispanics/Latinos of any race are 3.6% of RNs (15.4% of US population).
- Women outnumber men by more than 15 to 1 in the overall number of RNs, but among only those who became RNs after 1990, there is one male RN for every 10 women.
- One-third (33.7%) of RNs beginning their careers did so with a bachelor's degree, up from 31% in 2004 and twice as many as in 1980.
- Fewer RNs entered nursing with a diploma – just 20.4%, continuing the downward trend since 1980, when 63.7% of RNs entered the nursing workforce with a diploma.
- Significantly more RNs have advanced degrees – 404 163 in 2008, up from 275 068 in 2000.
- The average age of all licensed RNs increased to 47.0 years in 2008 from 46.8 in 2004; this represents a stabilization after many years of continuing large increases in average age.
- Nearly 45% of RNs were 50 years of age or older in 2008, a dramatic increase from 33% in 2000 and 25% in 1980.
- Although the number of RNs younger than 40 dropped steadily between 1980 and 2004, there was an increase in 2008 and they now comprise 29.5% of all RNs.

The shortage of nurses in the USA has been projected to be close to 1 million by 2020 (US Department of Health and Human Services, Health Resources and Services Administration 2010). The US Bureau of Labor and Statistics (2009) also projects that, as of 2008, there were 754 000 licensed practical nurses (LPNs) and/or licensed vocational nurses (LVNs).

Pharmacists

Projections of the number of pharmacists in the USA at present indicate that there are currently close to 270 000 pharmacists, and projections place the number to be 315 800 in 2018 (Bureau of Labor Statistics 2009). The Bureau of Labor Statistics projects that:

> the employment of pharmacists is expected to grow by 17% between 2008 and 2018, which is faster than the average for all occupations. The increasing numbers of middle-aged and elderly people – who use more prescription drugs than younger people – will continue to spur demand for pharmacists throughout the projection period. In addition, as scientific advances lead to new drug products, and as an increasing number of people obtain prescription drug coverage, the need for these workers will continue to expand.

Hawthorne and Anderson (2009), after an analysis of worldwide reports and papers dealing with pharmacist workforce issues, suggest that more coordinated monitoring and modeling of the pharmacy workforce worldwide (particularly in developing countries) are required.

Two pharmacists (Andersson and Snell 2010) wrote a book describing in detail what needs to be done, or how things should be done, when it is not possible to have a pharmacist available. These tasks range from managing medicines, how to order medications, store them, prepare them, dispense them, and use them safely and effectively. Their book is targeted at those who are doing the work of a pharmacist: anyone who sells, dispenses, prepares, manages, or explains to others how to use medicines.

Summary

Hagopian *et al.* (2010) suggest that active recruitment of health workers from developing countries to fill health staffing needs in developed countries has ethical implications. Physicians, nurses, and pharmacists have been actively recruited from developing countries for years. Hagopian *et al.* propose that well-established countries need to increase the training of health care workers within their own countries to stem the brain drain of such workers from developing countries, where they are needed more. They note:

> With 32 million uninsured Americans soon to be eligible for care, it's time to get serious about the fact that the US health work force is too

small and unevenly distributed across urban and rural areas. The Council on Graduate Medical Education has predicted the US will be short [of] approximately 85 000 physicians by 2020 (p. 1).

WHO (2010b) in May 2010 also passed a draft global code of practice resolution for international recruitment of health personnel in an attempt to place parameters around the practice in developed countries of recruiting health workers from developing countries.

Discussion questions

1 Within the chaotic environment of war-torn areas and those impacted by violence, how can health planning become a part of considerations before, during, and after conflict eras?

2 Women and children seem to be particularly vulnerable to the effects of violence. What can health planners consider when evaluating population needs during armed conflicts?

3 Emotional impacts of war affect combatants and civilians alike in differing ways. How should health policy considerations incorporate these impacts when discussing interventions, systems, and general health considerations?

4 Postwar Cambodia has experienced problematic issues related to drug distribution systems. How can health care channels of distribution be put into place with so many other competing demands readily apparent?

5 How should international NGOs address infectious disease outbreaks such as malaria epidemics and the emergence of drug-resistant strains of TB?

6 Lack of water, nutrition, sanitation, and health care system sophistication often occur in tandem. How should one go about addressing problems resulting from substandard or inadequate segments of each of these necessities?

7 Malaria was eradicated, so we thought, in the 1950s in the USA. How can reinfestations, infections, and transfusion-related transfers be occurring in the 21st century?

8 Why is there a link between HIV/AIDS and TB? What health policy impacts can be initiated to mitigate this deadly combination?

9 How can vaccinations be ethically rationed to provide coverage to infants and children on a preferential basis?

10 Do you think the vastly less than anticipated number of H1N1 influenza cases globally was due to superb surveillance or profiteering on the part of vaccine manufacturers?

References

Andersson S, Snell B (2010). *Where There are no Pharmacists, A Guide to Managing Medicines for all Health Workers*. Penang, Malaysia: TWN and Health Action International Asia Pacific.

Badjeck M-C, Allison EH, Halls AS, *et al.* (2009). Impacts of climate variability and change on fishery-based livelihoods. *Marine Policy* 34: 375–383.

Barer M (2002). New opportunities for old mistakes. *Health Affairs* 21: 169–171.

Barton H (2009). Land use planning and health and well-being. *Land Use Policy* 26 (suppl. 1): S115–S123.

Bashford A (2008). The history of public health during colonialism. In: Kris H (ed.) *International Encyclopedia of Public Health*. Oxford: Academic Press, pp. 398–404.

Bennett B (2009). Legal rights during pandemics: Federalism, rights and public health laws – a view from Australia. *Public Health* 123: 232–236.

Blanco H, Alberti M, Forsyth M, *et al.* (2009). Hot, congested, crowded and diverse: Emerging research agendas in planning. *Progr Planning* 71: 153–205.

Bureau of Labor Statistics (2009). Pharmacists. Occupational outlook, 2010–11. Available online at: http://www.bls.gov/oco/ocos079.htm (accessed 21 May 2010).

Burns J, Bond A (2008). The consideration of health in land use planning: Barriers and opportunities. *Environ Impact Assess Rev* 28: 184–197.

Cook IG, Dummer TJB (2004). Changing health in China: Re-evaluating the epidemiological transition model. *Health Policy* 67: 329–343.

Cooper RA, Getzen TE, McKee HJ, *et al.* (2002). Economic and demographic trends signal an impending physician shortage. *Health Affairs* 21: 140–154.

Council on Graduate Medical Education (1992). *Improving Access to Health Care through Physician Workforce Reform: Directions for the 21st Century*. Third report. Rockville, MD: United States Department of Health and Human Services.

Council on Graduate Medical Education (1994). *Recommendation to Improve Access to Health Care through Physician Workforce Reform*. Fourth report. Rockville, MD: United States Department of Health and Human Services.

Dummer TJB, Cook IG (2008). Health in China and India: A cross-country comparison in a context of rapid globalization. *Soc Sci Med* 67: 590–605.

Eastin J, Grundmann R, Prakash A (2010). The two limits debates: Limits to growth and climate change. *Futures*.(in press).

Friel S, Marmot M, McMichael AJ, *et al.* (2008). Global health equity and climate stabilisation: a common agenda. *Lancet* 372: 1677–1683.

Gage KL, Burkot TR, Eisen RJ, *et al.* (2008). Climate and vectorborne diseases. *Am J Prevent Med* 35: 436–450.

Gandy M, Zumla A (2002). The resurgence of disease: social and historical perspectives on the 'new' tuberculosis. *Soc Sci Med* 55: 385–396.

Giacaman R, Abu-Rmeileh N, Husseini A, *et al.* (2007a). Humiliation: the invisible trauma of war for Palestinian youth. *Public Health* 121: 563–571.

Giacaman R, Mataria A, Nguyen-Gillham V, *et al.* (2007b). Quality of life in the Palestinian context: An inquiry in war-like conditions. *Health Policy* 81: 68–84.

Gill M, Stott R (2009). Health professionals must act to tackle climate change. *Lancet* 374: 1953–1955.

GMENAC (1981). *Geographic Distribution Technical Panel, 3*. DHHS publication no. HRA-81-651. Washington, DC: United States Government Printing Office.

Green AT, Mirzoev TN, Kris H (2008a). Planning, for public health policy. In: Kris H (ed.) *Encyclopedia of Public Health*. Oxford: Academic Press, pp. 121–132.

Green AT, Heggenhougen K, Mirzoev TN (2008b). Planning, for public health policy. In: Heggenhougen K (ed.) *International Encyclopedia of Public Health*. St. Louis: Elsevier Press, pp. 121–128.

Grumbach K (2002). The ramifications of specialty-dominated medicine. *Health Affairs* 21: 155–157.

Hagopian A, Williams EB, DeRiel E (2010). Stemming the brain drain of health-care workers from developing countries. Available online at: http://seattletimes.nwsource.com/html/opinion/2011980262_guest29hagopian.html (accessed 1 June 2010).

Hanlon P, McCartney G (2008). Peak oil: Will it be public health's greatest challenge? *Public Health* 122: 647–652.

Hanson L, Robertson A-K, Bjersing J, *et al.* (2005). Undernutrition, immunodeficiency, and mucosal infections. In: Mestecky J (ed.) *Mucosal Immunology,* 3rd edn. Burlington: Academic Press, pp. 1159–1178.

Hart LG, Wagner E, Pirzada S, *et al.* (1997). Physician staffing ratios in staff-model HMOs: a cautionary tale. *Health Affairs* 16: 55–70.

Hawthorne N, Anderson C (2009). The global pharmacy workforce: a systematic review of the literature. *Hum Resource Health* 7: 48.

Health Resources and Services Administration (2006). Physician supply and demand: projections to 2020. Available online at: http://bhpr.hrsa.gov/healthworkforce/reports/physiciansupply-demand/default.htm (accessed 21 May 2010).

Heller DR (2006). The role of a paediatrician in a war zone. *Curr Paediatr* 16: 512–516.

Hinton Walker P, Garmon Bibb SC, Elberson KL, *et al.* (2009). Health system strengthening in Cambodia – A case study of health policy response to social transition. *Health Policy* 92: 107–115.

Hübler M, Klepper G, Paterson S (2008). Costs of climate change: The effects of rising temperatures on health and productivity in Germany. *Ecol Econom* 68: 381–393.

Institute of Medicine (1996). *Primary Care: America's Health in a New Era.* Washington, DC: National Academies Press.

Iqbal A (2010). *War and the Health of Nations.* Stanford, CA: Stanford University Press.

Iyengar GV, Nair PP (2000). Global outlook on nutrition and the environment: meeting the challenges of the next millennium. *Sci Total Environ* 249: 331–346.

Jordans F (2010). Expert panel to view confidential swine flu papers, expert panel examining WHO's swine flu handling to review confidential contracts with industry. Available online at: http://finance.yahoo.com/news/Expert-panel-to-view-apf-4171927666.html?x=0and.v=2 (accessed 20 May 2010).

Kaiser Family Foundation (2004). Women in conflict areas face sexual violence on 'massive scale', at risk for HIV, UNFPA Director tells Security Council. *Daily Reports* October 29.

Kaufmann SHE, Hussey G, Lambert P-H (2010). New vaccines for tuberculosis. Available online at: www.thelancet.com (accessed 19 May 2010).

Killeen GF, Fillinger U, Kichie I, *et al.* (2002). Eradication of Anopheles gambiae from Brazil: lessons for malaria control in Africa? *Lancet Infect Dis* 2: 618–627.

Kinney PL, O'Neill MS, Bell ML, *et al.* (2008). Approaches for estimating effects of climate change on heat-related deaths: challenges and opportunities. *Environ Sci Policy* 11: 87–96.

Kruk ME, Freedman LP, Anglin GA, *et al.* (2010). Rebuilding health systems to improve health and promote statebuilding in post-conflict countries: A theoretical framework and research agenda. *Soc Sci Med* 70: 89–97.

Kurtz L (2008). The effects of war and political violence on health services. In: Kurtz L (ed.) *Encyclopedia of Violence, Peace, and Conflict.* Oxford: Academic Press, pp. 933–943.

Leaning J, Kris H (2008). Disasters and emergency planning. In: Heggenhougen K (ed.) *International Encyclopedia of Public Health.* Oxford: Academic Press, pp. 204–215.

Levy BS, Sidel VW (2007). *War and Public Health,* London: Oxford University Press, chapter 1.

Malaria Facts (2010). UC Centers for Disease Control and Prevention. Available online at: http://www.cdc.gov/malaria/about/facts.html (accessed 20 February 2010).

Mamelund SE (2008). Influenza, historical. In: Kris H (ed.) *International Encyclopedia of Public Health.* Oxford: Academic Press, pp. 597–608.

Markovic M, Kesic V, Topic L, *et al.* (2005). Barriers to cervical cancer screening: A qualitative study with women in Serbia. *Soc Sci Med* 61: 2528–2535.

Martens P (2002). Health transitions in a globalising world: Towards more disease or sustained health? *Futures* 34: 635–648.

Mays N, Heggenhougen K (2008). Interest groups and civil society, in public health policy. In: Kris H (ed.) *International Encyclopedia of Public Health*. Oxford: Academic Press, pp. 650–658.

McCartney G, Hanlon P, Romanes F (2008). Climate change and rising energy costs will change everything: A new mindset and action plan for 21st century public health. *Public Health* 122: 658–663.

Miller KE, Rasmussen A (2010). War exposure, daily stressors, and mental health in conflict and post-conflict settings: Bridging the divide between trauma-focused and psychosocial frameworks. *Soc Sci Med* 70: 7–16.

Moszynski P (2010). Disappearance of drugs undermines Uganda's fight against malaria. *Br Med J* 340: c2611.

National Center for Immunization and Respiratory Diseases, CDC (2009). Use of Influenza A (H1N1) 2009 Monovalent Vaccine, Recommendations of the Advisory Committee on Immunization Practices (ACIP), August 21, 2009/58(Early Release). Atlanta, GA: US Centers for Disease Control and Prevention, pp. 1–8.

O'Neill MS, Carter R, Kish JK, *et al.* (2009). Preventing heat-related morbidity and mortality: New approaches in a changing climate. *Maturitas* 64: 98–103.

Paton C, Heggenhougen K (2008). Health policy: overview. In: Kris H (ed.) *International Encyclopedia of Public Health*. Oxford: Academic Press, pp. 211–225.

Reinhardt UE (2002). Analyzing cause and effect in the United States physician workforce. *Health Affairs* 21: 165–166.

Richardson J, Kagawa F, Nichols A (2009). Health, energy vulnerability and climate change: A retrospective thematic analysis of primary care trust policies and practices. *Public Health* 123: 765–770.

Rickard J (2007). Meuse river–Argonne forest offensive, 26 September–11 November 1918. Available online at: http://www.historyofwar.org/articles/battles_meuse_argonne.html (accessed 23 May 2010).

Sandberg KI, Bjune G (2007). The politics of global immunization initiatives: Can we learn from research on global environmental issues? *Health Policy* 84: 89–100.

Santow G (2001). Mortality, epidemiological, and health transitions. In: Smelser NJ, Baltes PB (eds) *International Encyclopedia of the Social and Behavioral Sciences*. Oxford: Pergamon, pp. 10071–10075.

Selgelid MJ (2009). Pandethics. *Public Health* 123: 255–259.

Shea KM, Truckner RT, Weber RW, *et al.* (2008). Climate change and allergic disease. *J Allergy Clin Immunol* 122: 443–453.

Shin Y-J (2006). Policy context of the poor progress of the pro-poor policy: A case study on the Medical-Aid policy during Kim Dae-jung's Government (1998–2002) in the Republic of Korea. *Health Policy* 78: 209–223.

St. Louis ME, Hess JJ (2008). Climate change: Impacts on and implications for global health. *Am J Prevent Med* 35: 527–538.

Stephens C, Satterthwaite D, Kris H (2008). Urban health in developing countries. In: Kris H (ed.) *International Encyclopedia of Public Health*. Oxford: Academic Press, pp. 452–463.

Sutherland JR (1919). *In The World War 1917–1918–1919*. Tekamah, NE: The Burt County Herald, p. 34.

US Centers for Disease Control and Prevention (2010). A global perspective on tuberculosis. http://www.cdc.gov/tb/events/WorldTBDay/PDF/aglobal_perspective_onTB.pdf (accessed 2 February 2010).

US Department of Health and Human Services, Health Resources and Services Administration (2010). *The Registered Nurse Population: Initial Findings from the 2008 National Sample Survey of Registered Nurses*, Available online at: http://bhpr.hrsa.gov/healthworkforce/rnsurvey/initialfindings2008.pdf (accessed 21 May 2010).

US Government Accountability Office (2006). Health Professions Education Programs: Action Still Needed to Measure Impact. Washington, DC: US Government Accountability Office.

Weiner JP (1994). Forecasting the effects of health reform on the United States physician workforce requirements: Evidence from HMO staffing patterns. *JAMA* 20: 222–230.

Weiner JP (2002). A shortage of physicians or a surplus of assumptions? *Health Affairs* 21: 160–162.

World Health Organization (2006). New global alliance seeks to address worldwide shortage of doctors, nurses and other health workers. Available online at: http://www.who.int/mediacen-tre/news/releases/2006/pr26/en/index.html (accessed 21 May 2010).

World Health Organization (2010a). *Good Procurement Practices for Artemisinin-Based Antimalarial Medicines.* Geneva: WHO.

World Health Organization (2010b). International recruitment of health personnel: draft global code of practice. Sixty-third World Health Assembly, Agenda item 11.5, A63/A/Conf. Paper No. 11, 20 May 2010. Geneva: World Health Organization.

Yang M, Tao S, Guan S, *et al.* (2010). Chinese traditional medicine. In: Mander L, Hung-Wen L (eds) *Comprehensive Natural Products II.* Oxford: Elsevier, pp. 383–477.

Younger M, Morrow-Almeida HR, Vindigni SM, *et al.* (2008). The built environment, climate change, and health: Opportunities for co-benefits. *Am J Prevent Med* 35: 517–526.

Zwi AB, Ugalde A, Richards P (2005). Research issues in preparedness for mass casualty events, disaster, war, and terrorism. *Nurs Clin North Am* 40: 551–564.

Further reading

Alejos A, Weingartner A, Scharff DP, *et al.* (2008). Ensuring the success of local public health workforce assessments: Using a participatory-based research approach with a rural population. *Public Health* 122: 1447–1455.

Andre K, Barnes L (2010). Creating a 21st century nursing work force: Designing a Bachelor of Nursing program in response to the health reform agenda. *Nurse Educ Today* 30: 258–263.

Ball E, Regan P (2010). Change and the NHS workforce: Ambivalence, anxiety and anger. *Nurse Educ Pract* 10: 113–114.

Bangay C, Blum N (2010). Education responses to climate change and quality: Two parts of the same agenda? *Int J Educ Devel* 30: 359–368.

Bernholz CD (2009). Pestilence in paradise: Leprosy accounts in the annual reports of the governor of the territory of Hawaii. *Govern Inf Q* 26: 407–415.

Betancourt TS, Agnew-Blais J, Gilman SE, *et al.* (2010). Past horrors, present struggles: The role of stigma in the association between war experiences and psychosocial adjustment among former child soldiers in Sierra Leone. *Soc Sci Med* 70: 17–26.

Cohn S, Dyson C, Wessely S (2008). Early accounts of Gulf War illness and the construction of narratives in UK service personnel. *Soc Sci Med* 67: 1641–1649.

Degenhardt L, Mathers B, Guarinieri M, *et al.* Meth/amphetamine use and associated HIV: Implications for global policy and public health. *Int J Drug Policy* 21: 347–358.

Dhavan P, Reddy KS (2008). Public health professionals. In: Kris H (ed.) *International Encyclopedia of Public Health.* Oxford: Academic Press, pp. 432–439.

Dussault G, Vujicic M (2008). Demand and supply of human resources for health. In: Kris H (ed.) *International Encyclopedia of Public Health.* Oxford: Academic Press, pp. 77–84.

Ford JD, Pearce T, Duerden F, *et al.* (2010). Climate change policy responses for Canada's Inuit population: The importance of and opportunities for adaptation. *Global Environ Change* 20: 177–191.

Harris R, Bennett J, Davey B, *et al.* (2010). Flexible working and the contribution of nurses in mid-life to the workforce: A qualitative study. *Int J Nurs Studies* 47: 418–426.

Jenkins R (2008). Mental health policy. In: Kris H (ed.) *International Encyclopedia of Public Health.* Oxford: Academic Press, pp. 393–406.

Jenner D, Hill A, Greenacre J, *et al.* Developing the public health intelligence workforce in the UK. *Public Health* 124: 248–252.

Martin GP, Currie G, Finn R (2009). Reconfiguring or reproducing intra-professional bound-aries? Specialist expertise, generalist knowledge and the 'modernization' of the medical work-force *Soc Sci Med* 68: 1191–1198.

Mays N (2008). Interest groups and civil society, in public health policy. In: Kris H (ed.) *International Encyclopedia of Public Health.* Oxford: Academic Press, pp. 650–658.

Mearns K, Hope L, Ford MT, *et al.* Investment in workforce health: Exploring the implications for workforce safety climate and commitment. *Accident Anal Prevent* 42: 1445–1454.

Miller KE, Rasmussen A (2010). War exposure, daily stressors, and mental health in conflict and post-conflict settings: Bridging the divide between trauma-focused and psychosocial frameworks. *Soc Sci Med* 70: 7–16.

Rafferty AM, Clarke SP (2009). Nursing workforce: A special issue. *Int J Nurs Studies* 46: 875–878.

Richardson J, Kagawa F, Nichols A (2009). Health, energy vulnerability and climate change: A retrospective thematic analysis of primary care trust policies and practices. *Public Health* 123: 765–770.

Sim F, Mackie P (2009). Tomorrow's workforce for health: Assessing the impact. *Public Health* 123. 293–294.

Tarantola D, Gruskin S (2008). Human rights approach to public health policy. In: Kris H (ed.) *International Encyclopedia of Public Health*. Oxford: Academic Press, pp. 477–486.

Tollefsen P, Rypdal K, Torvanger A, *et al.* (2009). Air pollution policies in Europe: efficiency gains from integrating climate effects with damage costs to health and crops. *Environ Sci Policy* 12: 870–881.

Ungar S (2008). Total war, social impact of. In: Kurtz L (ed.) *Encyclopedia of Violence, Peace, and Conflict*. Oxford: Academic Press, pp. 2121–2129.

Zwi AB, Ugalde A, Harris P (2008). The effects of war and political violence on health services. In: Kurtz L (ed.) *Encyclopedia of Violence, Peace, and Conflict*. Oxford: Academic Press, pp. 933–943.

Case Study

Methicillin-resistant Staphylococcus aureus (MRSA)

Introduction

From the initial discovery of the first wonder antibiotic, penicillin, in the 1930s, through to today, a major concern has been the adaptation of bacteria and subsequent development of strains resistant to antibiotics. The initial term used to describe resistant strains of bacteria and the infections they caused was "blood poisoning." When resistance to penicillin emerged, an antibiotic, methicillin, which was a penicillin analog, was developed and shown to be effective in treating *Staphylococcus aureus* (McKenna 2010a).

It is no wonder that resistant strains of *S. aureus* began appearing in the 1950s. Penicillin was sold freely from 1940 to 1951 without prescription as an over-the-counter product (McKenna 2010a).

Perhaps the most infamous of the resistant strains of bacteria is that of *S. aureus*. At present in the USA, *S. aureus* is carried by 30% of the US population (McKenna 2010b). Methicillin-resistant strains of *S. aureus* are now termed methicillin-resistant *S. aureus* or the abbreviated term, MRSA. It has been estimated that MRSA is currently carried by at least 1.5% of the US population.

Interestingly, when methicillin was introduced in 1960 it was presented with the caveat that this would be an agent that would not suffer from the ignominy of resistance that other antibiotics have met. This has turned out not to be the case. Another agent, vancomycin, was then developed to treat *S. aureus*. This agent too has been ineffective in cases of resistance, and now strains of vancomycin-resistant *S. aureus* (VRSA) have emerged, much to the chagrin of infectious disease specialists and public health practitioners and advocates. The present scenario when treating *S. aureus* is that there are only one or two agents that may show effectiveness in assaulting the bacterium (McKenna 2010b). This portends the death of the so-called series of "magic bullet" antibiotics theory that the discovery of the next best antibiotic is just around the corner.

Seriousness of the MRSA threat

The startling evidence for the seriousness of the MRSA threat is as follows:

- There are close to 20 000 deaths annually due to MRSA (Klevens *et al.* 2007). In comparison, there were 12 000 suspected deaths due to swine flu in 2009 worldwide (McKenna 2010b).
- It is estimated that there are 370 000 annual MRSA-related hospitalizations in the USA (McKenna 2010b).
- There are an estimated 7 million emergency room visits due to MRSA (McKenna 2010b).
- And finally, it is estimated that there is an annual expenditure of $38 billion annually in additional health care expenses for MRSA-related sequelae in the USA (McKenna 2010b).

MRSA is multifaceted

McKenna (2010a, b) notes that there are currently three overlapping epidemics of MRSA at play:

1 Hospitals: Many facilities have no accepted practices institution-wide for dealing with MRSA or suspected cases of MRSA.
2 Everyday life: in 1998 the first known community-acquired MRSA was highlighted.
3 In livestock: beginning in 2004 strains of MRSA were found in pigs.

These three scenarios for the overlapping nature of the epidemic are frightening. A startling factor presented by McKenna (2010b) is that a total of 70% of antibiotics used in the USA are for agricultural purposes (e.g., as food additives in fowl, bovine, and porcine populations).

What health policy actions need to be implemented?

McKenna (2010a) suggests that pronounced health policy actions are necessary from three groups:

1 for individuals, personal protection, and the responsible use of antibiotics
2 for health care institutions, institutional action: increase surveillance and monitoring
3 governmental: change agricultural practices via legislation to decrease antibiotics in foodstuffs, increase funding for MRSA-related research. Encourage the production of new, novel antibacterial agents.

Panchanathan and colleagues (2010) present a study examining the use of computer modeling, including sensitivity analysis to help guide decision makers in making policy decisions concerning MRSA outbreaks and necessary interventions. They reach the conclusion that, through building a high-quality simulation model and the validation of this model against population data, more effective conclusions may be reached in the future.

Overview of healthcare-associated MRSA

The following was released in 2010, and is adapted from the US Centers for Disease Control and Prevention:

Methicillin-resistant *Staphylococcus aureus* (MRSA) is a type of staph bacteria that does not react to certain antibiotics and will normally cause skin infections, but MRSA can also cause other infections – including pneumonia. MRSA can be fatal. In 1974, MRSA infections accounted for 2% of the total number of staph infections; in 1995 it was 22%; in 2004 it was 63%. CDC [Centers for Disease Control and Prevention] estimated that 94 360 invasive MRSA infections occurred in the United States in 2005; 18 650 of these were associated with death. MRSA is resistant to antibiotics including methicillin, oxacillin, penicillin, and amoxicillin. Since these strong drugs are not effective with MRSA, these infections are sometimes called multidrug-resistant organisms (MDROs). Staph infections, including MRSA, occur most often among people in hospitals and health care facilities (such as nursing homes and dialysis centers) who have weakened immune systems. The infection can be spread by skin-to-skin contact, sharing or touching a personal item with someone with infected skin, or touching a surface or item that has been in contact with someone with MRSA.

MRSA infections that occur in otherwise healthy people who have not been recently (within the past year) hospitalized or had a medical procedure (such as dialysis, surgery, catheters) are known as community-associated MRSA (CA-MRSA) infections. These infections are usually skin infections such as abscesses, boils, and other pus-filled lesions, but these infections may also lead to more serious illness, such as pneumonia.

Klevens *et al.* (2007), in a study examining the extent of MRSA, found that invasive MRSA infection affects certain populations disproportionately. They state:

It is a major public health problem primarily related to health care but no longer confined to intensive care units, acute care hospitals, or any health care institution (p. 1763).

Sir Arthur Fleming's salient warning about misuse of antibiotics

Sir Arthur Fleming (1945), the discoverer of penicillin, in his acceptance remarks for his Nobel Prize ceremony, sounded an alarm about misuse of penicillin and its resultant effects. These remarks are every bit as salient today as they were upon delivery on December 11, 1945:

But I would like to sound one note of warning. Penicillin is to all intents and purposes non-poisonous so there is no need to worry about giving an overdose and poisoning the patient. There may be a danger, though, in underdosage. It is not difficult to make microbes resistant to penicillin in the laboratory by exposing them to concentrations not sufficient to kill them, and the same thing has occasionally happened in the body.

The time may come when penicillin can be bought by anyone in the shops. Then there is the danger that the ignorant man may easily underdose himself and by exposing his microbes to non-lethal quantities of the drug make them resistant. Here is a hypothetical illustration. Mr. X has a sore throat. He buys some penicillin and gives himself not enough to kill the streptococci but enough to educate them to resist penicillin. He then infects his wife. Mrs. X gets pneumonia and is treated with penicillin. As the streptococci are now resistant to penicillin the treatment fails. Mrs. X dies. Who is primarily responsible for Mrs. X's death? Why, Mr. X, whose negligent use of penicillin changed the nature of the microbe. Moral: If you use penicillin, use enough (pp. 84–94).

Summary of MRSA health policy considerations

MRSA and its threat and the need for action are prime examples of the need for health policy impacts to be brought to the forefront of individual, collective, and governmental action. This example and the influence on so many aspects of health care, patient well-being, and dire consequences is not isolated: there are other similar stories that could have been presented in this case study. Health care, agriculture, and individual responsibilities are not mutually exclusive: with the MRSA epidemic and threat, they can be seen to be closely overlapping constructs.

Discussion questions

1 What responsibilities do pharmaceutical manufacturers have regarding MRSA outbreaks/epidemics?
2 Why do you suppose it is so difficult for health care groups and public health groups to grasp the seriousness of the MRSA invasion?
3 What health policy influencers do you feel would be the most significant in stemming this public health issue?
4 How can global effects be implemented to affect MRSA and VRSA?
5 How can the US federal government become more proactive regarding MRSA outbreaks?
6 In your mind, should MRSA or VRSA infections be a mandatory reportable illness to state sources (it is not at this point)? If yes, explain how this could be implemented. If no, why not?
7 Why is the golden age of antibiotic development by pharmaceutical manufacturers on the decline?
8 How can health policy influences impact rational antibiotic use?
9 What individual responsibilities can be influenced by health policy when it comes to issues such as MRSA and VRSA?
10 As a product manager for a new antibiotic, how would you proactively deal with MRSA potentials for your new penicillin-derived analog?

References

Fleming A (1945). Nobel Prize in physiology or medicine, acceptance comments. Available online at: www.Nobelprize.org/nobel_prizes/medicine/laureates/1945/fleming-lecture.pdf (accessed 12 February 2009).

Klevens RM, Morrison MA, Nadle J, *et al.* (2007). Invasive methicillin-resistant *Staphylococcus aureus* infections in the United States. *JAMA* 298: 1763–1771.

McKenna M (2010a). *Superbug: The Fatal Menace of MRSA.* New York: Free Press (Simon and Schuster).

McKenna M (2010b). *Not Imagining the Worst: The Advance of MRSA.* Atlanta, GA: Emory University Models of Excellence Lecture.

Panchanathan SS, Petitti DB, Fridsma DB (2010). The development and validation of a simulation tool for health policy decision making. *J Biomed Inform* 43: 602–607.

US Centers for Disease Control and Prevention (2010). Healthcare-associated methicillin resistant *Staphylococcus aureus* (HA-MRSA). Available online at: http://www.cdc.gov/ncidod/dhqp/ar_mrsa.html (accessed 27 May 2010).

Further reading

Andersen BM, Tollefsen T, Seljordslia B, *et al.* (2010). Rapid MRSA test in exposed persons: Costs and savings in hospitals. *J Infect* 60: 293–299.

Creamer E, Dorrian S, Dolan A, *et al.* (2010). When are the hands of healthcare workers positive for meticillin-resistant staphylococcus aureus? *J Hosp Infect* 75: 107–111.

Cuny C, Friedrich A, Kozytska S, *et al.* (2010). Emergence of methicillin-resistant staphylococcus aureus (MRSA) in different animal species. *Int J Med Microbiol* 300: 109–117.

Forward KR (2010). The value of multiple surveillance cultures for methicillin-resistant *Staphylococcus aureus. Am J Infect Control* 38: 596–599.

Gagné D, Bédard G, Maziade PJ (2010). Systematic patients' hand disinfection: Impact on meticillin-resistant *Staphylococcus aureus* infection rates in a community hospital. *J Hosp Infect* 75: 269–272.

Gilligan P, Quirke M, Winder S, *et al.* (2010). Impact of admission screening for meticillin-resistant *Staphylococcus aureus* on the length of stay in an emergency department. *J Hosp Infect* 75: 99–102.

Goldfain A, Smith B, Cowell LG (2010). Towards an ontological representation of resistance: The case of MRSA. *J Biomed Inform* (in press).

Hulscher MEJL, van der Meer JWM, Grol RPTM (2010). Antibiotic use: How to improve it? *Int J Med Microbiol* 300: 351–356.

Keen EF, III Robinson BJ, Hospenthal DR, *et al.* (2010). Prevalence of multidrug-resistant organisms recovered at a military burn center. *Burns* 36: 819–825.

Lee BY, Ufberg PJ, Bailey RR, *et al.* (2010). The potential economic value of a *Staphylococcus aureus* vaccine for neonates. *Vaccine* 28: 4653–4660.

Loeffler A, Pfeiffer DU, Lloyd DH, *et al.* (2010). Meticillin-resistant *Staphylococcus aureus* carriage in UK veterinary staff and owners of infected pets: New risk groups. *J Hosp Infect* 74: 282–288.

Ludlam HA, Swayne RL, Kearns AM, *et al.* (2010). Evidence from a UK teaching hospital that MRSA is primarily transmitted by the hands of healthcare workers. *J Hosp Infect* 74: 296–299.

Madeo M (2010). Efficacy of a novel antimicrobial solution (Prontoderm) in decolonising MRSA nasal carriage. *J Hosp Infect* 74: 290–291.

Mathews CJ, Weston VC, Jones A, *et al.* (2010). Bacterial septic arthritis in adults. *Lancet* 375: 846–855.

Morris-Downes M, Smyth EG, Moore J, *et al.* (2010). Surveillance and endemic vancomycin-resistant enterococci: Some success in control is possible. *J Hosp Infect* 75: 228–233.

O'Leary FM, Price GJ (2010). Alcohol hand gel – a potential fire hazard. *J Plast Reconstruct Aesthetic Surg* (in press).

Otter JA, French GL (2010). Molecular epidemiology of community-associated meticillin-resistant *Staphylococcus aureus* in Europe. *Lancet Infect Dis* 10: 227–239.

Owens PL, Barrett ML, Gibson TB, *et al*. (2010). Emergency department care in the United States: A profile of national data sources. *Ann Emerg Med* 56: 156–165.

Peterson A, Marquez P, Terashita D, *et al*. (2010). Hospital methicillin-resistant Staphylococcus aureus active surveillance practices in Los Angeles county: Implications of legislation-based infection control, 2008. *Am J Infect Control* 38: 653–656.

Ransjö U, Lytsy B, Melhus A, *et al*. (2010). Hospital outbreak control requires joint efforts from hospital management, microbiology and infection control. *J Hosp Infect* 76: 26–31.

Sexton JD, Reynolds KA (2010). Exposure of emergency medical responders to methicillin-resistant *Staphylococcus aureus. Am J Infect Control* 38: 368–373.

Sheaff R, Benson L, Farbus L, *et al*. (2010). Network resilience in the face of health system reform. *Soc Sci Med* 70: 779–786.

Shelton CL, Raistrick C, Warburton K, *et al*. (2010). Can changes in clinical attire reduce likelihood of cross-infection without jeopardising the doctor–patient relationship? *J Hosp Infect* 74: 22–29.

Thibaut S, Caillon J, Huart C, *et al*. (2010). Susceptibility to the main antibiotics of *Escherichia coli* and *Staphylococcus aureus* strains identified in community acquired infections in France (MedQual, 2004–2007). *Médecine Maladies Infectieuses* 40: 74–80.

Weigelt JA, Lipsky BA, Tabak YP, *et al*. (2010). Surgical site infections: Causative pathogens and associated outcomes. *Am J Infect Control* 38: 112–120.

Willis-Owen CA, Subramanian P, Kumari P, *et al*. (2010). Effects of 'bare below the elbows' policy on hand contamination of 92 hospital doctors in a district general hospital. *J Hosp Infect* 75: 116–119.

12

Summary, global health, and global health policy

Introduction

This book has as its primary focus health policy and health policy decisions that have ethical considerations. Ruger (2006) presents a focus of ethics within global health inequalities. The concept of human flourishing is presented. Human flourishing suggests that shared health governance is essential for delivering health equity on a global scale (Ruger 2006). In this chapter issues will be touched on that deal with aspects that are of global concern. Health policy and/or health care cannot be extracted from these concerns because they are intertwined. Culture, society, and health have always been enmeshed with one another, and health policy interacts with each and has tremendous importance for each. Water quality, food availability, access to health care and health care commodities (pharmaceuticals, laboratory testing), and personal safety are important considerations. This chapter begins with these broad issues and then selectively narrows the focus of coverage for locally tailored considerations.

Global health in a global context

A definition of health was presented in the foreword to this book, and is reprinted below:

> Definition of "health" from the World Health Organization:
>
> Health is a state of complete physical, mental and social well-being and not merely the absence of disease or infirmity (World Health Organization 2010).

As has been previously noted, this definition has remained the same since its initial publication in 1948. As has been discussed, health and disease are global constructs. The rapid mobility of individuals means that outbreaks of diseases cannot be isolated as easily as they once were. Outbreaks spread quickly due to air travel.

Need for locally tailored interventions

Despite the point that global health policy and public health concerns are just that, global, the best ways to make an impact are locally based. As noted by Griffiths *et al.* (2005), several factors need to be incorporated in order for public health efforts to be successful. These must:

- be population-based
- emphasize collective responsibility for health, its protection, and disease prevention
- recognize the key role of the state, linked to a concern for the underlying socioeconomic and wider determinants of health, as well as disease
- have a multidisciplinary basis, which incorporates quantitative as well as qualitative methods
- emphasize partnerships with all of those who contribute to the health of the population, including individuals, communities, voluntary groups and the business sector (p. 908).

These tenets are important for broad-based efforts, as well as specific efforts aimed individually at diseases such as malaria (Kilama 2009).

Examples of transitions in developing countries

Examples of transitions from one condition through others can be found in Table 12.1, which includes epidemiological, demographic, and nutritional subsections.

Initially in a country's development, the main causes of morbidity and mortality are infectious diseases. As a health delivery system infrastructure emerges, and health policy decisions guide the evolution of health care delivery, people do not succumb to infectious diseases to the same extent. Water and sanitation practices emerge and become more advanced, and the resultant

Table 12.1 Examples of health transitions in developed countries

Epidemiological

Infectious diseases → chronic diseases → emergent diseases

Demographic

High mortality → low mortality

High fertility → low fertility

Nutritional

Undernutrition → overnutrition

effect is an increase in longevity and more options available to treat infectious diseases. The availability of health workers and resources to treat disease or prevent disease impacts the ability of a country to succeed in overcoming the obstacle of infectious diseases. Access to antibiotics which are affordable, of high quality, and not counterfeit drug products allows for treatment of common bacterial infections. These levels of progress can be halted due to lack of funding, mismanagement of funds, or poorly designed systems of health care delivery based upon inadequate health policy formation and the carrythrough of sound policies and practices.

Demographic factors influence general levels of health and health conditions. Pregnancy rates can be high in undeveloped countries, leading to high birth rates and problems with prenatal, neonatal, and postnatal care. The year 2010 brought the 50th anniversary of the development of the oral contraceptive, the so-called birth control pill (Wood 2000). If access to birth control methods is restricted or not utilized due to low levels of literacy or education, women may not have access to proven methods of contraception. Lack of access to male condoms can lead to high birth rates, increased levels of sexually transmitted diseases, and problems due to condom unavailability. In addition, mortality rates fall as countries develop, with subsequent availability of health care and health resources. Health policy decisions favoring access to health care through policy decisions supporting widespread availability of services correlate directly with lower levels of mortality from any number of diseases.

From a nutritional standpoint, availability of safe food products enhances nutrition, but with these enhancements, populations in developing countries move from a state of undernutrition to overnutrition. Subsequently, higher rates of cardiovascular diseases and metabolic diseases (e.g., diabetes mellitus) increase in a corresponding fashion.

Global health initiatives and interrelated goals

Global health initiatives have overlapping and interrelated goals:

- saving lives
- reducing suffering
- building health care infrastructures
- investment in health for economic improvement
- improving education and understanding
- enhancing collaboration for common goals
- using technology to create security for a better future.

Global health advocates principles such as:

- real partnerships
- local capacity building

- need for substantial funding, such as the President's Emergency Plan For AIDS Relief
- community participation and involvement
- cooperative global disease surveillance: the US CDC now has the name Centers for Disease Control and Prevention and has offices throughout the world (e.g., China, Vietnam)
- a realization that "one size" health care does not fit all needs everywhere.

Current controversies in global health include difficult ethical dilemmas

Should funds be spent on expensive new technologies or less expensive, proven current technologies? Should funding be spent on research or interventions? Should treatment for infectious diseases be advanced over chronic diseases or vice versa? Finally, who sets these priorities – global, regional, national, or other entities? Success stories have emerged from these difficult questions.

Success stories

There have been major successes in global health initiatives, including the eradication of smallpox (Fenner et al. 1988). Over a decade, a physician with the CDC, Donald Ainslie Henderson, was responsible for the 1965–1966 planning of the western and central African smallpox eradication and measles control program, conducted with the support of the US Agency for International Development. Then from 1966 to 1977, he was chief of the smallpox eradication unit in the World Health Organization (Fenner et al. 1988). The success of the programs led by Dr. Henderson is a textbook example of how to plan, structure, and carry out interventions.

In addition, the revolution in child survival efforts, oral rehydration therapy, expanded vaccinations for communicable disease worldwide (polio, measles), and enhanced efforts to stimulate widespread adoption of breastfeeding have impacted children and families internationally.

There have also been successes in reducing polio (Senior 2010) and malaria (Plowe 2010) globally. Also, vitamin A and other nutritional interventions have been successful (Wedner and Ross 2008). And severe acute respiratory syndrome, feared to be a major pandemic, was less severe than it could have been (van Baalen and van Fenema 2009; Cleri and Ricketti 2010). And finally, the impact of H1N1 worldwide, although serious, was less severe than anticipated due to prompt and successful vaccinations and fowl eradication worldwide.

Vaccine makers sold $3.3 billion in H1N1 vaccines and were handsomely rewarded for their efforts to bring the product rapidly to market. Making such huge sales and profits for a vaccine raises ethical questions about profiting and public health needs and serving those who could not afford the vaccination. In fact, a group investigating the World Health Organization's response to the swine flu outbreak of 2009 requested documents and other types of confidential material sent between the agency and vaccine manufacturers. In an evaluative report released in May 2010 (Wilson 2010), Médecins Sans Frontières suggests there are multiple factors that make delivering vaccines to children in developing countries difficult. Wilson (2010) includes in the list of factors:

- high prices of newer vaccines
- lack of research and development for better-adapted and needed vaccines
- weak health systems with corresponding health worker shortages.

Newer vaccines are often prohibitively expensive, in part because of a lack of adequate competition in the market, hindering their use in developing countries (Wilson 2010). There is also little incentive for pharmaceutical companies to conduct research and development for diseases that affect populations with limited purchasing power. Some diseases continue to be unaddressed by vaccines altogether, while many vaccines are not well adapted for people in developing countries (Wilson 2010).

Ethical issues and vaccinations

Ethical issues affect vaccinations and determine who is vaccinated where there may be limited supplies (Silverstein 2006). Silverstein suggests that children under the age of 13 years should be in the priority group for vaccination, and if these are vaccine shortages, children should be the priority. When economic constraints are in place, these ethical dilemmas intensify. Resultant health policy decisions addressing these issues need to be carefully crafted and carried out.

The ethics and politics of compulsory human papillomavirus vaccination have been controversial (Colgrove 2006). Colgrove notes questions related to the acceptability of mandatory public health measures, scope of parental autonomy, and role of political advocacy. Messages promoting vaccines against sexually transmitted diseases and the efforts to send young women messages about the benefits of sexual abstinence until marriage may be diametrically opposed.

Impact of poverty and wealth on health status

A cause of health disparities and inequalities is extreme poverty. In the *International Classification of Diseases* version 10 (ICD-10) can be found under section Z59, Problems related to housing and economic circumstances, the following items:

- Z59.0 homelessness
- Z59.1 inadequate housing

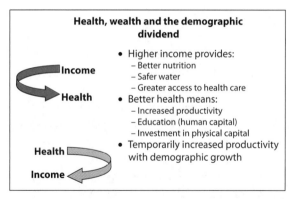

Figure 12.1   The relationship between health and wealth. Modified from Bloom DE, Canning D (2004). Global demographic change: Dimensions and economic significance. In: *Global Demographic Change: Economic Impacts and Policy Challenges,* proceedings of a symposium, sponsored by the Federal Reserve Bank of Kansas City, Jackson Hole, Wyoming, August 26–28, pp. 9–56.

- Z59.4 lack of adequate food
- Z59.5 extreme poverty
- Z59.6 low income.

Health status is directly proportional to wealth, and conversely, poverty is proportional to low levels of health status. The World Bank estimates that 3 billion people in the world live on less than $2.50 per day (Shah 2010).

The positive correlation between health and per capita income (Steckel and Rose 2002) is one of the most important indicators of modern development (Bloom and Canning 2004). Armelagos and Brown (2002) suggest: "Higher income provides better nutrition, safer water and greater access to health care." Bloom and Canning (2004) suggest the converse, in which development is linked to better health by increasing productivity, education, and investment in physical capital. Improved health is seen as a key to third-world development (Steckel and Rose 2002).

Figure 12.1 depicts the interrelatedness of wealth and health. Higher income provides better nutrition, safer water, and greater access to health care. Bloom and Canning (2004) suggest a converse in which development is linked to better health by increasing productivity, education, investment in physical capital and a "demographic dividend."

The primacy of basic needs for health considerations

People have fundamental needs, some of which have been described earlier, that are so crucial to achieving health that they bear repeating. Air, water, food safety, and sexual safety are taken for granted by many, and for others are unattainable. Unless they are attained, further discussions of health care and health care delivery seem to be unreasonable constructs to consider.

McKeown and Record (1962) and McKeown *et al.* (1975) decades ago indicated that the major determinants of health were access to food, proper sanitation and access to clean water, and birth spacing to control population growth. Water.org is a US-based non-profit organization committed to providing safe drinking water and sanitation to people in developing countries (www.water.org). Its website states: "We envision a day when everyone can have safe water." This is still a necessity for proper health, and remains an issue more than 50 years since McKeown and Record (1962) brought this concern to the forefront of health policy discussions.

These and other determinants of health are listed in Table 12.2. A description of each of these is presented below. This should not be considered an all-inclusive listing of all determinants of health: it is merely a sample.

Impacts from an air perspective on health include transmission of tuberculosis, acute respiratory infections, influenza, second-hand tobacco effects, air pollution, and fluctuating temperatures.

Water-borne illnesses include diarrhea, parasites, schistosomiasis, cholera, and malaria. Schistosomiasis, also known as bilharzia, is a disease caused by parasitic worms. Infection with *Schistosoma mansoni, S. haematobium,* and *S. japonicum* causes illness in humans. Although schistosomiasis is not found in the USA, more than 200 million people are infected worldwide (http://www.cdc.gov/ncidod/dpd/parasites/Schistosomiasis/factsht_schistosomiasis.htm).

Food-related morbidity and mortality include hunger, cardiovascular disease, diabetes mellitus, micronutrient malnutrition (Raynaud-Simon 2009; Zhao *et al.* 2009; Meenakshi *et al.* 2010), and protein-energy malnutrition (Haimamot 2009; Pavlovski 2009; von Haehling and Lainscak 2009; Longo and Fontana 2010).

Table 12.2 Partial determinants of health
Air
Water
Food
Shelter, safety, security
Social relations and sex
Medical services
Hope and meaning
Physical activity

Shelter, safety, and security factors are listed. Shelter includes housing and protection from exposures to fluctuations in temperature, wind, and sand. Also included are population density issues. Safety refers to protection from violence and the effects of war (O'Keefe and Rose 2008; Timothy and Teye 2009; Watson 2009).

Social relations and sex include acquired immune deficiency syndrome (AIDS), sexually transmitted infections, and sexually transmitted diseases. Domestic violence is listed as well.

Medical services refer to prevention, trauma care, and medical interventions (medical care, physicians, medications). Prevention includes smoking cessation and tobacco avoidance.

Hope and meaning allude to the increasing numbers of suicides, the incidence of depression and alcoholism, and the untoward effects of alcohol and alcohol abuse (Bácskai and Czobor 2009; Reutfors and Ösby 2009; Sublette and Carballo 2009; Zhang and Conner 2010).

Finally, physical activity refers to avoidance of cardiovascular disease through preventive physical activities.

United Nations Millennium Goals

In the early part of the 21st century, the United Nations developed The Millennium Project. The Millennium Project (http://www.unmillenniumproject.org) was commissioned by the United Nations Secretary-General in 2002 to develop an action plan for the world to achieve the Millennium Development Goals and to reverse the grinding poverty, hunger, and disease affecting billions of people. The Millennium Development Goals are listed in Table 12.3.

Table 12.3 The eight Millennium Development Goals	
Goal 1	Eradicate extreme poverty and hunger
Goal 2	Achieve universal primary education
Goal 3	Achieve gender equality and women's empowerment
Goal 4	Reduce child mortality
Goal 5	Improve maternal health
Goal 6	Combat HIV/AIDS, malaria, and other diseases
Goal 7	Ensure environmental sustainability
Goal 8	Develop a global partnership for development

Source: http://unstats.un.org/unsd/mdg/Data.aspx (accessed 10 April 2010).
HIV, human immunodeficiency virus; AIDS, acquired immunodeficiency syndrome.

Each of these goals is interrelated and affects health. From a health policy perspective, four of the goals, numbers 1, 4, 5, and 6 are directly related to health.

Infectious diseases and causation

Infectious diseases can be considered to have three levels of causation: biological, socioepidemiological, and political. The biological level includes the microbiological aspects of infections as well as interactions between host and parasite or infecting agent. The socioepidemiological level includes exposure due to social roles and associated disease exposure (Mayer 2008; Palsdottir *et al.* 2008; Sommerfeld 2008; Lönnroth *et al.* 2009). The political economic level reflects lack of access to medical resources, intellectual resources, and limits or constraints on behavior (Sommerfeld 2008; Budd *et al.* 2009; Gizelis 2009; Poland *et al.* 2009).

One of the significant US government agencies that plays a remarkable role worldwide is the US CDC. The CDC has a group of epidemiologists who travel the world investigating disease outbreaks and identifying causation. This group is the Epidemiologic Intelligence Service (McKenna 2004). These incredible individuals are probably unknown to populations anywhere, but serve all regardless of location.

Historic perspective and its importance to health policy

Table 12.4 lists the three distinct phases of international and/or global health in history (Fee 2003; Brown and Fee 2004): tropical medicine (1800–1950), international health (1950–1990), and, most recently, global health (1990 onwards). Fee (2003) noted:

In this general formulation, each era coincides with major epochs of international relations, marked by generally distinct forms of politics and international economics: tropical medicine corresponds to the eras of colonialism and imperialism; international health to the

Table 12.4 Stages of international global health

Tropic medicine	1800–1950, colonialism and imperialism
International health	1950–1990, Cold War
Global health	1990 to now, expansion of global economy

Source: adapted from Brown TM, Fee E (2004). A role for public health history. *Am J Public Health* 94: 1851–1853.

Cold War; and global health to the rapid advance of the global economy.

The switch in name also corresponds to changes in how public health policy and public health in general have evolved over time. Because of the fact that disease outbreaks are not easily contained due to enhanced mobility of the world's population, health problems are not just domestic but rapidly become global. Also, there has been a re-emergence of "controlled diseases" world-wide. Outbreaks of malaria, dysentery, polio, tuberculosis, and other trans-mittable diseases portend a dramatic need for health policy impacts on a global basis. Also, the entire globe becomes at risk due to outbreaks of H1N1 influenza, human immunodeficiency virus (HIV)/AIDS, drug-resis-tant strains of tuberculosis, and methicillin-resistant *Staphylococcus aureus* or health care-associated methicillin-resistant *Staphylococcus aureus*. The Bill and Melinda Gates Foundation was founded in 2000 with a stated mission to impact "global health" because of such outbreaks and their rapid emergence.

Historical antecedents to global health

Historical antecedents to global health are listed in Table 12.5; five move-ments have melded into international or global health. Although some, like military medicine and hygiene, have histories going back to the formation of professional armies, the crucial period for the development of international health was the 19th century. International cooperation and treaties were involved in the regulation of trade and travel, particularly in relation to quarantine systems. Disaster and war victim relief requires international cooperation regarding rules of war for safe transport of the wounded and the delivery of humanitarian aid. Tropical medicine, as a scientific field, has historical roots in the maintenance of health for troops in colonies in the aftermath of imperialism and colonization. Finally, missionary medicine involves the delivery of health care as part of a more general goal of "civilizing" and converting local people, while medical missions have a more

Table 12.5 Historical antecedents to international health

Regulation of trade and travel

Disaster and war victim relief

Tropic medicine

Military medical science

Missionary medicine and medical missions

secular motivation to bring modern health care and medicine throughout the world.

Need for cross-cultural collaboration

Public health, and the impact of health policy on public health, must have an approach that recognizes the key importance of cross-cultural collaborations. Peter Brown and colleagues (Armelagos *et al.* 2005) present health and public health in an anthropologic orientation. Anthropologists do not focus on the individual but rather on the group and they argue that human cultures are shaped by, as well as actively shape, the environment. The environment includes diseases. In general, the dual system of inheritance of human groups – that is, through genes and culture – is affected by evolutionary processes of evolution. This includes the development of public health and medical systems which decrease morbidity and mortality rates (Armelagos *et al.* 2005). But cultural practices can also exacerbate disease transmission. Public health interventions, especially those with health education components, are aimed at effecting cultural change.

Importance of recognizing culture and its role in health policy-driven public health initiatives

In 1955 Benjamin Paul wrote about the need to incorporate local communities within health policy-driven public health interventions. In the introduction to this classic collection of case studies, Paul quotes Gorgas, the public health hero of the building of the Panama Canal, as saying: "If you want to kill mosquitoes, you have to think like a mosquito." In other words, mosquito control strategies were dependent upon local species and the ecology associated with their habitat. It has been known that *Anopheles* populations have exhibited variability since the 1920s.

Paul applied Gorgas's observations, stating: "it is even more important to know how to think like the people if one wants a public health program to be accepted and effective." Health policy programs must be appropriate and acceptable to the local community and/or society where they are to be implemented.

Successful malaria control programs must be adapted to the local ecology, including the culture of the local people, the culture of the local health system, and the culture of the larger public health program.

Global health and the pandemic of tobacco use

In research conducted by Jha *et al.* (2002), globally, 29% of persons aged 15 years or older were regular smokers in 1995. During the timeframe of this study, four-fifths of the world's 1.1 billion smokers lived in low- or middle-income countries. East Asian countries accounted for a disproportionately high percentage (38%) of the world's smokers. Males accounted for 80% of all smokers, and prevalence among males and females was highest among those aged 30–49 years (34%). Jha *et al.* (2002, 2006) concluded that future decades will see dramatic increases in tobacco-attributable deaths in low- and middle-income regions. Although much of this excess mortality can be prevented if smokers stop smoking, quitting remains rare in low- and middle-income countries (Jha *et al.* 2002, 2006).

Peto and colleagues (2003) estimated that, between 1901 and 2000, there were 100 million tobacco-related deaths globally in mostly developed countries. These researchers extrapolate that there will be 1000 million deaths due to smoking from 2001 to 2100 and most of these deaths will be in developing countries. A total of 500 million of these deaths will occur in people living today.

HIV/AIDS

The occurrence and views toward HIV/AIDS vary because of context-based global and regional differences. In the USA, HIV/AIDS was considered to be solely a homosexual and/or intravenous drug user concern. This view of AIDS and of those affected was dramatically changed when two patients receiving transfusions were tragically infected: Arthur Ashe, the tennis great, received infected transfusions during the second of two heart surgeries, and Ryan White, an adolescent with hemophilia treated with infected transfusions placed a different face on patients with AIDS. Arthur Ashe began the Arthur Ashe Foundation to Defeat AIDS after he went public with the announcement that he had acquired AIDS during his heart surgeries and necessary transfusions.

In Thailand, Cambodia, and Vietnam HIV/AIDS is associated with the organized sex industry. In Africa, AIDS is a heterosexual component of transactional sex that is greatly impacted by myths and fallacies.

Summary

Global health, and health policy and implementation efforts resulting from health policy interventions, must adapt to local cultures. After all, local people are experts on local culture. Global health has a cultural component as well. For optimal effects, groups internal and external to a specific culture must work together.

Discussion questions

1　What local culture and mores need to be considered when developing health policy interventions?
2　Why do you feel the World Health Organization definition of "health" has not been revised after 60 years?
3　Discuss the importance of water and sanitation in developing countries, and why they are so crucial from a health policy standpoint.
4　Why are food and food safety primary concerns for health policy decision-makers?
5　Where did the term "tropical medicine" originate? Is it still a viable construct in the 21st century?
6　Discuss the health policy considerations related to methicillin-resistant *Staphylococcus aureus* on a global level.
7　Discuss the ethical issues surrounding the development, marketing, and sales of new, novel pediatric vaccines and their commercial availability.
8　Why has the Bill and Melinda Gates Foundation been successful in global outreach efforts in a decade of existence?
9　Why does the US CDC maintain offices in Beijing and Hanoi and elsewhere?
10　Why are health care, health policy, and the ethical ramifications of health policy decision-making so crucial at this point?

References

Armelagos GJ, Brown PJ (2002). The body as evidence; the body of evidence. In: Steckel RH, Rose JC (eds) *The Backbone of History, Health and Nutrition in the Western Hemisphere*. Cambridge: Cambridge University Press, p. 600.

Armelagos GJ, Brown PJ, Turner B, *et al*. (2005). Evolutionary, historical and political economic perspectives on health and disease. *Soc Sci Med* 61: 755–765.

Bácskai E, Czobor P (2009). Suicidality and trait aggression related to childhood victimization in patients with alcoholism. *Psychiatry Res* 165: 103–110.

Bloom DE, Canning D (2004). Global demographic change: Dimensions and economic significance. In: *Global Demographic Change: Economic Impacts and Policy Challenges*, proceedings of a symposium, sponsored by the Federal Reserve Bank of Kansas City, Jackson Hole, Wyoming, August 26–28, pp. 9–56.

Brown TM, Fee E (2004). A role for public health history. *Am J Public Health* 94: 1851–1853.

Budd L, Morag B, Brown T (2009). Of plagues, planes and politics: Controlling the global spread of infectious diseases by air. *Political Geogr* 28: 426–435.

Cleri DJ, Ricketti AJ (2010). Severe acute respiratory syndrome (SARS). *Infect Dis Clin North Am* 24: 175–202.

Colgrove J (2006). The ethics and politics of compulsory HPV vaccination. *N Engl J Med* 355: 2389–2391.

Fee E (2003). Examining a framework: The three phases of international health. American Public Health Association, 131st annual meeting, abstract #74493, 3249.0.

Fenner F, Henderson DA, Arita I, *et al.* (1988). *Smallpox and its Eradication.* History of International Public Health, No. 6. Geneva: World Health Organization.

Gizelis T-I (2009). Wealth alone does not buy health: Political capacity, democracy, and the spread of AIDS. *Political Geogr* 28: 121–131.

Griffiths S, Jewell T, Donnelly P (2005). Public health in practice: the three domains of public health. *Public Health* 119: 907–913.

Haimamot RT (2009). Neurological complications of malnutrition. In: Dobbs MR (ed.) *Clinical Neurotoxicology.* Philadelphia: WB Saunders, pp. 614–620.

Jha P, Ranson MK, Nguyen SN, *et al.* (2002). Estimates of global and regional smoking prevalence in 1995, by age and sex. *Am J Public Health* 92: 1002–1006.

Jha P, Chaloupka FJ, Moore J, *et al.* (2006). Tobacco addiction. In: Jamison DT (ed.) *Disease Control Priorities in Developing Countries,* 2nd edn. New York: Oxford University Press, pp. 869–886.

Kilama WL (2009). Health research ethics in public health: Trials and implementation of malaria mosquito control strategies. *Acta Trop* 112 (suppl. 1): S37–S47.

Longo VD, Fontana L (2010). Calorie restriction and cancer prevention: Metabolic and molecular mechanisms. *Trends Pharmacol Sci* 31: 89–98.

Lönnroth K, Jaramillo E, Williams BG, *et al.* (2009). Drivers of tuberculosis epidemics: The role of risk factors and social determinants. *Soc Sci Med* 68: 2240–2246.

Mayer JD (2008). Emerging diseases: overview. In: Kris H (ed.) *International Encyclopedia of Public Health.* Oxford: Academic Press, pp. 321–332.

McKenna M (2004). *Beating Back the Devil, on the Front Lines with the Disease Detectives of the Epidemiologic Intelligence Service.* New York: Free Press. (Simon and Schuster).

McKeown T, Record RG (1962). Reasons for the decline of mortality in England and Wales during the nineteenth century. *Populat Studies* 16: 94–122.

McKeown T, Record RG, Turner RD (1975). An interpretation of the decline of mortality in England and Wales during the twentieth century. *Populat Studies* 29: 391–422.

Meenakshi V, Johnson NL, Manyong VM, *et al.* (2010). How cost-effective is biofortification in combating micronutrient malnutrition? An ex ante assessment. *World Develop* 38: 64–75.

O'Keefe P, Rose J (2008). Relief operations. In: Kris H (ed.) *International Encyclopedia of Public Health.* Oxford: Academic Press, pp. 506–513.

Palsdottir B, Baker SH, Neusy A-J (2008). International organizational response to infectious disease epidemics. In: Mayer KH, Pfizer HF (eds) *The Social Ecology of Infectious Diseases.* San Diego: Academic Press, pp. 426–448.

Paul BD (1955). *Health, Culture, and Community; Case Studies of Public Reaction to Health Programs.* New York: Russell Sage Foundation.

Pavlovski CJ (2009). Screening for essential fatty acid deficiency in at risk infants. *Med Hypotheses* 73: 910–916.

Peto R, Lopez AD, Boreham J, *et al.* (2003). *Mortality from Smoking in Developed Countries,* 2nd edn. Oxford, UK: Oxford University Press.

Plowe CV (2010). Malaria eradication. *Int J Infect Dis* 14 (suppl. 1): e180–e181.

Poland GA, Jacobson RM, Tilbyrt J, *et al.* (2009). The social, political, ethical, and economic aspects of biodefense vaccines. *Vaccine* 27 (suppl. 4): D23–D27.

Raynaud-Simon A (2009). Virtual clinical nutrition university: Malnutrition in the elderly, epidemiology and consequences. *e-SPEN* 4: e86–e89.

Reutfors J, Ösby U (2009). Seasonality of suicide in Sweden: Relationship with psychiatric disorder. *J Affect Disord* 119: 59–65.

Ruger JP (2006). Ethics and governance of global health inequalities. *J Epidemiol Commun Health* 60: 998–1002.

Senior K (2010). Polio eradication within 5 years now a real possibility. *Lancet Infect Dis* 10: 148–149.

Shah A (2010). Causes of poverty. Global Issues Organization. Available online at: http://www.globalissues.org/issue/2/causes-of-poverty (accessed 17 December 2010).

Silverstein RP (2006). The ethics of influenza vaccination. *Science* 313: 758.

Sommerfeld J (2008). Social dimensions of infectious diseases. In: Kris H (ed.) *International Encyclopedia of Public Health*. Oxford: Academic Press, pp. 69–74.

Steckel RH, Rose JC (eds) (2002). *The Backbone of History, Health and Nutrition in the Western Hemisphere*. Cambridge: Cambridge University Press.

Sublette ME, Carballo JJ (2009). Substance use disorders and suicide attempts in bipolar subtypes. *J Psychiatr Res* 43: 230–238.

Timothy DJ, Teye VB (2009). *Safety and Security Issues in a Globalizing World. Tourism and the Lodging Sector*. Oxford: Butterworth-Heinemann, pp. 101–115.

van Baalen PJ, van Fenema PC (2009). Instantiating global crisis networks: The case of SARS. *Decision Support Systems* 47: 277–286.

von Haehling S, Lainscak M (2009). Cardiac cachexia: A systematic overview. *Pharmacol Ther* 121: 227–252.

Watson V (2009). 'The planned city sweeps the poor away...': Urban planning and 21st century urbanisation. *Progr Plann* 72: 151–193.

Wedner SH, Ross DA (2008). Vitamin A deficiency and its prevention. In: Kris H (ed.) *International Encyclopedia of Public Health*. Oxford: Academic Press, pp. 526–532.

Wilson P (2010). *Giving Developing Countries the Best Shot: An Overview of Vaccine Access and R&D. Campaign for Access to Essential Medicines*. Geneva, Switzerland: Médecins Sans Frontières.

Wood C (2000). Shopping at the contraceptive supermarket. *Lancet* 355: 763.

World Health Organization (2010). Frequently asked questions. What is the WHO definition of health? Available online at: http://www.who.int/suggestions/faq/en/ (accessed 17 December 2010).

Zhang Y, Conner KR (2010). Alcohol use disorders and acute alcohol use preceding suicide in China. *Addict Behav* 35: 152–156.

Zhao FJ, Su YH, Dunham SJ, *et al.* (2009). Variation in mineral micronutrient concentrations in grain of wheat lines of diverse origin. *J Cereal Sci* 49: 290–295.

Further reading

Bayer R (2008). Stigma and the ethics of public health: Not can we but should we. *Soc Sci Med* 67: 463–472.

Benatar SR (2002). Reflections and recommendations on research ethics in developing countries. *Soc Sci Med* 54: 1131–1141.

Cain JM (2000). A global overview of ethical issues in women's health. *Int J Gynecol Obstet* 70: 165–172.

Crane BB, Dusenberry J (2004). Power and politics in international funding for reproductive health: the US global gag rule. *Reprod Health Matters* 12: 128–137.

Duff C (2004). Drug use as a 'practice of the self': is there any place for an 'ethics of moderation' in contemporary drug policy? *Int J Drug Policy* 15: 385–393.

Fitchett JR (2009). Ethical considerations of clinical trials in the developing world. *Transact R Soc Trop Med Hygiene* 103: 756–760.

Fry CL, Cvetkovski S (2008). The regulation of drugs and drug use: Public health and law enforcement. In: Kris H (ed.) *International Encyclopedia of Public Health*. Oxford: Academic Press, pp. 501–505.

Gilson L, McIntyre D (2008). The interface between research and policy: Experience from South Africa. *Soc Sci Med* 67: 748–759.

Harper I (2007). Translating ethics: Researching public health and medical practices in Nepal. *Soc Sci Med* 65: 2235–2247.

Hsin DH-C, Macer DRJ (2004). Heroes of SARS: professional roles and ethics of health care workers. *J Infect* 49: 210–215.

Huish R (2009). How Cuba's Latin American School of Medicine challenges the ethics of physician migration. *Soc Sci Med* 69: 301–304.

Irwin KS, Fry CL (2007). Strengthening drug policy and practice through ethics engagement: An old challenge for a new harm reduction. *Int J Drug Policy* 18: 75–83.

Jennings B (2008). Foundations in public health ethics. In: Kris H (ed.) *International Encyclopedia of Public Health*. Oxford: Academic Press, pp. 660–669.

Johnstone M-J (2007). Patient safety ethics and human error management in ED contexts: Part I: Development of the global patient safety movement. *Australas Emerg Nurs J* 10: 13–20.

Kessel AS (2003). Public health ethics: teaching survey and critical review. *Soc Sci Med* 56: 1439–1445.

Kickbusch I (2000). The development of international health policies – accountability intact? *Soc Sci Med* 51: 979–989.

Lázaro P, Azcona B (1996). Clinical practice, ethics and economics: the physician at the crossroads. *Health Policy* 37: 185–198.

Magnusson RS (2009). Rethinking global health challenges: Towards a 'global compact' for reducing the burden of chronic disease. *Public Health* 123: 265–274.

Martin R (2008). Law, and public health policy. In: Kris H (ed.) *International Encyclopedia of Public Health*. Oxford: Academic Press, pp. 30–38.

Molyneux S, Geissler PW (2008). Ethics and the ethnography of medical research in Africa. *Soc Sci Med* 67: 685–695.

Ruger JP (2004). Ethics of the social determinants of health. *Lancet* 364: 1092–1097.

Schrecker T, Labonté R, De Vogli R (2008). Globalisation and health: the need for a global vision. *Lancet* 372: 1670–1676.

Stewart KA (2008). Anthropological perspectives in bio-ethics. In: Kris H (ed.) *International Encyclopedia of Public Health*. Oxford: Academic Press, pp. 184–193.

Street JM (2008). New technologies: Ethics of genomics. In: Kris H (ed.) *International Encyclopedia of Public Health*. Oxford: Academic Press, pp. 528–532.

Valdez-Martinez E, Trumbull B, Garduño-Espinosa J, *et al.* (2005). Understanding the structure and practices of research ethics committees through research and audit: a study from Mexico. *Health Policy* 74: 56–68.

Vian T (2008). Corruption and the consequences for public health. In: Kris H (ed.) *International Encyclopedia of Public Health*. Oxford: Academic Press, pp. 26–33.

Yong Kim J, Shakow A, Mate K, *et al.* (2005). Limited good and limited vision: multidrug-resistant tuberculosis and global health policy. *Soc Sci Med* 61: 847–859.

Index